‘As interconnected risks further compound into humanitarian crises, readers will find inspiration and practical guidelines on how to anticipate and mitigate these risks so that we can embark on a collective journey toward resilience.’

Mami Mizutori, *Former Special Representative of the UN Secretary General for Disaster Risk Reduction*

‘The types, patterns, and dynamics of threats to people’s security and survival are constantly changing. The millions who already experience high risks face ever more complex challenges. Meeting their needs asks for more skills and ingenuity from development practitioners who decide what approaches to embrace and what to jettison. They need trusted companions and mentors. Come in Randolph C. Kent whose landmark book on *Humanitarian Futures: Challenges and Opportunities* clearly sets the direction and lights up ways to get there.’

David Nabarro, *Co-founder and Strategic Director, 4SD Foundation, Geneva, Switzerland*

‘Dr. Randolph C. Kent’s *Humanitarian Futures: Challenges and Opportunities* masterfully blends deep intellectual rigour with practical insights, drawing on his unparalleled experience to illuminate future humanitarian crises and challenge current conventions and paradigms. In our world of perpetual crises, this is a vital, visionary work for leaders, policymakers and practitioners alike.’

Ben Ramalingam, *Author of* Aid on the Edge of Chaos *and Director of Strategy and Innovation, British Red Cross*

‘Randolph C. Kent offers a compelling vision of the complexities that will define a future humanitarian landscape and the imperative of drawing from an imagined future of the “what might-be’s” to prepare for threats outside today’s zones of organisational comfort. This book is a *must read* for those seeking to develop a capacity to anticipate uncharted humanitarian terrains.’

’Funmi Olonisakin, *Vice-President (International Engagement & Service) and Professor of Security, Leadership & Development, King’s College London*

Humanitarian Futures

Humanitarian Futures: Challenges and Opportunities explores the increasing types, dimensions and dynamics of crises threatening the world in the twenty-first century, and argues that those with humanitarian roles and responsibilities can only meet such challenges if their approaches to strategic and operational planning undergo fundamental paradigmatic shifts. Strategically and operationally, such shifts must begin by planning *from* the future, *for* the future.

Author Randolph C. Kent, the UN's first Humanitarian Coordinator, with experience in some of the most complex crises of modern times, including Rwanda, Ethiopia, Kosovo, Sudan and Somalia, provides a blueprint for dealing with ever greater complexity on planet Earth and beyond. That blueprint is not about upgrading existing tools or relying upon tried precedence. Rather, it points to a new paradigm for meeting crises. It begins by looking at the changing nature of humanness and governance, and then turns to plausible future crises based on such changes, before concluding with practical steps for dealing with ever more complex humanitarian threats, now and in the future.

This book will be an essential read for humanitarian policymakers and practitioners as well as for humanitarian and global studies researchers and students who are and want to be engaged in understanding and preparing for ever more complex and unpredictable humanitarian challenges.

Randolph C. Kent is Visiting Professor, African Leadership Centre, King's College London; Honorary Professor at the Institute for Risk and Disaster Reduction, University College London; Senior Associate Fellow, Royal United Services Institute and Director of the Humanitarian Futures Programme [www.humanitarianfutures.org]

Routledge Humanitarian Studies Series

The Routledge Humanitarian Studies series in collaboration with the International Humanitarian Studies Association (IHSA) takes a comprehensive approach to the growing field of expertise that is humanitarian studies. This field is concerned with humanitarian crises caused by natural disaster, conflict or political instability and deals with the study of how humanitarian crises evolve, how they affect people and their institutions and societies, and the responses they trigger.

We invite book proposals that address, among other topics, questions of aid delivery, institutional aspects of service provision, the dynamics of rebel wars, state building after war, the international architecture of peacekeeping, the ways in which ordinary people continue to make a living throughout crises, and the effect of crises on gender relations.

This interdisciplinary series draws on and is relevant to a range of disciplines, including development studies, international relations, international law, anthropology, peace and conflict studies, public health and migration studies.

Young Children in Humanitarian and COVID-19 Crises
Innovations and Lessons from the Global South
Edited by Sweta Shah and Lucy Bassett

Authoritarian Practices and Humanitarian Negotiations
Edited by Andrew J Cunningham

Depoliticising Humanitarian Action
Paradigms, Dilemmas, Resistance
Edited by Isabelle Desportes, Alice Corbet and Ayesha Siddiqi

Humanitarian Futures
Challenges and Opportunities
Randolph C. Kent

For more information about this series, please visit: www.routledge.com/Routledge-Humanitarian-Studies/book-series/RHS

Humanitarian Futures

Challenges and Opportunities

Randolph C. Kent

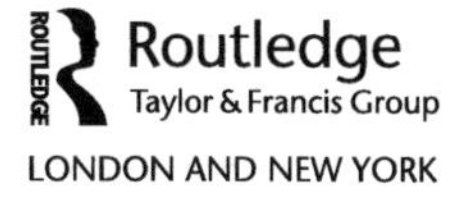

LONDON AND NEW YORK

Cover image: © Getty Images

First published 2025
by Routledge
4 Park Square, Milton Park, Abingdon, Oxon OX14 4RN

and by Routledge
605 Third Avenue, New York, NY 10158

Routledge is an imprint of the Taylor & Francis Group, an informa business

British Library Cataloguing-in-Publication Data
A catalogue record for this book is available from the British Library

ISBN: 9781032748016
ISBN: 9781032747996
ISBN: 9781003471004

DOI: 10.4324/9781003471004

Typeset in Times New Roman
by Newgen Publishing UK

Contents

Preface

I began this book just before the outbreak of the 2019 Covid-19 pandemic, and now am completing it as conflicts continue in Gaza and Ukraine, Sudan and on the Red Sea. At the same time, crises are mounting in Ethiopia and Tigray, hunger is intensifying in Afghanistan and the Uyghurs continue to be exploited by the Government in Beijing.

Of course, these are just some of the more evident humanitarian threats and crises across the globe. There are many more which in 2022 directly have driven at least 362 million people to the brink of survival.

These figures, however, do not include those people in many countries in the Americas, Europe and East and South Asia where inadequate food, lack of employment, poor healthcare and housing perpetuate profoundly unjust social divides. Then, too, there are the victims of so-called 'natural disasters' in a growing number of high-income countries, including the United States where an estimated 3 million people have been displaced due to growing numbers of incidents such as wildfires, increasingly intense storms and heat waves.

These dystopic views of the present, however, is not what this book is about. To the contrary, *Humanitarian Futures: Challenges and Opportunities* is about practical steps which can be taken to significantly reduce the human consequences of ever more complex humanitarian threats. It is focused on ways that those who are willing to assume humanitarian roles and responsibilities can identify, monitor and mitigate disasters and emergencies in ways hitherto unprecedented.

You, the reader, will see that the odyssey which I propose to take you on to arrive at this objective covers a very circuitous route. It begins with lessons from my past that I learned from involvement, principally in Africa, about the strengths and weaknesses of humanitarian action. Many of those remain today and need to be understood.

The journey then veers towards portraits of the future with few precedents. These portraits are fictional, though plausible, and generally do not reflect the realities of the contemporary world order. The purpose of taking the reader along this part of the journey is to see how relevant present approaches to humanitarian threats and crises would be when it comes to dealing with ever greater complexity and impacts. Then, finally, the reader arrives at the intended destination, which is to propose ways that those committed to humanitarian action can prepare to deal with the future by planning from the future.

As I reflect on the journey that I am proposing, I am all too aware that I owe this opportunity to so many – to colleagues in the United Nations and its agencies and programmes from whom I had learned so much over two decades pro; to officials in a wide range of regional organisations, including the Association of Southeast Asian Nations, the Economic Community of West African States, the European Union, the North Atlantic Treaty Organization, the Organisation of African Unity, the Organization of American States and the Southern African Development Community.

Similarly, my sincerest thanks goes to the many officials in 29 governments, several of whom funded and all of whom participated in this effort. There are too many to list here by name, but I do hope that those who contributed their time, insights and resources to the programme I established after leaving the UN – the Humanitarian Futures Programme at King's College, London – will feel that their involvement will prove to be of substantial benefit to the vulnerable.

And, as for the Humanitarian Futures Programme, itself, the list of those to whom I am enormously grateful is also extensive. I do hope that each one knows, how grateful I am for all their efforts, particulalrly Joanne Burke, who now has stayed with HFP for two decades.

There, too, is a wide range of non-governmental organisations to whom I owe so much. While once again, the numbers are too many to mention here, I do have to thank the 19 local NGOs and the 22 international NGOs for sharing their experiences and providing such relevant insights, both conceptual and operational.

It is perhaps self-evident to say this, but I must recognise what I learned from those people who suffered from the crises in which I had become involved. Ironically, perhaps paradoxically, it was with those affected that I engaged least on a one-to-one basis, but learned most. The true nature of vulnerability, the heroic sacrifices that were made to save their children, their willpower and extraordinary poise in such uncertain conditions, the squalor that in so many ways they were forced to tolerate – and on and on.

Out of these involvements came one abiding lesson – humanitarian crises ultimately have to be understood in terms of the nature of humanness. Of course, cultures, economic circumstances, traditions, social structures may differ – but those who want to assist others must begin by recognising that those who are trapped in humanitarian crises, like those who try to assist them, are individuals and must be recognised and treated as such. Those with humanitarian roles and responsibilities must begin by understanding the very nature of being human, and that it is every human's right to be in a place where he or she feels safe.

Now, the opportunity to conclude my humanitarian odyssey also has very personal dimensions. I would like to thank Valerie Kent who for so many years had been so supportive and tolerated my prolonged absences with such kindness and understanding when I worked for the UN in Ethiopia, Sudan, Rwanda, Kosovo, Somalia and UN headquarters.

I, too, would like to dedicate this book to my children and to my wife. To my wonderful children – Toby and Tim – I hope that *Humanitarian Futures: Challenges and Opportunities* will have positive relevance to them, their children and their children's children and beyond.

To my wife, Laura Sandys, I dedicate this book to her – truly the love of my life, whose energy, vision, creativity and deeply held commitments to others have been an inspiration to me over the past 20 years.

Oh yes, by the way, the phrase, *planning from the future* was actually hers…

Introduction

Cassandra's Challenge and the Helenus Alternative

The Copernican Vision[1]

Sometime around 1510, Nicholas Copernicus, the Renaissance mathematician and astronomer, announced his theory that the Earth was not at the centre of the universe but actually rotated around the sun. This proposition, though resisted initially by the establishment, ultimately formed an alternative basis of knowledge and understanding about our universe that continues today.

Just before the 2016 World Humanitarian Summit, a group of academics and researchers – all with considerable experience in the humanitarian sector – came together to launch a project, entitled, *Planning from the Future*. Led by the Humanitarian Futures Programme at King's College, London, the initiative intended to identify the strengths and weaknesses of the past and present humanitarian architecture and conclude with some prognostications about what will be required to meet the challenges of the future.

The project suggested various ways of understanding the contexts and factors which underpinned crisis threats. It reviewed the loosely defined humanitarian sector's capacities for dealing with ever more complex and uncertain humanitarian crises, and in so doing warned that the sector was essentially ill-equipped to deal with such future challenges:

> Circumspection, self-reflection and self-criticism are ingrained in the humanitarian psyche. Evaluations have a well-established role within the humanitarian system: the sector publishes hundreds of formal evaluations and lessons learned studies each year and pages upon pages of grey literature exist as internal documents within humanitarian organisations. However, despite the wealth of critical reflection and self- examination, the sector has difficulty applying the lessons learned from its mistakes. This is, in part, due to the fact that it is decidedly a-historic, as humanitarians operate in a perpetual present… Such a-historicism also maintains a short-term view of the humanitarian role, when today's recurrent and protracted crises demand that humanitarian practice must be grounded in long-term analytical perspectives.[2]

DOI: 10.4324/9781003471004-1

The point was so very important for setting the scene for the *Planning from the Future* project. Yet, at the same time it created a degree of tension among the project's contributors. If the sector is not fit for the future, plausible solutions may emerge for improving it through institutional change and methodologies that reflect our present understanding of the nature of crisis threats and mitigation. Or, alternatively, the assumptions that are made about crisis threats and appropriate action may stem from different understandings about the nature of crises as well as profoundly different approaches to crisis identification, prevention, preparedness and response.

What were the parameters of our approach to humanitarian action? In light of the all too evident poverty and limited resources in developing countries, should the geopolitical focus remain principally on them? Were we suggesting ways to improve the capacities and expand the vision of that sector, or were we saying that something far more fundamental was required? Were we proposing a paradigmatic shift that would reflect inherently different perspectives on the nature of humanitarianism and humanitarian motivation, the boundaries of humanitarian action, the construct of systems capable of dealing with ever more complex threats and who in the final analysis was a 'humanitarian actor'?

In the most basic sense, the contending perspectives were really never reconciled, though an acceptable compromise was agreed. Now, however, that compromise for at least some of us became increasingly inadequate to deal with threats that were clearly emerging. A new humanitarian paradigm was needed.

The underlying assumptions upon which knowledge and the search for knowledge are based are generally referred to as *paradigms*. The search for alternative paradigms is intended to improve both understanding and explanations by challenging the assumptions that underpin present conceptual constructs. It is not about improving understanding and explanation by building upon existing assumptions, but rather by proposing alternative assumptions that might provide different frameworks for ordering evidence that leads to knowledge.[3]

Cassandra's Challenge and the Helenus Alternative

The original title of this book was to be *Cassandra's Challenge: Planning from the Future*. It was a title intended to suggest that – like the tragic figure from ancient Greek mythology – few things can be more frustrating than having a sense of what the future might hold, and which is ignored by all. Of course, it is more than presumptuous for me as author to assume that I can predict the changing nature of humanitarian crises, and that few if anyone will listen. Nevertheless, for reasons that are explained in this book, all too often, those who have responsibilities to deal with plausible and actual humanitarian crises are reluctant to go beyond the immediate – the world and set of assumptions that they know. All too rarely, do they look beyond their comfort zones to deal with the prospect of ever more complex humanitarian crises.

Writing this book began well before the outbreak of the Covid-19 pandemic in 2020. Nevertheless, as the final version of this effort suggests, Covid-19 has substantiated the book's main themes. As the pandemic made very clear, the sorts of global systems, institutional structures and leadership needed for anticipating and responding to plausible and actual crisis threats all too often appear, if they even do, at the brink of chaos. Decision-makers, strategists, policy planners adjust for the evident, but all too rarely choose to explore the *what might be's* – factors that could well have transformative consequences beyond the immediately obvious. This is certainly the case for what is generally referred to as 'the humanitarian sector' – those institutions and individuals who to date have major roles and responsibilities for preventing, preparing for and responding to disasters and emergencies.

With this in mind, *Humanitarian Futures: Challenges and Opportunities* has three objectives. The first is to warn that those with humanitarian roles and responsibilities appear trapped in a state of conceptual and operational stasis. The time is ripe to consider emerging patterns and assumptions that could result in a hitherto underexplored humanitarian paradigm, which in turn could dramatically enhance the relevance and impacts of humanitarian action.

Despite myriad efforts to reform, those institutions that presently comprise the sector are transfixed on a set of assumptions that have less and less relevance to the dynamics and dimensions of new types of vulnerabilities and, hence, increasingly plausible humanitarian crises. These in turn may require a new set of assumptions about the nature of humanitarianism, humanitarian crisis drivers and action and the 'humanitarian sector', itself. Therefore, the book's second objective is to set the parameters of an alternative humanitarian paradigm to meet the challenges of the future.

The third objective is to propose a global agenda based upon that emerging humanitarian paradigm – for a different architecture, systems, networks as well as institutions – which this author believes will be vital for identifying and mitigating ever more complex and uncertain crisis threats.

Together, the book's three objectives will suggest what needs to be done to save large swathes of humanity from emerging humanitarian threats. If these perspectives and solutions are ignored, like Cassandra's truths, failure to listen could well lead to life-threatening chaos across the globe. Alternatively, if those concerned with the challenges which humanitarian threats do and increasingly will pose and are willing to act within the context of an evolving paradigm, then Casandra's brother – Helenus – becomes the symbol. It was he to whom many writers ascribe not only his prediction about the fall of ancient Troy, but also anticipating the practical and certainly unconventional means that it would be achieved – the Trojan Horse.

The route towards achieving these objectives begins with Chapter 1 *An Odyssey*. This first chapter uses incidents in the author's career as triggers for identifying a specific set of humanitarian challenges which he believes has persisted certainly since the mid-1980s, and will need to be addressed to deal with ever more complex humanitarian crises in the future. Much of what is covered in Chapter 1 is not new. There are many analyses that have described the evolution and strengths and weaknesses of 'the humanitarian sector'. However, the musings here focus on a set of conceptual and operational factors that will form the basis of a new humanitarian paradigm proposed in Chapters 5, 6, 7 and 8, which discuss the theme, *Destination – Planning from the Future.*

The incidents that guide Chapter 1 are intended (i) to explore the motivations that underpin 'humanitarianism', using Ethiopia in 1984 as a starting point, (ii) to reflect on the increasingly fluid parameters of humanitarian action that were made so evident in decisions made in 1991 at UN headquarters in New York, (iii) to recall the disconcerting degree to which humanitarian priorities are all too often determined by narrow inter-organisational interests, so evident in the Sudan in 1990 and in a related vein, (iv) how conventional organisational behaviour too often stimies effective collaboration, as was so evident in the response in the aftermath of the Rwandan genocide in 1994–1995, (v) to consider the definition of a 'humanitarian actor', an issue that challenged me during operations in Kosovo in 1999 and (vi) as Somalia made so clear in 2001, to rethink the ways that innovation and innovation practices are identified and implemented.

In no sense are these musings intended to ignore the considerable accomplishments of the sector – as presently defined – then and in subsequent years. However, the issues and perspectives that were triggered then led me eventually to believe that the humanitarian sector, specifically, and the international community more generally needed to rethink its assumptions about humanitarian motivations, the nature of humanitarian crises and the ways they anticipated and responded to them.

The relevance of the 'Western-oriented' humanitarian paradigm was becoming less so in the transformative age of the 21st century. Its assumptions about the 'aberrant nature' of humanitarian crises, interpretation of humanitarian principles and compliance, the dynamics of humanitarian crisis drivers, attitudes about the crisis affected and types of assistance required, partnerships and organisational and inter-organisational behaviour have all too often narrowed its perspectives, approaches and ultimately its impact.

As with other industries, there comes a moment when systems and organisations, no matter how successful and well intentioned, fail to adapt to fundamental change that inevitably will determine their survival. To a significant extent, what is normally referred to as the humanitarian sector continues to appear relatively insensitive to some fundamental transformations underway. Such transformative factors – internal and external – could well, perhaps to the peril of the sector's presumed status, undermine those very assumptions and baselines that many feel define it.

That is not to say that such factors are not frequent subjects of discussions, studies, workshops and conferences. Rather it is to say that all too often those perspectives and insights result in tactical adjustments, and do not result in the necessary conceptual, perceptual and strategic transformations that may determine the present sector's relevance in the future.

At the core of *Humanitarian Futures* lies the prospect that the global system will have to move into a humanitarian paradigm that is dramatically different, conceptually and operationally, from the one that frames humanitarian action today. The precedents of the past and the perspectives of the present will be less relevant for understanding the future. The global community and those within that community who assume humanitarian roles and responsibilities will have to assess their competencies for dealing with potential threats in terms of '*what might be's*' and not in terms of where we were and are today.

Its purpose and approach define what is meant by *planning from the future.*

However, underpinning *planning from the future* and the journey towards a new paradigm, is a proposition that reflects humanitarian crises in any age – past, present and future. That is that humanitarian crises are reflections of normal life, the ways that societies structure themselves and allocate their resources. They generally are not aberrant phenomena. Hence, whenever assessing the past, attempting to understand the present or anticipating the future, this assumption is fundamental to the journey upon which readers have embarked.

If a key objective of *Humanitarian Futures* is to have those with relevant roles and responsibilities think differently about an emerging humanitarian paradigm, one way is to take them to into a world that is rarely if ever considered from a humanitarian perspective. Here, the starting point is Chapters 2, 3 and 4, which cover the theme *Portraits of the Future.*

These chapters take the reader on a voyage focused on different but interrelated aspects of 'normal life' towards the end of the 2050s. Each examines plausible futures – those 'what-might-be's' – but none are intended to be predictions. To the contrary, the purpose of this section is to take those with humanitarian interests and concerns into a world normally not part of professional planning. The future is used as a test to assess their capacities to anticipate and adapt to changes in unfamiliar contexts. How relevant would their organisational systems be? What might be the motives for humanitarian action and how would one pursue collaboration and innovation and innovative practices in anticipating and responding to crisis threats?

The first step towards that longer-term future begins with Chapter 2 *The Changing Dimensions of Human Agency.* The assumption that underpins this chapter is that whoever we might be, wherever we are, whatever we may do, our lives and the ways we live will be dramatically different in a generation's time. And as the transformations that drive such changes intensify, human agency – our sense of who we are within ourselves and our capacities for interacting beyond ourselves – will also change dramatically.

Myriad factors could affect what the chapter refers to as 'human agency'. The impacts of climate change, ecological erosion and population growth, new religious and political movements: these could all affect how human beings see themselves and relate to others. This chapter, however, focuses in large part on how scientific and technological transformations will affect, and be affected by human capacities and perspectives on planet Earth and beyond. It looks at the upsides and downsides of those drivers of change affecting human agency, and suggests what impacts these might have on the ways that individuals, various types of groupings and societies as a whole can benefit from or be victims of profound societal change.

Clearly societal constructs reflect the ways that societies and those within them are governed and clearly this links to the ways that resources are prioritised and distributed.

Chapter 3 *Governance and Resource Prioritisation from a Futures Perspective*, therefore, explores how possible changes in human agency could affect and be affected by alternative forms of governance and processes affecting resource allocation. It begins with reflections on the types of overarching global architecture which may increasingly frame systems and behaviour patterns across the planet – and beyond – by mid-century.

Within that global architecture, the very nature of the state may undergo fundamental transitions. To what extent might states become increasingly 'virtual', and geopolitical boundaries lose much of their significance? Will states become co-dependent upon a growing number of non-state actors that have no operational or geographical boundaries? What means of enforcement might states have to assert their purpose, and might these be the same as those of other actors on Earth and elsewhere? In other words, what might be alternative, longer-term perspectives on the nature of governance?

Governance and organisational behaviour clearly interrelate, and so this chapter will explore not only possible organisational behaviour patterns in the future, but also how transformative technologies could well change the very dynamics of policy analysis, prioritisation and decision-making.

In turn, answers to these questions clearly lead to the issue of governance and resource distribution. How might resources be prioritised? Who might be the beneficiaries and who might not? And, if crises are generally a reflection of the ways that societies structure themselves and allocate their resources, what might that prioritisation process suggest about future vulnerabilities and their humanitarian consequences?

So far, readers will have explored future types of societal dynamics in order to get them inducted into worlds that they most likely will never have experienced. They will have been able to envision *portraits of the future* – by no means hard predictions, but contextualised imagination.

Yet, where does all this lead for those concerned with humanitarian issues? The answer is that it will take them to the edge of chaos and catastrophes. In other words, the last chapter in this section – Chapter 4 *Towards the Brink* – paints portraits of future crisis threats that have few if any precedents. Clearly climate change is a threat of potentially catastrophic proportions as are nuclear confrontation and nuclear winters. However, the *portraits of the future* in this chapter are intentionally far less familiar.

The humanitarian consequences of synchronous failures, social fragmentation in an interplanetary context, collapse of the Earth's ecological bandwidth, cognitive manipulation of communities, bacterial invasion from outer space, mass displacement as a violent continuum: these are all examples of threats that have received little if any consideration as triggers of humanitarian crises and are the sorts of threats that will be explored in this chapter.

For those readers who might wonder why such portraits have never found themselves in national and international risk registers, the answer hopefully will be clear. They are intended to provide a 'clean slate' for policy planners and decision-makers to test how effective their present approaches would be when it comes to dealing with the totally unanticipated. Are their organisations sufficiently anticipatory and agile to deal with events with few precedents, and in a related vein, to what extent will international systems as presently configured be adequate to respond?

Speculative *portraits of the future*, therefore, raise some fundamental questions about what needs to be done now to prepare for a rapidly changing humanitarian future. How will our understanding of crisis threats, humanitarian action and what defines a humanitarian actor have to change? How will myriad institutions across the globe play effective monitoring and mitigation roles, and what changes in organisational behaviour will be vital for identifying, monitoring and responding to crisis threats, now as well as in the future? And, are there practical measures that you, the reader, can take now to test your and your organisation's capacities and indeed to improve them?

These questions underpin the final chapters of the book, which look at the theme *Planning from the Future*. Chapters 5, 6, 7, and 8 take you, the reader, back from the future to the present. Each in various ways point to assumptions that are made about the present world order, international systems and organisations, and each proposes ways that those concerned with the increasing types, dimensions and dynamics of humanitarian threats can begin to prepare now for future uncertainties.

Chapter 5 *The Entanglement Nexus* begins this segment of the humanitarian odyssey by moving away from the perspective that humanitarian crises can be divided into those that are local, regional and global. Rather, it proposes that most crises are not only complex but that their direct and indirect consequences are already increasingly global. In an intensifying, interconnected and interdependent world, crisis threats and impacts are spilling across borders and boundaries at virtually all levels.

This emerging reality poses two interrelated questions. In the first instance, who has humanitarian roles and responsibilities in such an interdependent and interconnected world? Second, what would be the motivations for assuming such roles and how could one build upon them?

The cross-societal impacts of global crises means that the traditional assumptions about those deemed to be vulnerable and resilient are already losing their relevance. And, as the nature of vulnerability and resilience change, so, too, are those who feel increasingly compelled to identify, monitor and mitigate humanitarian threats. From that perspective, the standard motivations for taking on a humanitarian role – motivations of sympathy, empathy and personal self-interest – increasingly are giving way to one of *mutual self-interest*. Mutual self-interest may well become the dominant factor in global planning and response processes. If that arguably is the case, then the words of a distinguished observer of crises across the globe truly resonates: 'We're all humanitarians now.'

If the reader would like to see the operational implications of this perspective, there are very practical recommendations about how those with humanitarian roles and responsibilities can best capture and use the momentum of recognised mutual self-interests as a basis for dealing with emerging global threats. Similarly the chapter that follows, Chapter 6, provides practical measures for using a growing number of collaborative systems, alliances, coalitions, networks and social movements to manage humanitarian threats.

As the chapter's title suggests, *Managing Global Threats in a Polylateral World*, the underpinnings of the present world order are already moving away from state-based multilateralism to a more polylateral world order. That is not to dismiss the relevance of 'the state', *per se*, and its related institutions and processes. However, one must acknowledge that states are increasingly overburdened. Their capacities and will to fulfil conventional, let alone new types of commitments and responsibilities, seem constrained, and a plethora of alternative collaborative systems, alliances, coalitions, networks and social movements are emerging. Some will be state-dominated, others not. Some will include states, but not be dominated by them, and others may not include states at all.

In that sense, so it will be argued, humanitarian action will reflect a situationally mixed and multidimensional set of actors who will form *clusters, webs and swarms* when it comes to anticipating and dealing with humanitarian crises. This is by no means to suggest that polylateralism will continue over time. It may well be replaced by another governance paradigm in the future. However, as the recommendations suggest at the chapter's conclusion, those with humanitarian roles and responsibilities should be sensitive to the implications of polylateralism as they look to the foreseeable future.

One of the principal difficulties of adjusting effectively to emerging realities stems from organisational behaviour. In fact, a group of senior policy planners and decision-makers who had come together towards the end of 2020 to discuss ways to manage global threats agreed that 'one of the most serious global hazards which the world faces now and most likely will in the future are the very institutions that have responsibility for dealing with such threats'.[4] Organisations responsible for managing global threats, it was felt, failed to think beyond the immediate in consistent and coherent ways.[5]

With that perspective in mind, Chapter 7 *The Humanitarian Organisation for the Future* first has to clarify what types of organisations might fit within a humanitarian framework. To some extent that issue was explored in the previous chapter when the clusters, webs and swarms metaphors were used to suggest degrees of random organisational diversity in achieving interrelated objectives. Given such diversity, it can certainly be argued that there are behavioural differences that have to be recognised. Conversely, it can also be argued that the very concept of 'the organisation' inevitably suggests all too evident commonalities – sometimes positive, sometimes disconcerting, sometimes negative.

This penultimate chapter will touch on both – organisational differences and commonalities – in order to draw lessons about organisational strengths and weaknesses which are certainly relevant when it comes to humanitarian action. The lessons to be drawn will be based upon five factors, each essential for organisational effectiveness.

The capacity of an organisation to be *anticipatory* is the first. This is not to suggest that prediction is essential. No. However, it does suggest how organisations should have the capacities to explore plausible futures not necessarily based upon the past or present, but based upon the 'what might be's'. A willingness to go beyond precedence in anticipating possible futures clearly relates to a second essential feature of an effective organisation, namely, its *adaptive* capacities. In other words, will the responses of an organisation deemed to be humanitarian depend principally upon well engrained standard operating procedures, siloed responses, an unwillingness to abandon its 'comfort zones' and an abiding concern with institutional survival?

Alternatively, will the organisation realise the importance of operational flexibility, cross-departmental collaboration, shared resources and more integrated decision-making processes? The answer to these questions leads in turn to the third, fourth and fifth factors. The third concerns *collaboration*, or, the willingness of organisations to share information, data, resources, strategies and operational programmes with those across the organisation as well as outside it?

An organisation that is anticipatory, adaptive and collaborative will also actively seek *innovations* and *innovative practices* to enhance its impact. This fourth issue is not about adopting and adapting to the evident but instead to see the search for the unconventional and a willingness to explore its potential applications as an essential component for achieving organisational objectives. There are always better ways to do better things.

However, all too often this aspiration is stymied by conventional organisational processes. And, this last point leads to the issue of *leadership*, the fifth factor. Earlier, reference was made to a group of experts' views that 'the organisation', itself, was all too often 'a global threat'. The reason in part were leaders' seeming reluctance to speculate about the future. 'The challenge though isn't lack of vision but short-term time frames, competing priorities and flawed delivery', concluded the experts.[6]

An ethos of effective anticipation, adaptation, collaboration and innovation all link to the ability of a leader to limit those sorts of recognised organisational dynamics. Rather, leaders will need to see their roles as facilitators and mentors as much as being 'the boss'. They will be willing to promote new ways of working and a commitment to fostering greater internal and external collaboration. They will understand and support decisions which need to be made at the right strategic as well as operational levels and not presume that decisions only can be made top down.

With that in mind, Chapter 7 points to the types of challenges most leaders have to face, and also suggests ways that leaders can overcome at least some of the challenges that in various ways limit organisational performance – in this case, those that impact upon humanitarian strategies and perspectives.

Humanitarian Futures: Challenges and Opportunities arrives at the end of its journey with Chapter 8 *The Helenus Alternative: Planning from the Future*. Over the previous chapters, the reader will have had opportunities to explore many of the strengths and weaknesses of the humanitarian construct as it began to emerge in the mid-1980s. Whether that construct as it has evolved could now deal with the hypothetical but not implausible portraits of future humanitarian threats poses a very fundamental challenge. Already, faced with increasing types of humanitarian crisis drivers often with unprecedented impacts, what steps should be taken to begin to introduce and implement vitally needed change?

Recommendations about such steps have been proposed in Chapters 5, 6 and 7. However, there will be those who remain unconvinced that such transformations are actually needed for their own organisations or for the humanitarian construct as a whole. To a significant extent, this uncertainty and perhaps scepticism underscores the purpose of this book's final chapter. For example, to what extent do those who are uncertain or sceptical understand and appreciate the implications of an increasingly entangled world construct? How would they identify, monitor and mitigate complex humanitarian crises in an increasingly polylateral world? Who will they presume to be 'a humanitarian' and why? And, whatever the organisation, are those upon whom so many of the potentially crisis threatened will depend, adequately anticipatory, adaptive, innovative and collaborative and has its leadership broken away from the conventional?

It is for this reason that Chapter 8 offers a series of practical measures offered as first steps towards testing the capacities of those individuals, organisations and systems with humanitarian roles and responsibilities. These measures are based upon 'tools' and processes that have been developed in collaboration with governments, intergovernmental, regional and non-governmental organisations in Africa, the Americas, Europe, South and Southeast Asia and the Pacific region between 2004 and 2020.

So, what will *Humanitarian Futures: Challenges and Opportunities* have given the reader by the end of this humanitarian odyssey? The author hopes that you, the reader, will ultimately have recognised the strengths and weaknesses of the systems that now determine and implement approaches for dealing with vulnerability and resilience on a cross-societal scale. He, too, hopes that if the reader will be willing to step back from a humanitarian world that is familiar into a world that is dramatically different, and others will begin to ask if present systems and approaches – for all their strengths and weaknesses – are really adequate for dealing with ever more complex humanitarian threats? If not, what are the ways forward? And, with that last question in mind, has the book identified opportunities to meet future humanitarian challenges?

At the outset of this introductory chapter, the tragic figure, Cassandra, was used to say that there are few things more frustrating than having a sense of what the future might hold, which she did, but which was ignored by all. Of course, as also emphasised earlier, the author would not presume to be able to predict – except in one sense. Based upon the actions of those with roles and responsibilities to monitor and mitigate crisis threats and the likelihood that crisis drivers, their dimensions and dynamics, will be increasingly complex, paradigmatic change is needed.

The author hopes that those with humanitarian roles and responsibilities will make the effort to consider such vital changes; and like those who agreed with Cassandra's brother, Helenus, not only will they begin to listen but also to act – starting by *planning from the future* now – for the future.

Notes

1 The Copernican Vision perspective is based upon work supported by the Danish and Swedish governments in 2016 for the *Planning from the Future* project led by the Humanitarian Futures Programme at King's College, London, and partnered with the Overseas Development Institute and Tufts University. (See: www.planningfromthefut ure.org). This author also owes very sincere thanks to Amanda Taylor and Joanne Burke, who supported his work in developing what was entitled, An Alternative Humanitarian Paradigm. See: www.humanitarianfutures.org

2 A history of game changers, Chapter 1, *Planning from the Future* project www.humanita rianfutures.org, Library section, p. 18.

3 Two key figures in the understanding of paradigms and the assumptions that sustain or challenge them are Thomas Kuhn, *The structure of scientific revolutions*, University of Chicago Press, 50th Anniversary Edition, 2012, and Imre Lakatos, *Proofs and refutations: The logic of mathematical discovery*, Cambridge University Press, 1976.

4 This analysis stemmed from a project undertaken by the UK's Royal United Services Institute, supported by King's College, London, *Towards an International Architecture for Managing Global Threats.* Over a period of ten months, 68 experts in the natural sciences, international relations, foresight, and organisational behaviour met to discuss ways to anticipate and deal with a wide range of plausible crisis drivers. The 30 June 2022 report can be found on Royal United Services Institute website, under RUSI – *Towards an International Architecture for Managing Global Threats.*

5 'Some of the greatest mistakes are made when dealing with a complex mess, by not seeing its dimensions in their entirety, carving off a part, and dealing with this part as if it were a complicated problem, and then solving it as if it were a simple puzzle, all the while ignoring the linkages and other connections to other dimensions of the mess.' Ben Ramalingam and H. Jones with T. Reba and J. Young, *Exploring the science of complexity: Ideas and implications for development and humanitarian efforts*, Working Paper 285, ODI, London, 2008.

6 Op. cit., #4. See also Richard Dobbs et al., *No ordinary disruption: The four global forces breaking all the trends*, Public Affairs, McKinsey & Co., 2015.

Bibliography

Dobbs, Richard, Manyika, James and Woetzel, Jonathan, *No ordinary disruption: The four global forces breaking all the trends*, Public Affairs, McKinsey Global Institute, 2015.

Kent, Randolph, *Towards an international architecture for managing global threats*, Royal United Services Institute, June 2022.

Kent, Randolph, Donini, Antonio, Bennett, Christina and Maxwell, Dan, *Planning from the future: Is the humanitarian system fit for purpose?*, 2016. www.humanitarianfutures.org – Library section.

Kuhn, Thomas, *The structure of scientific revolutions*, University of Chicago Press, 50th Anniversary Edition, 2012.

Lakatos, Imre, *Proofs and refutations: The logic of mathematical discovery*, Cambridge University Press, 1976.

Ramalingam, Ben and Jones, Harry with Reba, Toussaint and Young, John, *Exploring the science of complexity: Ideas and implications for development and humanitarian efforts*, Working Paper 285, ODI, 2008.

1 An Odyssey

With the palm of his hands firmly on the desk in front of him, the aid official summed up his experience in the 1970 East Pakistan Bhola cyclone in five words – 'it was pandemonium run riot'.

It was a telling statement, and clearly fit into one of the central themes of a book I was to complete almost a decade and a half later, *Anatomy of Disaster Relief: The International Network in Action*. My research had concluded that the crisis in East Pakistan had generated an international response deemed at the time to be unprecedented. It was the beginning of a loose-knit though identifiable humanitarian network.

Of course, it was by no means the first humanitarian crisis to have gained the attention of the international community during those times. The horror of the Biafran famine from 1967 to 1970, resulting in over one million victims, the 1970 Peruvian earthquake in which 66,000 people lost their lives in a matter of hours, and the two million refugees fleeing in the face of the Cambodian civil war between 1965 and 1970: these were among a growing number of crises that had captured the attention of the media and many governmental and non-governmental organisations around the world.

In various ways, each of these crises had resulted in well-intentioned responses, each reflecting the complex balance between humanitarian concerns and political objectives, and each revealing the interplay between the media, politics and finance, including priority-setting, planning and decision-making processes, as well as organisational and inter-organisational behaviour.

However, that devastating Bhola cyclone and subsequent refugee crisis that had defined the East Pakistan tragedy began by the mid-1970s to frame the dimensions and dynamics of that loose-knit humanitarian network. And, though not intended, it also had begun to provide greater insights into the dynamics and dimensions of threats and subsequent crises more generally.

Soon after *The Anatomy of Disaster Relief* was finished, I joined the United Nations and took up an assignment in the midst of the 1984 Ethiopian famine. By then a degree of predictability had emerged in the humanitarian sector. More and more international non-governmental organisations were engaging in disaster and emergency response, the United Nations finally assumed a highly relevant role

DOI: 10.4324/9781003471004-2

as did some of the UN's key agencies and programmes and a growing number of governments, principally Western-based, became part of a loose-knit network that today is labelled 'humanitarian'.

As a United Nations official from the mid-1980s through to 2004, I was part of that humanitarian sector. Over those years, I was able to work with a wide range of governments – recipients as well as donors, inter-governmental and non-governmental organisations, and on occasion the private sector, the military and religious bodies, all of whom were engaged in various ways in efforts to save the lives and livelihoods of millions threatened by humanitarian crises.

Each of the operations in which I was involved had left me with a variety of impressions, and eventually 'lessons learned'. That said, most of these operations have been very well described and analysed by others. However, the ensuing lessons from those analyses are frequently not applied, and that failure will grow in significance when it comes to dealing with radically changing types, dimensions and dynamics of humanitarian crises in a very uncertain future.

As I try to convey in this book, those with humanitarian roles and responsibilities need to appreciate the fact that historic precedence and short-term strategies are in and of themselves inadequate to prepare for the prospect of future crises. Greater attention has to be given to the importance of anticipating potential crises and the methodologies for doing so.

Organisations that are committed to dealing with humanitarian threats need also to be far more adaptive than has been the case to date. And, in a related vein, they, too, will require new approaches for identifying innovations and innovative practices for monitoring, mitigating and, in the worst case, responding to ever more complex crisis threats. Similarly, the very concept of what is a 'humanitarian actor' and what are humanitarian roles and responsibilities will also need to reflect a fundamental change in how vulnerability will be defined as well as an appreciation of how mutual self-interests will change the very nature of future collaboration.

So many of these fundamental transformations will depend upon new types of leadership. The assumptions that have for millennia defined leadership based upon hierarchies and top-down decision-making will have undergone profound changes over the next generation. Those organisations fit for an ever more complex future will have to adjust accordingly in a world in which more anticipatory and adaptive organisations will in a humanitarian context determine human survival.

To what extent are these transformative aspirations fully understood by those that are and who in the future may well be involved in humanitarian action? And, to what extent would they be willing to implement them?

As one looks to the uncertainties which will inevitably underpin humanitarian futures, these questions must be answered.

Defining the Nature – Types, Dimensions and Dynamics – of Crisis Threats

It was October 1987 in Ethiopia's capital, Addis Ababa. I, as the Emergency Prevention and Preparedness Coordinator for the United Nations Prevention and Preparedness Group, had an appointment with the country director of the US Agency for International Development. The USAID representative was highly regarded and totally committed to providing disaster relief to a country which, three years before, had suffered a famine that had been described as 'a biblical famine in the 20th century... the closest thing to hell on Earth'.[1]

That biblical famine had left an estimated 1.2 million dead, 2.5 million internally displaced and 400,000 refugees over three years. Those horrors were blamed as much on the Ethiopian government's resettlement and 'social transformation' priorities as on the changing pattern of rainfall – 'natural hazards' – that had affected key agricultural areas of the country. The former were driven by the socialist policies and civil war conflicts of the Derg leadership, which covered the period following the overthrow of Emperor Haile Selassie a decade before. The latter, those presumed natural causes, were seen as the results of inadequate and deviant patterns of the belg *rains (from February to April) and the* kerempt *rains (July to September). It was the combination of the two that resulted in approximately 5.8 million people becoming increasingly dependent upon food aid. Long gone were the days when the international community accepted that famines in Ethiopia were unfortunate 'Acts of God'.*

Despite the Derg's priorities, a growing number of senior civil servants and some government ministers were aware that the present situation could not continue, that recovery programmes would have to be introduced as quickly as possible if levels of starvation were to be reduced. Trapped between government priorities and a sceptical international community, they turned to the United Nations Development Programme – at the time the in-country UN co-ordinating body – to ask it to push for much more international assistance to provide tools and seeds, transportation and storage for vital recovery programmes.

That was the reason for my meeting with the USAID official, and I had assumed that the compelling rationale would be positively received. But the answer to the request I was asked to deliver was 'that will be difficult. You see, this sort of aid is not disaster relief; it's development. And we're not here to do development. We're here to deal with the emergency.'

He knew that the Ethiopian request made sense, but he also knew that it would be difficult to sell to USAID under the present Reagan administration in Washington. We discussed the issue from various perspectives – the humanitarian logic, US political opportunities in the Horn of Africa, financial savings and 'definitional' considerations. It was those last – what does one mean by 'humanitarian' and what is meant by 'humanitarian assistance'? – which were perhaps the most interesting and most difficult part of the conversation.

'OK,' he finally said, 'we'll call it "emergency development."'

Looking back, I recall how uncertain the definition of 'humanitarian' was at the time, how seemingly fluid were its boundaries. As the types, dimensions and dynamics of crisis drivers have increased in number and complexity since then, it is interesting to speculate how the concept and operational boundaries of humanitarian action have changed since that discussion a generation ago. Is there really clarity now?

The one thing that perhaps was not generally accepted then, though it is increasingly acknowledged since, is the direct relationship between humanitarian crises and the ways that societies structure themselves and allocate their resources. In Ethiopia at the time, some of the causes of the famine – but by no means all – were regarded as 'natural disasters'. The assumption was that, while conflicts were 'man-made' phenomena such as droughts, volcanic eruptions, floods and earthquakes were not. The impacts of the latter went beyond society's ability to control: in that sense, they were perceived as 'aberrant phenomena'. Even so-called 'man-made disasters', stemming for example from conflict and technological failures, were regarded by many policymakers as being divorced from normal societal contexts. They, too, were seen as 'aberrant'.

In that famine of Biblical proportions, there was considerable reluctance to mesh the 'man-made' and the 'natural', but the reality was that both were reflections of Ethiopian society more generally. What was driving the famine was a combination of social and socio-economic systems that were only beginning to emerge from a kind of neo-feudalism, with an economy that was dominated by 'landlords' who controlled the land and (for all intents and purposes) its produce. It was a society gravely torn by ethnic conflict, and one that lacked an infrastructure or commercial system that could maximise the country's few resources.

As it has proved over time, a distinction between natural and man-made crises was a convenience for donors, and that in turn spilled over into aid operations. To provide assistance to those affected by natural phenomena was regarded as generally acceptable both to domestic publics and internationally. To do so in conflict situations could create political dilemmas which might (in different ways) alienate both. Hence the demarcation between natural and man-made was a convenience, though not a reflection of the true nature of humanitarian crises more generally.

Political dilemmas further complicated another core issue in the humanitarian portfolio, namely humanitarian principles. To a significant degree, international responses to humanitarian crises were supposed to be underpinned by a set of core principles, namely humanity, impartiality, neutrality and independence. They were intended to ensure that all in need could receive assistance regardless of their race, ethnic group, religion, gender, age, nationality or political affiliation. These principles were the basis of the Red Cross and Red Crescent Movement,[2] reaffirmed in UN General Assembly resolutions, and enshrined in numerous humanitarian standards and guidelines.

The reality that emerged, however, was that (more often than not) the principles were merely aspirations, not seeming to be applied in intra-state (e.g. in the Democratic Republic of the Congo) or inter-state (e.g. in Ukraine) conflicts. Lack of predictability and inconsistencies underscore the link between principles and practice. For example,

> ...there is not a consensus on what neutrality looks like in practice. These gaps in common understanding are being used in some contexts to deny local organizations access to funds. In contexts where communities are living in areas

controlled by non-state armed groups, the requirement for organizations to demonstrate 'neutrality' may be effectively meaningless.[3]

The challenges that continue to be confronted when applying humanitarian principles also lead to the issue of the boundaries of humanitarian action more generally.

When the USAID official in Addis Ababa suggested that the term 'emergency development' might provide a solution to the dilemma we had faced, the purpose of that ambiguity was clear. More generally, however, it was also symptomatic of a more persistent problem – agreeing on the conceptual as well as operational boundaries of humanitarian action. Then as today, efforts were made to reach agreement on humanitarian and development boundaries. Is humanitarian assistance solely about meeting the survival needs of the disaster-affected, or should humanitarian assistance also include measures to prevent, prepare for and even recover from disasters?

Take, for example, the situation in Somalia in 2022. Humanitarian organisations had provided health and food aid, but such aid could not prevent the collapse of livelihoods and economic activities, and the risk of further humanitarian crises. As Afghanistan during this same period illustrated, functions that were crucial for the maintenance of economic activity, and for health, education and social protection systems to be effective, needed to include electricity and telecoms as well as payment systems.

From an operational perspective, the boundary between development and humanitarian action depends upon very pragmatic negotiations and arrangements with a wide array of actors (who can include those who have obtained power unconstitutionally, or who are accused of corruption, or whom donor states do not recognise or have prohibitions against). In other words, determining humanitarian-development boundaries remains at best uncertain and situationally dependent.

From a more conceptual perspective those boundaries had been framed in terms of a 'disaster-development continuum'. In other words, those factors that triggered a crisis could – for the continuum-oriented – be used as the basis for targeted development. But, this perspective was countered by a contending view, in which development and disaster prevention and response, rather than relying on a continuum, could be accomplished in parallel. Neither, according to those adhering to this sort of parallelism, should constrain the other.

As the number of conflicts and accompanying humanitarian crises increased substantially by 2016, the means for reconciling conflicts and humanitarian assistance took other forms. The 'triple nexus' was one such example, being created to bring together peacebuilding, development and humanitarian assistance to interact with each other in conflict-driven crises.[4] The OECD, among others, had also been urging donors to promote social protection, humanitarian preparedness and development more generally, in addition to humanitarian response.

As I look back more than a quarter of a century later, the dimensions and dynamics of the Covid-19 pandemic suggest disconcerting parallels with key aspects of the

Ethiopian crisis. For both there was a plethora of contending perspectives on the nature, source and parameters of the crises and solutions for dealing with them.

As other OECD studies have made clear, there were very fundamental differences in interpretations between scientists and governments about the causes of the crises and solutions for addressing them. At the same time, there were inconsistent interpretations among the scientists themselves, and certainly between the natural and social sciences. The latter were particularly concerned that even scientific data all too often reflected subjective assumptions about those being analysed. Such 'data inequality' and 'exclusion' posed profound threats to evidenced-based policy planning and decision-making.[5]

More generally, the technical knowledge of the sciences was subject to contending interpretation: experts on many occasions did not speak with one voice. In many countries, conflicting expert advice was the norm, not the exception.

In part, as in the Ethiopian famine, the boundaries of the Covid-19 crisis remained uncertain and, for example, international organisations such as the World Health Organization provided inadequate guidance about the nature and parameters of the threat. Some argued that the WHO was too diplomatic and hence too slow, prioritising consensus over tough choices. Others accused it of having been too close to China, and thus unable to provide impartial advice in a timely manner, to prevent an epidemic from becoming a pandemic.[6]

In any event, similar to that 'emergency development' solution proposed in Addis Ababa, there was little agreement about the parameters of the Covid-19 threat. There were various reasons why. Frequently, there were contending interpretations about the reasons and nature of crises that all too often ignored essential aspects of their contexts. Furthermore, extensive analysis has made it very evident that not only do emergencies often amplify pre-existing conditions in economic and political systems but can also aggravate divisions such as racial and economic disparities, political hyper-partisanship and distrust of governing elites.

In that sense, outcome measures were always value-laden, that is to say that theories concerning the source of the pandemic and who was to blame distorted objective responses to it. Out of Covid-19 emerged a 'geography of blame' that would stigmatise Asian and Asian-American peoples, neighbourhoods and communities. As was noted by anthropologists in the midst of the crisis, a 'fortress mentality' of controlling borders did not translate into effective disease control strategies.[7] Covid-19, like the Ethiopian famine, resulted in a resurgence of such divisions. For example,

> within the Dominican Republic officials became concerned with regulating Haitians as 'dangerous' bodies rather than responding to the public health threat. During the Covid-19 pandemic, these ethnographic accounts alert us to the likelihood that social surveillance and political exclusion will intensify stigmas associated with domestic or international border/ boundary-crossers – migrants, immigrants, refugees, and tourists. Viruses know no borders, so violent political discourses and social measures generate conditions for viruses to replicate,

moving from body to body regardless of what side of a border someone finds themselves.[8]

Back in the mid-1980s, many of Ethiopia's Tigrayan and Eritrean populations in the north of the country would recognise many of those factors that blurred an understanding of the causes, nature and boundaries of the famine. So, too, would many of those observers of the dimensions and dynamics of Covid-19, for example, in Brazil, India and the United States some 25 years later.[9]

Now, reflecting on that meeting so many years ago in Addis Ababa, I wonder if my USAID counterpart would have been able to convince his Washington headquarters that 'emergency development' was justifiable within the boundaries of humanitarian action. In reality, I doubt that the definitional issue ever arose. There might have been political ramifications discussed and, of course, the cost of implementation, and would anyone in USAID's Office for Foreign Disaster Assistance want to venture into the institutional maze of the Office of Management and Budget, let alone relevant committees in the US Congress?

Anyway, that official soon left Addis Ababa in the normal course of rotation, and his successor had little time for what, a few weeks previously, had been called 'emergency development'.

Crises from Organisational Perspectives

At long last, it seemed as if we were going to get the breakthrough. The UN agencies, along with various NGOs, had been pressing the Government of Sudan to permit access into the south to assist the tens of thousands of civilians caught up (once again) in a conflict between the Sudanese Patriotic Liberation Army and government forces. It was 1991, two years after Operation Lifeline Sudan (OLS) had brought UN agencies, principally UNICEF and the World Food Programme, and approximately 35 NGOs together to provide assistance throughout the war-torn and drought-afflicted regions in the South, during the second Sudanese civil war.

Now the heads of UN agencies, along with myself as Chief of the UN Emergency Unit, were crowded into the Commissioner's small office, with the hope that there would be a renewal of OLS, and that the Government would once again recognise the need to provide 'neutral' international assistance to the drought- and conflict-affected.

The Commissioner was welcoming and, as always, dignified. He began on a very upbeat note. The Government, he said, had agreed to permit the UN agencies, along with the NGOs, to provide assistance to their 'Sudanese brothers in the south'. He went on to say that the Government fully recognised that the agencies knew as much as the Government about the needs of the affected and the best delivery routes, and clearly would have greater access to much-needed resources. The Government therefore trusted the international agencies completely, and they should know how grateful the Government and he, on behalf of the Relief and Rehabilitation Commission, were for the assistance that the agencies and NGOs would provide.

The agencies had climbed the mountain. Their roles were recognised. Though not overtly demonstrated, there was a sense of euphoria. 'However', continued the Commissioner, 'the Government only makes one request...' And, with the prospect of that 'one request', all the hopes of the agencies around the room began to deflate. There was a sense that 'that one request' would most likely be that all resources, or at least a significant portion, would have to go through the Government, or at least that the Government would assume overall responsibility for the operation.

To the contrary, the Commissioner made no mention of the Government's involvement. There was a resurgence of optimism among the agencies, and, just before concluding, the Commissioner said that 'The Government's only other request – which shouldn't be a problem – is that all resources and all aspects of the relief operations should go directly through one single body – the office of the United Nations in Khartoum.'

There was shock throughout the room. Disbelief. The agency representatives looked at each other aghast. Didn't the Commissioner understand? There was no way that the resources for the operation, provided to individual agencies, could be filtered through one single organisation. Surely he didn't understand... or did he?

Certainly, since the 'pandemonium run riot' that marked the initial response to the 1970 East Pakistan cyclone, the aid agencies that were assembled to meet with the RRC Commissioner reflected a more organised and structured network of actors. And, despite the fluctuating boundaries of humanitarianism, a sector was emerging that was increasingly responsive, and with recognised competencies when it came to humanitarian crises, the drivers of which were deeply intertwined.

However, collaboration and integrated operational planning and response to meet these challenges were by no means predictable. Though increasingly the sharing of information became the norm, it was often self-serving and not necessarily transparent. Rarely were there planned responses that reflected a sense of interdependence, or (from an operational perspective) a willingness to come together for reasons of common interest, or even of accepted mutual self-interest. There was, in other words, little reason to assume that, when it came to responding to the prospect of humanitarian threats or crises, the sector would come together in ways that reflected recognised, interdependent and integrated objectives. Whether for the purposes of a single time-bound objective or of objectives over time, little suggested the emergence of a coherent, consistent and predictable network that might be regarded as a *system*.

This is not to imply that there were not determined efforts to improve the humanitarian sector, to focus on better approaches and institutions for response and coordination, to expand the sources of support and utilise innovative practices to respond to the perceived needs of the crisis-affected. Nor is it to say that the sector did not have well-intentioned critics as it evolved, or that within relevant organisations and across them, there were not considerable efforts to prompt change and to strengthen coordination and collaboration. It is, though, to say that with all the dynamism and commitments to improve and reform the sector, it was trapped in a kind of stasis – which in this instance failed to turn the ostensible willingness for reform into truly systemic collaboration.

Despite the initiatives to bring UN agencies and NGOs together in harmonious ways to seek humanitarian funding for specific issues (e.g. via the Common Appeals Process), to promote more timely and reliable humanitarian assistance (e.g. via the Central Emergency Response Fund), or to create a 'cluster approach' to promote more coherent and coordinated operational action, neither strategic nor technical commitments ultimately could be relied upon when institutional survival was at stake.[10] All too often, what one saw were increasing and discordant scrambles for resources that were deemed essential for institutional survival.

Of course, it could be argued that such competition should in theory result in enhanced specialisations, that could make humanitarian response more effective and (perhaps paradoxically) a more interactive system. That might well be the case if donor funding were provided in a practical and rational manner. Sadly, it was not and is not. It had become, in the words of one highly experienced UN official, 'a marketplace', and in the words of another, 'a humanitarian *souk* in which institutional independence and self-absorption belie a seeming increase in relative cooperation and predictability'.[11] And, as one senior NGO staff member stressed, 'a good emergency can keep an agency running in the black for months'.[12]

Such projects might well have been worthwhile and well-intentioned, yet the fluid boundaries defining humanitarian action also continued to intensify competition among humanitarian actors. All too often, those with humanitarian roles and responsibilities were tempted to go beyond their recognised expertise and adopt an 'I can-do-that-too' attitude that collided with the acknowledged expertise of others. Inter-organisational competition may have filled the coffers of individual actors, but it clearly spoiled the terrain for a system's approach to humanitarian action.

Frequently this competitive aid environment also distorted the assessment of beneficiary needs, and the international appeals for assistance to meet such needs. According to one generally well-received study, the process by which needs were determined was not based upon a systematic approach to data collection and prioritisation but all too often was determined 'by the resource-mobilisation process'.[13] As for efforts to monitor the impact of humanitarian interventions, the study concluded that accountability in this respect is determined (more often than not) by humanitarian organisations' delivery calculations for donors, rather than upon the effects that aid has had upon those in need.[14]

If principles become fungible, if beneficiary needs are time and again determined by donors' interests and organisations' own fixation on institutional survival, if aid becomes a witting or unwitting accomplice in political and military strategies, then the moral and practical significance of humanitarianism will have been lost. Certainly what was clearly lost is an enduring commitment to any interactive systems for the survival of the crisis-affected, as well as for those institutions that were ostensibly there to assist them.

As many who have looked at the consequences of organisational and inter-organisational behaviour will attest, the reactions of those humanitarian bodies during their meeting with the Commissioner were not untypical. Across the institutional spectrum, whether in organisations in the private or the public sector, the tendency to perceive organisational survival as a legitimate driving force is by no means unusual. It is a reality reinforced by the very constructs of 'the organisation': who are the experts, who are the planners and decision-makers, and what are the processes and procedures that lead them to decisions?

A quarter of a century later, a group of 41 experts from the public and private sectors came together in a series of Zoom meetings to discuss the sorts of systems that are required to manage global threats. Some 54 per cent of the discussants noted that one of the most serious global threats which the world faced then, and most likely will do in the future, are the very institutions that have responsibility for dealing with such threats.[15]

Governments, it was felt, failed to think beyond the immediate in consistent and coherent ways. Sometimes specific types of threats and responses were seen as being so embedded in their own processes that governments do not welcome alternatives that might change those processes. This assumption is reinforced by the ways that organisations all too often fail to search for what has been described as the 'butterfly effect', where the proverbial flapping of that butterfly's wings can eventually be the triggering factor responsible for a storm in some other part of the world. There, too, is the compelling though disconcerting 'black swan theory' where an event reflects a situation deemed to be totally anticipatable, though generally with severe consequences.[16] And, of course, there, too, are those 'unknown unknowns'…[17]

Deep uncertainties further reflect the ways that planners and decision-makers define hazards. All too often it is only shocks that generate change, and those changes all too often create unanticipated vulnerabilities.

When dealing with what was described as 'longer-term threats', the experts felt that planners and decision-makers tend to suggest that these threats are far away, and that their plausibility and 'practical relevance' are therefore significantly reduced. A better term, it was felt, would be 'hidden threats'.

The belief that institutions that are responsible for addressing threats were all too often threats themselves was reflected in the ways that hazards were analysed.[18] A person will view and interpret an event largely in terms of what he or she has been led to expect: therefore, the more familiar a particular phenomenon, the more quickly it will be recognised, and even rare occurrences, given the force of previous experience, may lead one to mistake them for the usual. Furthermore, information that is consistent with expectations is rated by observers as more accurate, and is better remembered, than information that is inconsistent with the expectations of the observer.

These observations all too often lie at the core of organisational behaviour. Warnings missed, relief delayed, insensitivity to victims, inappropriate relief – all of these were accusations laid at the doorsteps of an increasing number of organisations, governmental, inter-governmental and non-governmental. For many observers, organisations with their preoccupation with institutional survival and mechanistic approaches to complex problems inevitably had to bear the opprobrium of the callousness and inefficiency that marked all too many relief efforts.

When it comes to the ways that goals are defined, no matter how clear are the 'formal goals' an organisation cannot operate in a realm of ambiguity, and it deals with ambiguity by focussing on those issues that it recognises, and that it can extract as definable and tangible issues from ambiguous situations. What the organisation can handle are essentially those matters to which the experts are attuned. When executives talk about getting to grips with the 'immediate problem', more often than not they are talking about the organisational propensity to deal with problems that they recognise and that are readily definable in their own terms.

Where and how information comes into the organisation is also a paramount consideration in determining the process by which organisations define problems. The very fact that disaster information has so many unpredictable and inconsistent entry points means that information may be screened in different ways, or indeed even screened out, depending upon how and where the information enters into the organisation.

Once specialists have focused on their particular component of a problem, the organisation needs to group its various standard operating procedures (SOPs) into an overall organisational solution. This grouping or coordinating process results in a 'programme', and, a programme, too, becomes standardised, reflecting an overall organisational approach to any particular problem. Given that an organisation continually confronts problems – some perceived as similar and others as different – an organisation has an arsenal of programmes that it can apply to a variety of matters that fall within its purview.

This accumulation of programmes is the organisation's 'repertoire', and it is from repertoires of pre-programmed responses that the organisation normally picks and chooses what it deems to be the best solution for any particular response. Of course, SOPs and repertoires can be modified or even abandoned, and alternatives sought – but all too often only at the edge of chaos when so-called 'tried and tested means' are clearly irrelevant.

In light of the increasing numbers and complexity of global threats, overcoming such organisational weaknesses should be high on the list of organisational priorities. Yet, though the word is out, major gaps between theory and application seem to continue unrelenting. This would seem to be the case when it comes to those in the corporate sector who are all too often perceived as being comfortable taking risks which they can control, but are far less so when confronted 'with new and severe non-financial risks that challenge status quo assumptions about control effectiveness'.[19]

Similarly, reflecting on the rapid upsurge of the Covid-19 pandemic in 2019, the Independent Panel on Climate Change noted that there were two worlds at play. The first was the world of fast-paced information and data-sharing, constantly updating and sharing outbreak information. The second was the slow and deliberate pace with which information is treated, with organisational step-by-step confidentiality, verification requirements and threshold criteria, and with greater emphasis on action that should not be taken, rather than action that should.[20]

And, this is true well beyond the boundaries of pandemics. Even in a world in which systems more generally are being transformed by an upsurge in data and AI, there is either a reluctance to share such potentially transformative outputs or a lack of designated responsibility or capacity to promote 'shared intelligence'.[21]

This message was further reinforced in a study focused on Collective Intelligence for humanitarian organisations, which concluded that when it comes to putting AI in the hands of frontline humanitarian actors, organisational inertia and lack of leadership come into play.

> Slow adoption of new tools and innovative methods is often a result of a lack of senior advocacy within major humanitarian organisations. Many of these organisations have traditional structures and approaches that have been ingrained through decades of practice, often resulting in "organisational inertia." Persistent scepticism about the value of community or frontline derived knowledge and data has resulted in top-down preference for traditional data sources and a lack of process shift and/ or willingness to include participatory approaches into the workflows.[22]

Such reluctance, too, goes back to that meeting in Khartoum in 1989 when the group of humanitarian organisations resisted effective collaboration in no small part due to financial self-interests. It was an attitude that was reflected in a survey of leaders in the INGO sector over 30 years later, in which one interviewee noted that 'money unfortunately speaks very loudly, certainly in my organisation and I think in many of the others'. There are matters that may for some at the organisation transcend all other organisational interests, such as Black Lives Matter:

> and we also have other members (I'm sad to say), where it's like it's not real for them. I mean they see it and they empathise, I'd say, and intellectually they go on part of the journey, but to really get to the point where they have to change and their part of the organisation has to change, I've not seen that fully.[23]

In a related vein, 'collaborative advantage', a by-product of interconnectedness, reflects a growing awareness that 'organisational success is born out of fostering an optimal relationship with the entire external environment that maximises the combined total value-creating process and generates benefits for the organisation'.[24] In other words, it would appear that effective systems reflect a perception that their value is based not only upon recognised interdependencies, but also that such interdependencies rely on ecosystems far more extensive than any single sector.

After our meeting with the RRC's Commissioner, I returned to the UN's compound to meet with an old friend and expert on disasters and emergencies.[25] *He wanted to propose an interesting approach for dealing with the famine crisis affecting large parts of Sudan's western province, Darfur. He asked me what the UN was going to do about the situation, and I replied that among other initiatives, the World Food Programme would soon be distributing over a quarter of a million tonnes of food that was awaiting delivery from the warehouse in Port Sudan.*

He didn't look impressed. 'Why would you do that?' he asked. 'What you want to do is to take about 15 tonnes to a couple of local markets, and that would be enough to force the traders to lower their prices, and those lower prices would make food far more accessible. Dumping a quarter million tonnes of food in the area will destroy the market and leave those poor people totally dependent upon food aid.'

'Good point,' I replied, 'but though it makes sense, I could never get WFP to agree to that.' But what I didn't bother saying was that there was little that could be done to adjust the situation. The agencies would most likely object if we tried to interfere in any single organisation's operations.

The Politicisation Process and Humanitarian Implications

'You see, we just can't call what's happening in Bosnia a "man-made emergency": it's a "complex emergency",' insisted the New York Director of the United Nations Department for Humanitarian Affairs [now the Office for the Coordination of Humanitarian Affairs]. 'We must avoid giving the sense that domestic conflict was the principal factor that led to the emergency. We know that they're principally "man-made", but if we describe them as such, the government [of the disaster-affected peoples] will just slam the door in our face. It is more than likely that the government will become extremely suspicious and will just not accept our assistance. I think the term "complex emergencies" is better under the circumstances.'

It was difficult to ignore the logic. Clearly, so many of the crises that were emerging were politically driven. Bosnia was certainly one. In April 1992, a bloody conflict broke out in Bosnia-Herzegovina when it declared independence from Yugoslavia – pitting Bosnia's three main constituent communities – ethnic Serbs, Croats and Muslims – against each other. The war resulted in massive displacement and forms of genocide. As for the former, the number of Bosnian refugees and internally displaced persons reached 2.6 million. Regarding the latter, ethnic cleansing resulted in the deaths of at least 8,000 Bosnian Muslims.

Even though the term 'complex emergency' had begun to gain operational definition by 1994, for some it still suggested a degree of convenient vagueness, which in turn provided political latitude and flexibility. The official term meant that a humanitarian crisis stemmed from multiple causes which normally would require the intervention of UN peacekeeping forces. Unofficially, the term was used to bypass confrontations that otherwise would stir political pots. Politics to depoliticise politics.

At this stage a few of my seniors in the department didn't want to over-emphasise that fact. That was their call. If relief organisations were going to get access to a country's crisis-affected populations, then the last thing that was needed was to have a government refuse access, assistance or both. Finding ways to avoid these sorts of confrontations, and to bring contending parties together, seemed to me justification enough for the UN's involvement in humanitarian crises.

'You see, that's why we call them "complex emergencies,"' he reminded me. 'They're not "natural"; they're not "man-made". They're just "complex".' And at the time, I agreed. Around the office I sensed a kind of subtle winking or perhaps

wincing among a few of my colleagues whenever the term "complex emergency" was used.[26]

In the midst of the East Pakistan crisis in 1971, a distinguished Indian civil servant, P. N. Haksar, commented that in international relations 'there is no system which can move in a humanitarian rather than a political fashion. There are two streams in society: emotions of conscience and the state system. The first is prevented by the second.'[27] An equally telling perspective was that of former UN Secretary-General Kurt Waldheim, who was quoted as saying that 'four years ago [1974], I believed that humanitarian relief was above politics. Now I know that humanitarian relief is politics.'[28]

Those reflections, as well as what was happening during my two-year stay at New York headquarters, really did seed that perspective in a couple of interrelated ways. One was that it was evident that for aid providers, as well as recipients at institutional levels, humanitarian action was shrouded in self-interested politics, more often than not. Another was that political constraints reinforced short-termism at the expense of more considered perspectives.

Complex emergencies from the UN perspective – be it in Bosnia, Sudan or Somalia – reflected the reluctant but inevitable acceptance that more and more humanitarian crises were due to overt political failures. At the same time, the more evident the political drivers the more obvious were the politically defined responses of the international community. This recognition, difficult for the United Nations to parade too publicly, appeared to pit humanitarian principles against the UN's more overtly political and judgemental responsibilities, particularly when it came to issues affecting sovereignty and peacebuilding.

That political calculations permeated humanitarian assistance – in this case, international assistance – was by no means a new theme. As humanitarian crises moved to centre-stage in governmental interests, they were increasingly imbued with high levels of political significance, both domestically and internationally. While the survival of a government of a crises-affected country may depend upon the way it responded to a humanitarian crisis, the ways that other governments and international actors responded to that crisis will have increasingly political consequences as well.

The political consequences of external support for a beleaguered state are as old as humanitarian response itself.[29] What was new and increasingly significant was the ever more overt politicisation of humanitarian engagement. It was not merely the type of assistance that was provided, but the context – the perceived public relations support or overt or implied criticism – that came with assistance. For both sides – recipient and donor governments – this context clearly affected wider interests, including commercial relations and common security arrangements.

This meant in no small part that how and who provides assistance would weigh heavily on recipient and donor government decision-makers, and that decisions would be more and more influenced by the abiding political interests linked to the provision of assistance. What is referred to as the 'instrumentalisation of humanitarian assistance',[30] where assistance is used often in surreptitious ways to achieve 'non-humanitarian objectives', was becoming more overtly calculated and more obviously political.

An emerging reality, closely tied to the increasingly politicised nature of humanitarianism, was a general reluctance to go too far beyond what were deemed to be immediate convenience. Longer-term perspectives were generally sacrificed to the more immediate. Capturing lessons-learned arising from past operations, let alone anticipating future challenges, were not priorities for a sector which worked in a perpetual present, a present that inhibited or limited creative thinking, and narrowed horizons to recognisable experiences – ignoring the possibility that there might be a different, let alone, bigger picture.

Such limitations were reflected in ever-more-cumbersome bureaucracies throughout the humanitarian sector, including governmental, inter-governmental and non-governmental organisations. Intensified centralisation and an increasing focus on organisational priorities and competition mirrored political constraints and opportunities. All too often the well-being of those in need was 'distanced' by the priorities of donors' political agendas.

Caution, too, seeded a focus on the immediate. A growing number of policy-planners, decision-makers and even supposedly impartial analysts were becoming collectively short-sighted, succumbing to a kind of political blindness in which the implications of transformative change and complexity were being ignored. As organisations they appeared to be reluctant to go beyond acceptable political limits, perhaps symbolised in the post-9/11 world by the strictures of compliance, or donors' insistence that organisations receiving their support will be held responsible for any aid falling into the hands of those deemed to be politically unacceptable.

Clearly political acceptability and unacceptability take many forms, but perhaps what is most disconcerting is the extent to which – despite rhetoric to the contrary – both were rarely determined by longer-term interests and objectives. The need for policymakers to accommodate contending interests within their own state systems and related alliance structures generally meant that the longer term was all too often sacrificed for the immediate. This obvious home-truth was particularly evident at the UN Climate Change Conference (COP 26) in November 2021 in Glasgow, and its follow-on (COP 27) one year later in Sharm el-Sheik. In different ways, except in a few instances, the global futures rhetoric was not truly reflected in practical measures to achieve the goals that the organisers sought, as evidenced once again at COP 28 in Dubai.[31]

Despite the fact that scientists from around the world warned of the perils of not addressing climate change by 2030, few governments went beyond broad aspirational rhetoric,[32] and few committed themselves to setting tangible targets in the immediate future.

> What countries didn't do is commit to taking the emissions-cutting actions needed to achieve this. They didn't have to, because under the agreement [the 2015 Paris Climate Change Agreement], it is up to each country to say what it will do to tackle climate change by 2030.[33]

More and more, however, there were dimensions of politically driven state control that by the 2020s reflected an alternative political reality, namely, that the assumptions underpinning the drivers of politics were undergoing varying degrees of fundamental change. *Functional* inter-dependencies and interests in principle were running in parallel with those of short-term political interests, and actors and political motivations were perceived as changing.[34]

The divisions between the political and functional were distinct but were becoming increasingly blurred at the edges. In various ways, as the World Health Organization knew all too well, the political could certainly override the functional. Increasingly, however, functional interests were determining the political, or frequently influencing political agendas, and those pursuing such functional interests increasingly reflected an amalgam of actors that were not necessarily dominated by those of the state.

That rebalancing might also have reflected another emerging reality, described as *polylateralism*, in which 'agents of global civil society and subnational governments are taking up the slack of faltering nation-states'.[35] The traditional multilateral construct may increasingly have lacked the capacities of dealing with complex problems.[36] Even in some of the richest states in the world there were signs that opaque, drawn-out processes, combined with contending bureaucratic interests, all too often reflect(ed) pervasive dysfunctionalities.[37] Governance within the foreseeable future, so it was suggested, may well be more distributed and will reflect 'diverse constituencies from across the world with common interest and values [which] can act effectively alongside creaking sovereignty'.[38]

This is not to suggest that states had abandoned their involvement in issues of potentially global consequence. Rather it is to suggest that as one looks towards systems for managing global threats, the functional may more and more determine the political. Pandemics, cyber vulnerabilities, climate change, the growing dependence upon outer space for communications and eventually for mineral resources, all reflect functional issues which increasingly framed political agendas.

The upsurge of international and global non-state and multisectoral institutions and networks, many but by no means all including states, rose by 46 per cent between 1992 and 2021. Some 44 per cent of this was accounted for by institutions and networks involved in environmental issues, which would seem to point to a more polylateral international architecture.[39] Such institutions and networks spanned a considerable range of global concerns. From the GAVI Vaccine Alliance, the International Science Council, the World Benchmarking Alliance and the Research Data Alliance, all attempted to support global initiatives that are essential, broadly speaking, for human survival, and that are not determined by conventional political agendas. They are not inherently against the nation-state construct, but rather attempt to guide it, or compensate for its failings, or further support it. In that sense, they fall naturally into a governance paradigm that is deemed to be polylateral.

Those who see that multilateralism will give way to polylateralism often begin with the potential impacts of technological transformations. They suggest, for example, that the proliferation of communications technologies will be a key factor in moving the concentration of power away from states and state-based institutions, and transferring it to alternative virtual and physical networks, organisations, local communities and individuals.[40] To a very significant degree, sheer complexity will force fundamental structural change. 'We have to be able to hardwire an ability to adapt and see things that we'd otherwise ignore because they don't fit our old conditions,' noted two well-respected proponents of more globalised perspectives.[41]

Over the next two decades, the pace and reach of technological developments are likely to increase ever faster, transforming a range of human experiences and capabilities, and they will have a major influence in determining the political dynamics that will influence and be influenced by political systems, now and certainly in the longer term.

As I prepared to leave UN headquarters for Rwanda in September 1994, I recall a chat I had in a colleague's office about the challenges which the international community faced in the aftermath of one of the worst genocides in recent history. We were discussing why the international community had responded so slowly to that genocidal horror, despite a plethora of warnings. We both concluded that a critical factor was that the US didn't want to get embroiled in another UN peace-building exercise, in the wake of its disastrous raid in the Somali capital, Mogadishu, in October 1993.

The White House was most likely concerned that the public would not want to witness what might be regarded as yet another wasted intervention on the turbulent African continent.

That disinterest seemed to spill over into the attitudes of many other governments. Whatever the implications or the reputation of the UN, for international human rights which had been so grotesquely violated by this most recent genocide, and for peacebuilding in the future, political immediacy would be the principal determinant. It's the way states normally did things, so we concluded.

Confronting Complexity in Humanitarian Contexts

No one was quite sure of the numbers killed between 18 and 23 April 1995. Estimates ranged from 260 to 8,000. Nor was anyone ever sure about the incidents that immediately precipitated the massacre, although it eventually became the subject of an international inquiry. Most eyewitnesses agree that large numbers of internally displaced persons (IDPs) in a camp called Kibeho in southwest Rwanda just panicked. Deprived of food, shelter and basic sanitation for almost four days, and uncertain about the future that lay before them, a large group of the camp's occupants tried to break out of the cordon created by the Rwandese Patriotic Army; and, the army, under-trained and on edge, let loose with volleys of automatic weapons and rocket grenade-launchers into the terrified crowds.

The new Government of Rwanda that had taken over in July 1994 was determined to see the IDP camps closed. It saw them as safe havens for those predominantly Hutu genocidaires responsible for the death of approximately 800,000 people in four months as well as an affront to Rwanda's sovereignty – 'little Rwandas within Rwanda' – which posed a security problem.

The humanitarian sector's responses to the Kibeho assault had for all intents and purposes been quite effective. Though very ad hoc, there was good coordination and delivery of assistance and, at the insistence of the government, also transport to return the IDPs to their villages. Those who refused to return, the government would assume, were perpetrators of the genocide.

Not long after Kibeho, I was invited to have lunch with the recently appointed Vice President and Minister of Defence for Rwanda, General Paul Kagame, and his wife. It could at best be described as a business luncheon. It certainly wasn't social.

'You know,' said General Kagame, 'I'm not convinced that the international community is fully aware of the profound changes that have occurred in the country since the genocide. Do you appreciate, for example, the number of women who have become heads of households since July [the end of the genocide]? How much does the international community understand about what the country has suffered?'

My host was clearly frustrated by many aspects of the international community's response to the abhorrent events that had befallen the country – a point that he underscored in more than one instance. The government was 'disappointed' at the relatively slow response of the aid sector, and was particularly upset that an estimated 900,000 internally displaced persons were receiving international assistance in such camps as Kibeho, many of whom were genocidaires. He was more than perplexed that the United Nations peacekeeping force – UNAMIR – had been given a relatively wide-ranging responsibility for protection, which in the aftermath of the genocide reflected a deeply cruel irony.

Nevertheless, to some extent several of the international community's perceived failings were being addressed. The UN Special Representative of the Secretary General, Shaharyar Khan, had begun discussions with the Government about ways to close down the displaced persons camps, and certainly by September over 130 NGOs had come to provide assistance, along with the ICRC and UN agencies. Despite very positive progress on a variety of fronts, the Government remained an uneasy partner, and in light of the traumas which the nation had experienced, its suspicions about the trustworthiness of the international community were clearly understandable.

As someone whose family was forced to leave Europe prior to the Second World War, I was not insensitive to the plight of the Rwandan people. In that sense, my role as UN Humanitarian Coordinator had particular meaning for me. And, yet, as I recalled my stay in Rwanda a few years later, I realised something that I so unfortunately had failed to see at the time. In a country in which an estimated 800,000 people were slaughtered in four months, we had provided significant amounts of assistance to those who had survived. Food, clothing, shelter, medical assistance – all those things that the aid community deemed essential.

Where, however, was the psychological support, the social-psychological assistance to those who had survived the worst genocide since the Second World War? What did this say about our sensitivity to the context in which we were operating? Even when we ostensibly shared common objectives with the crisis-affected, we failed to take into account their perspectives and perception of needs. Together – the international community and those whom it was there to assist – failed to understand each other's motives, assumptions and capacities.

When General Kagame had condemned what he saw as the international community's insensitivity in the ways that it responded in the aftermath of the genocide, he might have been right on two counts. The first was in relation to the sorts of assistance that Rwanda was receiving, which probably owed as much to organisational dynamics as they did to adequately sensitive assessments and understanding of need. Organisations unintentionally – but inevitably – responded within their comfort zones.

A second issue, closely related to the first, was that this same gulf (between the international community's understanding of the Rwandan situation and that of the Rwandan Government) also undermined various attempts at collaboration. There were of course a plethora of factors, well beyond organisational standard operating procedures, that widened that gulf. There was, for example, the very contentious issue of what the UN and the ICRC deemed to be unjust and overcrowded prisons for those whom the Government regarded as genocidaires. There, too, were persistent fears among the authorities that UN-supported refugee camps in what was then Zaire would pose a threat to communities on the Rwandan borders. Also, there was that all-too-recognisable and understandable competition for international resources among recently established Government ministries. And, then there was that seemingly insurmountable divide between those from the international community who tried to provide assistance, and those Rwandan officials who believed that too many 'outsiders' did not truly understand the impact of a late-twentieth-century 'holocaust'.

The list of differences and conflicting interests and perspective was extensive. However, in retrospect what it also demonstrated was that neither side really appreciated what it would take to generate effective collaboration. Neither was able to listen with sufficient sensitivity to the other's case. There were so many routes which together could have been tested to foster a sense of common cause, even if core issues remained contentious. In retrospect, the failure to open doors for joint undertakings was all too evident.

Different approaches to information and processes, and different professional 'languages' and ways to assess problems and determine solutions, may not have resolved immediate, core concerns. Jointly exploring differences and commonalities for purposes that were not immediately contentious might have led to levels of collaboration which, sadly, were never achieved.

In May 2016 a World Humanitarian Summit was held in Istanbul, bringing together over 9,000 participants from 173 countries, including 55 heads of state, private sector and civil society representatives, as well as those from a wide range of intergovernmental and non-governmental organisations. Its purpose, according to the UN's Secretary-General at the time, Ban Ki-moon, was to establish common best practices among the increasingly wide spectrum of organisations involved in humanitarian action.

Perhaps one of the most substantive results of that two-day meeting was the 'Grand Bargain' which consisted of 55 commitments – one of which was a call for *localisation*. The term localisation was vague when it came to precise definition, let alone implementation. Yet, at least it was a recognition by some of the world's largest aid donors that too little attention had been given to recognising and (where required) enhancing the participatory roles of local authorities and communities when it came to humanitarian responsibilities. This was by no means to ignore the vital role of international actors, but at the same time it was a recognition that the determination of needs and distribution should be 'local' whenever and whenever possible. These were intended to be positive steps towards substantive collaboration.

Despite such good intentions, implementation had proven to be difficult. The conclusions of a study, undertaken five years after the Grand Bargain was launched, would have been recognised by many officials in Rwanda in the aftermath of the genocide.

The participation of affected populations appeared to be more of an 'add-on' than an integral approach to achieving the improved humanitarian outcomes that were envisaged. Efforts at localisation were recognised in principle, but in practice they fell far short of a system-wide shift towards ensuring that humanitarian responses were more demand-driven. The data available at the time of the review, including from four years of perception surveys, suggested that aid continued to be provided on the basis of what agencies and donors wanted to give, rather than what people said they wanted and needed. The study's authors concluded that 'in the absence of any genuine incentives to change, and in the context of increasing risk intolerance among donors, progress under this workstream is likely to remain incremental at best'.[42]

Of course, as noted earlier in this chapter, donors' political and related financial priorities became (as they continue to be) intertwined with the humanitarian 'marketplace' and explain in part the limited success of localisation. In addition to these factors has been another equally enduring theme so relevant and consistent with the hurdles to collaborative localisation, namely, the presumption of a 'Resilient North' and a 'Vulnerable South' which pervades the attitudes of many in the humanitarian sector.

Some scholars trace this division to the roots of colonialism, with the humanitarian culture of the present reflecting the unequal power dynamics of humanitarianism.[43] Others, such as the Dunantists, reflecting the principles underpinning the International Committee of the Red Cross, are seen as the source of a type of morality imposed by the 'North' upon the 'South', while others just assumed that the wealth and presumed stability of the former justified philanthropic interventions upon the relatively unstable and under-resourced latter.

Whatever the explanation, it had become increasingly evident that – up though the first quarter of the 21st century – power hierarchies persisted. Expatriate humanitarian aid providers tended to be in charge of interventions, and local experts' roles were largely to implement rather than to lead.[44] Even when it came to the transformative implications of artificial intelligence for facilitating local data collection and dissemination, it all too often bypassed local investigators.

> [The failure to put AI in the hands of frontline humanitarian actors can be explained by] organisational inertia and lack of leadership buy-in. Slow adoption of new tools and innovative methods is often a result of a lack of senior advocacy within major humanitarian organisations. Many of these organisations have traditional structures and approaches that have been ingrained through decades of practice, often resulting in 'organisational inertia.' Persistent scepticism about the value of community or frontline derived knowledge and data has resulted in top-down preference for traditional data sources and a lack of process shift and/ or willingness to include participatory approaches into the workflows.[45]

Yet even in cases where efforts had been made to have truly collaborative systems and methods, insensitivity to the 'local' differences were all too apparent. For example, in 2012 the Intergovernmental Science-Policy Platform on Biodiversity and Ecosystem Services (IPBES) was created, with a membership of 134 governments and four UN agencies, to promote more coordinated and interactive research on science and policy. Yet, even with these motives in mind, seven years later it had become evident that the IPBES had been deemed insufficiently inclusive. 'Expertise and regional gaps' were obvious, for example where representatives of non-Western regions were still under-represented. It was difficult to align views and contending interests and perspectives.[46]

Nevertheless, since 1994 (when my assignment began in Rwanda) there had been significant changes in lower- and middle-income countries that began to gnaw away at various presumptions sustaining the North/ South perceptual divide. Rwanda itself by 2016 had become the world's first country to offer commercial drone delivery, partnering with the US-based Zipline, to deliver life-saving medical supplies to remote rural areas.

Using other countries on the African continent as cases in point, it is interesting that by the early 2020s there was growing evidence of the continent's technological coming of age. For example, at least a quarter of the population had internet access, and by 2030 Africa had been forecast to achieve rough parity with the rest of the world, with three-quarters of Africans likely to be internet users. The economic potential was regarded as enormous. Throughout Africa, mobile technologies alone generated 1.7 million jobs and contributed $144 billion to the economy or roughly 8.5 per cent of GDP.[47]

So, too, alignments between low and middle income countries and Western 'developed countries' could no longer be presumed. An exponential increase in collaboration, trade and formal agreements, not necessarily instigated by or including Western governments, was more and more in evidence across geographies – North–South, South–South, East–West. More and more dependencies were becoming interdependencies. And, in a period in which the Covid-19 pandemic, the Ukraine invasion, severe economic recession, eroding post-Second World War institutions and alignments and raging populism had such global impacts, it could well be argued that the distinction between a Resilient North and a Vulnerable South has declining relevance. Even before then, a number of organisations from the South had come to assist those in the North. Not many, not often, but an indicative pattern, nonetheless.

Towards the beginning of April 1995, I had a meeting with one of General Kagame's close assistants – someone who in the British context would have been referred to as his SPAD or Special Advisor. We came together to review the overall humanitarian situation and how and where assistance was being distributed. I, of course, made reference to camps for the internally displaced, though I hadn't mentioned Kibeho specifically.

Only two weeks later, as troops began to surround that camp, did I realise that she had never asked me about our assistance to the displaced. Nor, for that matter did the acting Force Commander of the United Nations Assistance Mission for Rwanda (UNAMIR) ever share with me the information that he had, namely, that the Rwandan army was about to launch its operation to shut down that camp, come what may. Despite the fact that earlier in the year we had set up an Integrated Operations Centre to share information with the military – UNAMIR – this unusual (though initially welcomed) form of collaboration proved irrelevant.[48] *No one seemed to take into account the fact that from an international perspective we had common interests, and neither side was willing to understand the potential mutuality of interests.*

However, in retrospect what was even more evident was that when it came to the needs of the people of Rwanda, we assumed that not only did we know what we needed to do, but also how to do it. Whether it affected villagers or IDPs, the government (out of sheer necessity) would ultimately accede to our plans. How wrong we were.

Who Is the Humanitarian and Where Is the Action?

By June 1999 Slobodan Milosevic, the President of what had been the Federal Republic of Yugoslavia, had finally agreed to the terms laid down by NATO forces. The Serbian and Yugoslav army would withdraw from what would now be the liberated state of Kosovo, and NATO's Kosovo Force (KFOR), as of 11 June, would occupy the country and attempt to restore stability and eventually some kind of normality.

Prior to that agreement, an extensive bombing campaign by NATO from March to June and violent human rights abuses – 'ethnic cleansing' – by Milosevic's armed forces had resulted by the end of May in 1.5 million people having fled their homes – 90 per cent of Kosovo's population. Now, with the signing of the agreement, almost a million of those who had become refugees returned to Kosovo. Within Kosovo itself hunger was rife, and as for government, Kosovo's capital, Pristina, was virtually barren of any effective governance structure.

A few international aid agencies were in country before June of that year. A few months later, there would be approximately 250 in both Kosovo and neighbouring

Albania to deal with returning refugees, the displaced and people lacking livelihoods. However, in the immediate aftermath of the conflict there were insufficient resources to deal with any of those humanitarian crisis drivers nor adequate means for distribution, even for the relatively small amounts of assistance that were available.

In June 1999, I had been appointed the UN's Humanitarian Coordinator and had entered Pristina as part of the United Nations Interim Administration in Kosovo. We had hoped that we could use the airport in the capital as a base for our humanitarian operations, but Russian troops had taken over the airport just before we arrived in the capital. The alternative was a warehouse and a handful of trailers that would serve as our temporary base of operations.

Dealing with a major emergency in Europe was for me a strange, if not disconcerting, experience. Of course, I was well aware that there had been a plethora of natural, conflict-created and technologically induced crises along that geographical fringe of the so-called developed world. But, the nature and the degrees of violence, the increasing lack of food and basic supplies more generally, and the growing levels of displacement had so many parallels with Ethiopia, Sudan and certainly Rwanda. That all this was happening in Europe was a totally unanticipated event in my career.

One evening in early July, a German officer (a deputy commander in KFOR) and I were discussing the overall situation in the country. He clearly knew a great deal about the area, and as we both looked out on to the Goljak mountains that bordered Kosovo's capital, I remarked on this. He knew it, he said, because his PhD thesis was about German military involvement during the Second World War in Yugoslavia, and European history continued to be one of his main interests.

KFOR had from its inception justified its existence and role in terms of a 'humanitarian war' that might be 'illegal but moral'. However, despite its supposed moral underpinnings, various humanitarian organisations were gravely concerned that this sort of initiative violated humanitarian principles. Their point was more than understandable; but there in the midst of this crisis, I was relieved that KFOR was providing substantial assistance – dealing with refugees and displaced persons, offering logistic support and demonstrating an active interest in our relief interests by participating in daily briefings. In so many ways they were unexpected humanitarian actors.

Kosovo was a roller-coaster when it came to interpreting humanitarian objectives. Sometimes degrees of common understanding were arrived at, sometimes they were not. Compounding various interpretations of humanitarian objectives were other hurdles such as lack of common institutional language, criticisms about operational inefficiencies (mainly from the military), failure to coordinate and differing interpretations of what was meant by 'humanitarian action'. Yet, when it worked it really worked.

One couldn't help but wonder what actually determines a humanitarian actor. How might actors such as the military or private sector contribute to humanitarian action? Who else should be there and what justifies their presence at the humanitarian table? In the final analysis is the question really 'who is a humanitarian actor', or instead 'who undertakes humanitarian action, and why?'

In various ways the Western-oriented humanitarian sector that emerged during the 1970s began by the mid-1980s to guard its evolving role from those who were presumed to lack the capacities, objectives and ostensible commitment to principles which defined the sector; and few outside that sector seemed interested or willing to replicate its role. By 1985, however, that assumption began to fray at the edges. Initiatives such as Band Aid and the Live Aid concerts raised public awareness of suffering in Ethiopia and eventually Sudan to new heights, and that growing awareness resulted in more and more private-sector organisations feeling compelled to enhance their public image with donations under the banner of 'Corporate Social Responsibility' (CSR).

While seemingly well-intentioned, many in the private sector had made it clear that CSR was not the same as altruism. It could generate many benefits for the community, but its ultimate purpose was to help the company (no matter how indirectly) and as one Canadian businessman pointed out, 'corporations feel no sense of responsibility for solving the world's problems. It's just not their role.'[49]

In various ways that CSR perspective of many major large corporations, and particularly that of the multinational corporations (MNCs), began to recede. In its place grew a sense of greater mutual self-interest between affected communities and corporate interests. The main factor behind that trend was an obvious paradox – the greater the growing power of business, the greater was its sense of growing vulnerability. Businesses' sense of growth, particularly in the multinational sector, began to emerge at a time when state and state institutions, including inter-governmental organisations, began to appear overloaded. At the same time, corporate interdependencies and interconnectedness were increasing and intensifying, and it was increasingly recognised that a humanitarian crisis in one part of the world could affect the supply chains and markets in many other parts.

As evidenced in Firestone Corporation's response to the Ebola crisis in 2014, a growing number of states throughout the world were intentionally or unintentionally beginning to transfer their crisis response responsibilities to the private sector. As noted by the US Government's Center for Disease Control and Prevention, 'This redistribution of power between the three sectors of government, business and civil society has made it necessary for each of them to think about their roles and to renegotiate their relationships with the others.'[50]

In a related vein, the military's presence was increasingly in evidence in humanitarian crises.[51] UN peacekeeping forces had for at least five decades been tentative humanitarian actors, particularly when it came to logistics. More and more other militaries were becoming engaged in humanitarian operations, particularly those that stemmed from conflict, referred-to as 'military humanitarianism'.[52] The relatively rapid response to the 2013 Typhoon Haiya in the Philippines, the 2010 Haitian earthquake, foreign as well as domestic militaries' involvement in the 2005 earthquake and subsequent floods over the next two decades, were indications of a military presence that was not merely a spill-over from existing conflicts.

Organisations such as the Economic Community of West African States (ECOWAS) formally recognised the military's leadership role in disaster response, and the Association of Southeast Asian Nations (ASEAN) Agreement on Disaster Management and Emergency Response, that included member states' militaries, had been hailed as good practice – progressive, comprehensive and (unusually for a disaster instrument) legally binding. In a host of other non-OECD emerging powers, the importance of the military had become increasingly evident in responding not only to domestic disasters and those within their regions but also in situations where they were engaged in international humanitarian action further afield.

Of course, the military and the private sector often varied in operational styles. These differences were tolerated (and on occasion welcomed) by humanitarian organisations, but to varying degrees both were frequently concerned, if not frustrated, by the ways that many humanitarian organisations dealt with relief operations.

Few outside the humanitarian sector doubted that humanitarian organisations often had to deal with highly complex situations and operations. Nevertheless, there were often raised eyebrows among military and private-sector representatives when discussing humanitarian organisations' programming and logistics operations. Such criticisms focused on a lack of strategic planning, poor information management and ineffective operational integration. In a relief operation that should be managed as a single programme, military and private-sector observers noted that it was

> not unusual to find food and health inputs being administered separately, with little recognition of their inherent relationships to one another. This extends to the issue of incompatible assessments and numerous layers of administration for what should be treated as a simple task.[53]

At the same time, there were others who were increasingly recognised as kinds of humanitarian actors. The 'diaspora' was one. It was more and more apparent that those who had migrated from their original homelands (such as Somalia, Ethiopia, Sudan and the Philippines) to more developed countries were responding to crises in their countries of origin.[54] While people in these diasporas were often accused of taking ethnic or political sides in responding to humanitarian crises, and indeed of perpetuating social inequalities, they were often at the forefront of raising awareness and responding to crises in those countries from which they had originally come.

Resources from the diaspora steadily increased. For example, from 1988 to 2019, the flow of resources from high income countries – principally North America and Europe – to Africa, Asia, Central and South America and South Asia had grown from an estimated $20 billion to $613 billion, including what could be described as development assistance, but clearly also including contributions of food, medical supplies and shelter materials, as well as funds for recovery and reconstruction initiatives.[55] They, too, have been recognised for facilitating the work of INGOs and establishing local relief organisations and networks of trust.

In a related vein, 'social media' was also becoming a recognised humanitarian actor. And, though, as noted earlier, there had been a reluctance on the part of various IGOs and INGOs to share AI and related technologies, it is clear that what one study referred to as 'techno-optimist approaches' implied that social media at least was being accepted as a humanitarian actor: it was deemed to be a powerful tool for sharing information and engaging with hard-to-reach groups.[56] No doubt the downsides of social media were also evident. Hate speech, disinformation and misinformation were all accepted as potential hazards, but the fact of the matter was that as the use of iPhones increased exponentially, social media indeed was a tool, but its value in anticipating and responding to crises made it also a humanitarian actor.

It was a tool because among its many benefits, it also strengthened the capacities of local NGOs and government authorities to mitigate and respond to crises. It was a humanitarian actor because it was generally trusted as a source of warnings and solutions.

Over a decade after those complex operations in Kosovo, I was asked if I would collaborate with the World Food Programme in developing a workshop on humanitarian crisis preparedness. The workshop which took place in 2012 was designed for representatives of planning ministries from countries in the Southern African Development Community (SADC), and after extensive consultations, it was finally decided to use 'dealing with pandemics' as the workshop's theme.

Attending the workshop were various private-sector organisations based in the region, and (to my surprise) the United States Africa Command (US Africom) – one of 11 US combatant commands based in regions around the world – also offered to attend.

Partly because of my experience in Kosovo, I was pleased to see the interest that the military showed in the proposed event. In fact, throughout the workshop, Africom representatives proved to be active facilitators. But, why, I wondered did Africom seem so interested and committed to the event? In between one of the workshop sessions I recall approaching the senior officer, and asking why Africom seemed so engaged. With a touch of formality he replied: 'You have to understand, sir, pandemics are a direct threat to the security of the United States.'

Two years later, 3,000 US troops were deployed in West Africa to help deal with the Ebola crisis. Who was the humanitarian actor, and what should determine who should have roles and responsibilities for dealing with humanitarian crisis threats?

In Search of Innovation and Innovative Practices

At the time, it really did seem that Somalia was slowly emerging out of a decade of conflict and violence into something that bordered on societal normality and relative peace. Since the collapse of President Mohammed Siyad Barre's dictatorship in 1988, there had been approximately 13 efforts by various Somali groups and international organisations to arrive at a country-wide peace deal. Now, thanks in no small part to Djibouti's president, Ismail Omar Guelleh, the fourteenth such attempt took place in Arla, 30 km from the capital, in November 1999. It was to include the Somali Peace Alliance,[57] *and international organisations were invited to attend. Great care was taken to ensure that the meeting was successful, including requisitioned housing for conference participants and more than sufficient goat and camel meat and rice.*

Eventually even the Arta initiative did not live up to expectations, and by August of that year it seemed that its results would be 'disappointing'.

For the Representative of the UN Secretary General, David Stephen, and certainly for me as the UN's Resident and Humanitarian Coordinator, the results of the conference were far from perfect. There were clearly some positive results coming out of the meeting, such as a Transnational National Charter, and eventually the establishment of a Transnational Assembly and Government (TNG). However, it was all-too-evident that the differences between Somaliland and Somalia would not be resolved, that the full panoply of Somali society was not represented, and that there were suggestions being planted that the TNG would inevitably be allied to Islamist extremism.

Nevertheless, there were some reasons to be optimistic. One was the election of Abdiqassim Salad Hassan as the President of the TNG in August, becoming – whatever his strengths and weaknesses – the first Somali leader since 1991 to be at the helm of an internationally recognised government.

It was clear that to sustain the momentum of the peace process would require a concerted effort by the international community to move that process along. I suggested as much when I was quoted as saying that

> *the UN system should prepare itself for the outcome of the conference. [I] hope for a very positive result, but one way or another, we have to be ready to deal with the consequences of this initiative. The UN's humanitarian office has set up a Somali Peace Planning Team to prepare for a post-Djibouti scenario in partnership with the Somali Aid Coordination Body, an umbrella group of UN agencies, international NGOs and donors, and established technical committees in Somalia. [But] because of lack of confidence from the international community over the past decade, UN resources for Somalia are limited.*[58]

And, then soon after, Rift Valley Fever (RVF) struck. The RVF virus was a contagion which spread between livestock and humans, and for a country in which approximately 60 per cent of the population was dependent upon livestock, its implications were potentially catastrophic. A significant proportion of that livestock dependence was based upon exports to the Gulf States and Saudi Arabia. If Somali herders and traders could not get healthy livestock to the ports of Berbera in Somaliland and Bossaso in Somalia, the loss of livelihoods could be the first step towards a devastating famine and probably a resurgence of violence across the country. Rather than focusing the UN's energy on post-Djibouti education, health and agriculture programmes, the focus now had to be on dealing with the prospect of another humanitarian crisis.

Clearly, the UN's Food and Agriculture Organization would take the lead in dealing with the issue of the cattle disease and related concerns, but the rest of the agencies might well have to intensify their focus on food and non-food assistance, and not on what I had hoped would be the 'post-Djibouti scenario'.

The RFV crisis seemed to be expanding, and the flow of cattle from the ports to the Gulf States was rapidly declining. That seemed to be the case until about three months after the initial announcement. Now, reports were coming in that the flow of healthy cattle was increasing, that herds were moving in greater numbers to Berbera and Bossaso. Unbelievably good news, but why was this happening?

It transpired that a major factor was that in this country – synonymous with catastrophic governance, persistent conflict and poverty – an extraordinary and totally unforeseen initiative was underway. A large number of veterinarians, from the south of Somalia all the way to the north of Somaliland, had come together to monitor the health of the cattle as they were being herded to the ports. They exchanged essential information – prognoses and locations – from those vets who made themselves available in an informal system of stateless order and an informal economy.

They were able to do this because of something we had never anticipated. A private telecommunications company, Somali Telecom, which for over a decade had been developing a mobile network across the country, was now making it possible for the vets to communicate wherever they were. It was a totally unexpected initiative – so very innovative, and the results when it came to information flows were evident. Nevertheless I was concerned that the seemingly effective screening process would not necessarily lead to the reopening of the Gulf States' ports for cattle.

Concerned about the Saudi reaction in particular, I called on the Saudi ambassador in Nairobi to ask if Riyadh would now be willing to reopen its ports for cattle imports. I accepted that the monitoring system was informal, that no one could provide the official documentation normally required by governments. Much to my surprise and satisfaction, the ambassador said that his government would 'trust the expertise and innovative practices of the Somali doctors [sic] more than the bureaucrats sitting in some government office'.

I'm not sure if my meeting did have any impact on the Saudi decision eventually to open its ports to Somali cattle, but the whole episode was an interesting experience of bumping into solutions in totally unexpected ways.

Ten years later, 18 representatives of governments of states ranging from Ethiopia and Indonesia to Brazil and Ghana sat around a conference table in Kuala Lumpur to discuss their respective views of international humanitarian policy. This was a side event, one of several at that year's ALNAP's annual meeting.[59] The results of the discussion were intended to be used as material for inclusion in the British Government's Humanitarian Emergency Response Review.

The key question that was asked by the convenor was quite simple: 'What do you need when it comes to humanitarian response in your country?' The answer from virtually all the representatives followed a common line: 'We don't need your boots on the ground; we need innovations to help us prepare for disasters well before they happen.'

There can be little doubt that the traditional humanitarian sector has made uneven progress when it comes to identifying and implementing innovation in their operations. In part this has reflected the 'reactive nature' of many in the sector; in part what had earlier been referred-to as organisational unwillingness to go beyond established norms and procedures. Whatever the explanation or explanations, many organisations within the traditional humanitarian sector encountered difficulties when it comes to scaling-up innovation. This is by no means to suggest that, over the past few years, major innovations have not significantly and very positively enhanced humanitarian response.

However, it is intended to suggest that potential sources of innovations for those in the humanitarian sector were not adequately or consistently pursued, let alone implemented. Rather, that the 'search for innovation' all too often began at the wrong end. Very little efforts were made throughout the humanitarian sector to explore the innovations of other sectors in any kind of systematic way: not necessarily those that were concerned with humanitarian action but those coming from the military, from the private sector in general and technology companies in particular, or from academic institutions and research laboratories.

It is important at the same time to stress that the humanitarian sector had not been devoid of innovation. One of the most enduring symbols of the humanitarian sector, namely the Red Cross, was indeed an innovation in and of itself. There can be little doubt, either, that what has been described as 'digital humanitarianism' involving cash and cash transfers have been profoundly transformative in many ways.[60] It is likely that the list of innovations is longer than some critics of the humanitarian sector would acknowledge. Nevertheless, there are many areas where the humanitarian sector has failed to be as innovative as it could or should have been,[61] or where innovations have been too sporadic or have been unable to reach scale.

> The challenge is widely recognized: good ideas, demonstrated through pilots, often fail to reach scale at which they can maximize value. This is partially due to the general challenge posed by a voluntary, fluid humanitarian system that struggles to consistently adopt changes in policy and practice, particularly those that disrupt the status quo and balance of power.[62]

Beyond these organisational inclinations and related funding issues has been the lack of dedicated and routine resources devoted to the exploration and pursuit of the 'unconventional' – of those innovations and innovative practices that appear to have no direct relevance to humanitarian operational requirements. Nor, for that matter, has there been consistent or formalised processes within or across sectors to promote innovation.

The sector has been affected by a 'lack of policies and frameworks for raising issues and scanning for solutions and, few, if any, means to assess results'.[63]

Such analyses and comments pose significant challenges for those who recognise that ever more complex crises, combined with unprecedented technological and societal change, will demand innovative practices and innovations. Advances in technology have always disrupted the *status quo*, a leading group of analysts has noted, 'but they have never done so across so many markets and at the speed and scale that is being seen today'.[64] And this is only a foretaste of the speed of change in the foreseeable future.

Hence, the inherently haphazard and frequently hesitant approaches to innovation will fail to keep pace not only with the types of crises that will have to be faced, but also with the sorts of innovative solutions that will prevent or address such crises. As effective anticipation and adaptation must reflect the ethos of an organisation, so, too, must the search for, testing and application of innovation be part of an organisation's DNA.

That search, however, should not end merely with a recognition of that innovation, nor necessarily with the application of that innovation to existing approaches and practices. The full implications of transformative technologies must – as the word *transformative* suggests – test whether they open up opportunities for new ways of doing things, and new 'products'.

I remember, after leaving Mogadishu for the last time, checking into an hotel in Nairobi in anticipation of my flight to England the following day. The next morning I was having a cup of coffee at a table cluttered with magazines. I remember picking up a copy of a business magazine, and beginning to read an article that included comments on the Fortune 500. The rate of change of those companies that appeared in the Fortune 500 between 1955 and 2004 was considerable. As I recall, only 12 per cent remained in the list over that half century. What, however, I clearly remember was a reference to the Polaroid company, known as a sector leader since 1937 in film and camera production.

In 2001, Polaroid filed for bankruptcy, apparently because it was unable to anticipate the impact that digital cameras would have on the film business. Polaroid had dismissed the need to explore new territory and, in so doing, to enhance its long-term relevance and viability. It had failed to understand and apply the full potential of transformative innovation – a lesson for those responsible for anticipating, monitoring and mitigating crisis threats.

Leaving 'the Field'

I have always resisted using the term, 'the field', when referring to other people's countries. I know that the term has been and continues to be applied to many situations in the developed and developing worlds when and where 'operational' activities are underway. Yet, its use for me suggested a persistent sense of condescension, where there was an inherent assumption about what earlier had been referred to as Northern resilience in the face of 'the vulnerable South'.

In any event, I had a choice to make. I would accept an opportunity to move to another post for the UN or a position as a Senior Research Fellow at King's College, London. The former was compelling as usual, but I chose the latter for a variety of reasons, personal as well as professional: hence, my decision to leave 'the field'.

That choice, however, was in no way about abandoning my commitment to humanitarian issues and action. To the contrary, it afforded me an opportunity to step back from day-to-day operational commitments to think about humanitarianism in a wider context. Issues came to the fore that I had sensed but never really explored or articulated. Being at King's enabled me to consider the strengths and weaknesses of that very complex sector in which I had been involved for almost two decades – not only where that sector had been and was but also where would it have to be to deal with crises that were becoming more and more complex, their dimensions and dynamics ever greater.

The creation of the Humanitarian Futures Programme (HFP) at King's in 2004 gave me (and hopefully others) opportunities to explore a wide range of future-related issues that could result in humanitarian crises. From urban futures to the consequences of planetary exploration, from polylateral systems to the virtual state, how might their positive implications also be sources of vulnerability?

The venture took me into realms of investigation and thought which I might never have had. And, yet at the same time, it also reflected a set of issues and concerns that had emerged in various ways and at various times throughout my career. In a world in which the types, dimensions and dynamics of crisis threats were increasing, might there be at least broad themes from my own experiences, and humanitarian action more generally, that could be relevant when considering humanitarian crises in the future?

- How does and should one anticipate and plan for what seem to be ever more uncertain and complex crisis threats? In that sense, what does one mean by 'humanitarian crises' and how does one anticipate their causation and consequences?
- What sorts of structures might need to be in place to address such future challenges, and how should they be resourced? To what extent might conventional organisational and systems behaviour need to be overcome to deal with unprecedented complexity?
- To what extent might greater global interconnectedness and interrelatedness change assumptions about the nature of humanitarian action and who the 'humanitarians' are? Who should be responsible for anticipating, monitoring and mitigating ever-more-complex crisis threats?
- If innovations and innovative practices could be fundamental for dealing with future threats, how might they be identified, by whom and from where?

As the search for answers to these sorts of questions continued, there was an overarching theme that began to emerge. The present approaches and attitudes to humanitarian crises and response were inadequate to deal with plausible future challenges. New ways of thinking about the nature of threats and response were required. A new paradigm was needed – reflecting greater sensitivity to a growing number of plausible threats in the future. The starting point though was not to dwell on the lessons of the past, but rather to begin *planning from the future*.

Therefore, the next step in this humanitarian odyssey is to consider how adequate present approaches are for dealing with plausible humanitarian threats and crises in the future. It begins with a description of types of societal behaviour that *could* emerge in a generation's time – the changing nature of human agency – before asking how effective present approaches would be in dealing with plausible crises in the future.

Notes

1 'Ethiopian appeal', DEC Appeal, Michael Buerk, BBC, 1987.
2 The movement includes the International Committee of the Red Cross, the International Federation of Red Cross and Red Crescent Societies, and 192 National Red Cross and Red Crescent Societies.
3 Martin Barber, Mark Bowden, Armida van Rij and Rose Pinnington, *Applying humanitarian principles in armed conflict: Challenges and ways forward*, Royal Institute of International Affairs, International Security Programme, December 2023.
4 'While there is a 30-year history of efforts to increase collaboration between humanitarian and development actors, the idea of strengthening relations between humanitarians and peace actors has only surfaced on the international agenda in the last five years or so. The concept of the "triple nexus" stems to date from both the twin resolutions on Sustaining Peace in the UN Security Council and General Assembly and the Secretary General's inaugural speech in 2016.' Elizabeth Ferris, *The humanitarian-peace nexus*, Research Briefing Paper for UN Secretary-General's High-Level Panel on Internal Displacement, Georgetown University, August 2020.
5 OECD, *Covid-19 and policy for science*, OECD Science, Technology and Industry Policy Papers, No. 152, pp. 13–14, July 2023.
6 Karin von Hippel and Randolph C. Kent, 'In a world of pandemics and "black sky hazards," Can the UN be rendered fit for the 21st century?' Commentary, Royal United Services Institute, 25 March 2020.
7 Ibid.
8 Michael C. Ennis-McMillan and Kristin Hedges, 'Pandemic perspectives: Responding to Covid-19', *Open Anthropology*, 8 (1), April 2020.
9 Sheila Jasanoff et al., *Comparative Covid response: Crisis, knowledge, politics – interim report*, Harvard Kennedy School, 12 January 2021.
10 Christina Bennet, 'The Grand Bargain at two: Collapsing under its own weight', Overseas Development Institute, 19 July 2018.
11 Mark Bowden and Angela Penrose, *The evolution of the humanitarian marketplace and NGO financing models*. Unpublished Working Paper available at www.nuffield.ox.ac.uk/media/5567/the- evolution-of-the-humanitarian-marketplace-and-ngo-financing-models.pdf, July 2021. The latter from Randolph C. Kent, 'The UN's disaster and emergency roles and responsibilities', *Disasters: The Journal of Disaster Studies, Policy and Management, Overseas Development Institute*, 28 (2), 2004.
12 Michael Barnett, *Empire of humanity: A history of humanitarianism*, Cornell University Press, 2010, p. 42.
13 See for example John Holmes, in *The politics of humanity: The reality of relief aid*, Head of Zeus, Bloomsbury Publications, p. 401. He notes that 'progress has to be made irrespective of unworthy agency and NGO concerns about either competition with other agencies or worries that if they give "too much" information to donors or the media, their appeal funds might be challenged'.
14 Ibid.
15 Randolph C. Kent et al., *Towards an international architecture for managing global threats: Systems compendium annex*, Royal United Services Institute, 2021.

16 Nassim Nicholas Taleb, *The black swan: The impact of the highly improbable*, Penguin Books, 2008
17 'Reports that say that something hasn't happened are always interesting to me, because as we know, there are known knowns; there are things we know we know. We also know there are known unknowns; that is to say we know there are some things we do not know. But there are also unknown unknowns—the ones we don't know we don't know. And if one looks throughout the history of our country and other free countries, it is the latter category that tends to be the difficult ones.' Donald Rumsfeld, the US Secretary of Defence, in a 12 February 2002 press conference regarding the Iraq invasion.
18 Ben Ramalingam and H. Jones with T. Reba and J. Young, *Exploring the science of complexity: Ideas and implications for development and humanitarian efforts*, Working Group Paper 285, Overseas Development Institute, 2008.
19 Fritz Nauck, Thomas Poppensieke and Olivia White, *Meeting the future: Dynamic risk management for uncertain times*, McKinsey & Co., 17 November 2020.
20 Helen Clark and Ellen Johnson Sirleaf, *Covid-19: Make it the last pandemic*, The Independent Panel for Pandemic Preparedness and Response, 2 May 2021.
21 Geoff Mulgan, *Thinking systems: How the systems we depend on can be helped to think and serve us better*, Department of Science, Technology, Engineering and Public Policy, University College, London, 2021, p. 16.
22 Kathy Patch et al., *Collective intelligence for frontline humanitarian response*, NESTA, September 2021, p. 78.
23 INGOs & The Long Humanitarian Century, *Leadership survey report: What leaders of international NGOs think about the challenges they face, and the future of the aid and development sector*, University of Oxford, 2022, p. 39.
24 Paul Skinner, *Collaborative advantage: How collaboration beats competition as a strategy for success*, Little Brown Book Group, 2018, p. 33.
25 His name was Frederick C. Cuny. Fred was a humanitarian from Texas whose work spanned disaster relief, refugee emergency management, recovery from war and civil conflict, as well as disaster and emergency preparedness, mitigation and peacebuilding. He was first and foremost a practitioner but also a prolific author, an educator and a field-based researcher. When he came to my office he was wearing 'cowboy boots'. He normally did.
26 In this context, it is worth noting that during the same period that I was in New York, *An overview of disaster management* (Department of Humanitarian Affairs, United Nations Disaster Relief Office, United Nations Development Programme, Chapter 5, 'Compound and Complex Emergencies'), in a subsection on 'Socio/Political Forces' was noting that in 'a growing number of countries, complex disasters are becoming more evident. Essentially a complex disaster is a form of human-made emergency in which the causes of the emergency as well as the assistance to the affected are bound by intense levels of political considerations. [For example] the government becomes extremely suspicious or uninterested in afflicted people who have fled from non-government to government held areas. The government or opposition groups actually create or compound a disaster through actions that generate refugees and the mass displacement of people.' In addition, it is 'the obstacle of national sovereignty that limits outside agencies to assist this population'.
27 Randolph C. Kent, *Anatomy of disaster relief: The international network in action*, Pinter Publishers, 1987, p. 118.
28 Ibid.

29 Peter Walker and Daniel G. Maxwell, *Shaping the humanitarian world*, Routledge, 2009.
30 Dennis Dijkzeul and Dorothy Hilhorst, 'Instrumentalisation of aid in humanitarian crises' in *Humanitarianism and challenges of cooperation*, Routledge, 2016.
31 Nathalie Bernasconi, International Institute for Sustainable Development, 13 December 2023.

'COP 28 outcomes represent significant wins overshadowed by disappointments. While we celebrate the historic deal on financing for loss & damage and the commitment to transition away from fossil fuels—adopted for the first time—we can't ignore the heart-breaking let-downs on adaptation and the dangerous loopholes in mitigation. The decisions adopted today in Dubai will impact the most vulnerable communities on earth, leaving them underprepared, underfinanced, and exposed to the consequences of global warming breaching the 1.5°C threshold.'

32 See, for example, the 'Four Key Achievements' outlined by UN Climate Change Executive Secretary, Patricia Espinosa, on 24 November 2021: (1) a work programme exists to define the global goal on adaptation; (2) governments at COP26 agreed on the need for much greater support to developing countries; (3) the collective agreement by governments to explore ways of increasing actions to close the current emissions gap; and, finalising of guidelines for the full implementation of the Paris Agreement; the compromise reached on Article Six relating to carbon markets, which will ensure a level playing field for everyone; and the finalising of negotiations on the Enhanced Transparency Framework, which allows countries to continue building trust.
33 Michael LePage, 'Last shot', *New Scientist*, 29 October 2022, p. 38.
34 Will Moreland, 'The purpose of multilateralism: A framework for democracies in a geopolitically competitive world', Foreign Policy at Brookings, September 2019, p. 17.
35 Nathan Gardels. 'Planetary politics when the nation-state falters', *Noema*, 3 September 2021, www.noemamag.com/author/nathan-gardels/
36 John Micklethwait and Adrian Woolridge, *The wake-up call: Why the pandemic has exposed the weakness of the West, and how to fix it*, Short Books, 2020, p. 64.
37 In this context, Professor Martin Rees quotes the long-time scientific advisor to the UK government, Solly Zuckerman, as saying that 'the basic reason for the irrationality of the whole process [of the arms race] was shaped by technologists, not because they were concerned with any visionary picture of how the world should evolve, but because they were merely doing what they saw to be their job.' Martin Rees, *Our final century: Will the human race survive the Twenty-first Century?*, Basic Books, 2003, p. 32.
38 Op. cit., #35, Gardels.
39 Randolph C. Kent et al., *Towards an international architecture for managing global threats: Systems compendium annex*, Royal United Services Institute, 2021. In a related vein, see Randolph C. Kent, *Building an international architecture for managing global threats*, Royal United Services Institute, July 2022.
40 Eric Schmidt and Jared Cohen, *The new digital age: Reshaping the future of people, nations and business*, John Murray Publishers, 2013, p. 6.
41 Joi Iyto and Jeff Howe: *Whiplash: How to survive our faster future*, Grand Central Publishing, 2016, p. 250. See also, Oliver Letwin, *Apocalypse how: Technology and the threat of disasters*, Atlantic Books, 2020. This perspective also relates to the emergence of cryptocurrencies that by-pass so-called 'middle men', e.g. government treasuries, banks, etc. See Paula Vigna and Michael Casey, *Crypto currency: The future of money*? Vintage, 2016.

42 Victoria Metcalfe-Hough, Wendy Fenton, Barnaby Willitts-King and Alexandra Spencer, *The grand bargain at five years: An independent review*, Overseas Development Institute, June 2021, https://odi.org/en/publications/the-grand-bargain-at-five-years-an-independent-review

43 Agnieszka Sobocinska, author of *Saving the World? Western volunteers and the rise of the humanitarian-development complex*, suggested this theme in a talk entitled Humanitarianism versus Development: Historical Perspectives, at a York University, Toronto, and King's College, London, conference, 31 October 2022.

44 A. Benton, 'African expatriates and race in the anthropology of humanitarianism', *Critical African Studies*, 8 (3), 266–277.

45 Kathy Peach et al., *Collective crisis intelligence for frontline humanitarian response*, NESTA, 15 September 2021, www.nesta.org.uk report collective-crisis-intelligence

46 Anne-Sophie Stevance et al., *The 2019 review of IPBES and future priorities: Reaching beyond assessment to enhance Policy Impact*, December 2019, https//doi.org/10.1080/25395916.2019.1702590

47 Nathaniel Allan, 'The promises and perils of Africa's digital revolution', *Tech Stream*, Brookings Institution, 11 March 2021.

48 For specific details of the Integrated Operations Centre and relations between the humanitarian aid providers and UNAMIR, see Randolph C. Kent, 'The integrated operations centre in Rwanda: Coping with complexity', in Jima Whitman and David Pocock, *After Rwanda: The coordination of United Nations humanitarian assistance*, Macmillan Press, 1996, pp. 63 ff.

49 John Twigg, *Corporate social responsibility and disaster reduction: A global overview*, Benfield Greig Hazard Research Centre, University College, London. Funded by what was then the UK Department for international Development (DFID): ERSCOR award No. R7893.

50 The Centre for Disease Control reported that on 30 March 2014, the Ministry of Health and Social Welfare (MOHSW) of Liberia alerted health officials at Firestone Liberia Incorporated of the first known case of Ebola virus disease (Ebola) inside Firestone's rubber tree plantation. The patient, who was the wife of a Firestone employee, had cared for a family member with confirmed Ebola in Lofa County, the epicentre of the Ebola outbreak during March–April 2014. To prevent a large outbreak among Firestone's 8,500 employees, their dependents and the surrounding population, the company responded by (1) establishing an incident management system, (2) instituting procedures for the early recognition and isolation of Ebola patients, (3) enforcing adherence to standard Ebola infection control guidelines and (4) providing differing levels of management for contacts depending on their exposure, including options for voluntary quarantine in the home or in dedicated facilities. CDCP, *Morbidity and Mortality Weekly Report* (MMWR), 'Control of Ebola disease – Firestone District, Liberia 2014', 24 October 2014, 63 (42), 959–965.

51 The Guidelines on the Use of Military and Civil Defense Assets to Support United Nations Humanitarian Activities in Complex Emergencies – the MCDA Guidelines (OCHA 2006) – and the Use of Foreign Military and Civil Defense Assets in Disaster Relief – the 'Oslo Guidelines' – should be a last resort (and for a limited time only), when there is no comparable civilian alternative for meeting (critical and immediate) needs and where traditional humanitarian agencies can control and direct the use of assets. Yet the guidelines do not address how these agencies should relate to the military forces of affected states. See Samuel Carpenter and Randolph C. Kent, 'The military and the private sector', in Zeynep Sezgin and Dennis Dijkzeul, *The new humanitarians*

in international practice: Emerging actors and contested principles, Routledge, 2016, pp. 151 ff.

52 Thomas G. Weiss and Kurt Campbell, 'Military humanitarianism', *Survival*, 3 March 2008, https://doi.org/10.1080/00396339108442612

53 Humanitarian Futures Programme, *The virtuous triangle and the fourth dimension: The humanitarian, private and military sectors*, www.humanitarianfutures.org. In Key Findings.

54 Hammond et al., define 'diaspora' in terms of three characteristics: dispersal of a population from an original homeland, continued or reinvigorated orientation towards a real or imagined homeland, and identities based on boundary-maintenance vis-à-vis a host society. Referenced in Andrew Bostrom, Dayna Brown and Sarah Cechvala, *Humanitarian effectiveness and the role of the diaspora: A CDA literature review*, CDA Collaborative Learning Projects, May 2016, pp. 20–21.

55 John Bryant, *Remittances in humanitarian crises*, Humanitarian Policy Group, Overseas Development Institute, March 2019.

56 Oliver Lough, *Social media and inclusion in humanitarian response*, HPG Working Paper, Overseas Development Institute, May 2022.

57 The Somali Peace Alliance comprised representatives of the Somali region, Puntland, the Somali Consultative Body, the Rahanweyn Resistance Army and the Somali National Front.

58 ReliefWeb, IRIN Horn of Africa Update, 4 September 2000.

59 ALNAP, or, the Active Learning Network for Accountability and Performance in Humanitarian Action, is a global network of NGOs, UN agencies, members of the Red Cross/ Red Crescent Movement, donors, academics and consultants dedicated to learning how to improve response to humanitarian crises.

60 Peter Maier, *The rise of digital humanitarianism*, CRC Press, Taylor & Francis Group, 2015.

61 Op. cit., #21 and 46. Also see, Ben Ramalingam, Howard Rush, John Bessant, Nick Marshall, *Strengthening the humanitarian innovation ecosystem*, Ecosystem Research Project. Final Report, May 2015.

62 Paul Knox Clarke, 'Transforming change', as referenced in the *Global alliance for humanitarian innovation, untangling innovation: The many paths to scale*, www.thegahi.org

63 Op. cit., #61, Ben Ramalingam et al.

64 Richard Dobbs, James Manyika and Jonathan Woetzel, *No ordinary disruption: The four global forces breaking all the trends*, Public Affairs, McKinsey & Co., 2015, p. 583.

Bibliography

Allan, Nathaniel, 'The promises and perils of Africa's digital revolution', *Tech Stream, Brookings Institution*, 11 March 2021.

Barber, Martin, Bowden, Mark, van Rij, Armida and Pinnington, Rose, *Applying humanitarian principles in armed conflict: Challenges and ways forward*, Royal Institute of International Affairs, International Security Programme, December 2023.

Barnett, Michael, *Empire of humanity: A history of humanitarianism*, Cornell University Press, 2010.

Bennet, Christina, 'The Grand Bargain at two: Collapsing under its own weight', Overseas Development Institute, 19 July 2018.

Benton, Adia, African expatriates and race in the anthropology of humanitarianism,' *Critical African Studies*, 8 (3), 2016.

Bostrom, Andrew, Brown, Dayna and Cechvala, Sarah, *Humanitarian effectiveness and the role of the diaspora: A CDA literature review*. CDA Collaborative Learning Projects, May 2016.

Bryant, John, *Remittances in humanitarian crises*, Humanitarian Policy Group, Overseas Development Institute, March 2019.

Carpenter, Samuel and Kent, Randolph, 'The military and the private sector', in Zeynep Sezgin and Dennis Dijkzeul (Eds), *The new humanitarians in international practice: Emerging actors and contested principles*, Routledge, 2016.

CDCP, Morbidity and Mortality Weekly Report (MMWR), 'Control of Ebola disease: Firestone District, Liberia 2014', *The Morbidity and Mortality Weekly Report*, 63 (42), 24 October 2014.

Clark, Helen and Sirleaf, Ellen Johnson, *Covid-19: Make it the last pandemic*, The Independent Panel for Pandemic Preparedness and Response, 2 May 2021.

Dijkzeul, Dennis and Hilhorst, Dorothy, 'Instrumentalisation of aid in humanitarian crises' in *Humanitarianism and Challenges of Cooperation*, Routledge, 2016.

Dobbs, Richard, Manyika, James and Woetzel, Jonathan, *No ordinary disruption: The four global forces breaking all the trends*, Public Affairs, McKinsey & Co., 2015.

Ennis-McMillan, Michael C. and Hedges, Kristin, 'Pandemic perspectives: Responding to Covid-19', *Open Anthropology*, 8 (1), April 2020.

Ferris, Elizabeth, *The humanitarian-peace nexus*, Research Briefing Paper for UN Secretary-General's High-Level Panel on Internal Displacement, Georgetown University, August 2020.

Gardels, Nathan, 'Planetary politics when the nation-state falters,' *Noema*, 3 September 2021, www.noemamag.com/author/nathan-gardels/

Holmes, John, *The politics of humanity: The reality of relief aid*, Head of Zeus, Bloomsbury Publishing, 2013.

Humanitarian Futures Programme, *The virtuous triangle and the fourth dimension: The humanitarian, private and military sectors*, www.humanitarianfutures.org. In Key Findings.

INGOs & The Long Humanitarian Century, *Leadership survey report: What leaders of international NGOs think about the challenges they face, and the future of the aid and development sector*, University of Oxford, 2022.

Iyto, Joi and Howe, Jeff, *Whiplash: How to survive our faster future*, Grand Central Publishing, 2016.

Jasanoff, Sheila, Hilgartner, S., Hurlbut, J. B., Özgöde, O., and Rayzberg, M., *Comparative Covid response: Crisis, knowledge, politics – interim report,* Harvard Kennedy School, 12 January 2021.

Kent, Randolph, *Building an international architecture for managing global threats*, Royal United Services Institute, July 2022.

Kent, Randolph et al., *Towards an international architecture for managing global threats: Systems compendium annex*, Royal United Services Institute, 2021.

Kent, Randolph, 'The UN's disaster and emergency roles and responsibilities', *Disasters: The Journal of Disaster Studies, Policy and Management, Overseas Development Institute*, 28 (2), 2004.

Kent, Randolph, The integrated operations centre in Rwanda: Coping with complexity, in Whitman, Jima and Pocock, David (Eds), *After Rwanda: The coordination of United Nations humanitarian assistance*, Macmillan Press, 1996.

Kent, Randolph, *Anatomy of disaster relief: The international network in action*, Pinter Publishers, 1987.

Knox Clarke, Paul, Transforming change, as referenced in the Global Alliance for Humanitarian Innovation, *Untangling innovation: The many paths to scale*, www.thegahi.org

LePage, Michael, 'Last shot', *New Scientist*, 29 October 2022.

Letwin, Oliver, *Apocalypse how: Technology and the threat of disasters*, Atlantic Books, 2020.

Lough, Oliver, *Social media and inclusion in humanitarian response*, HPG Working Paper, Overseas Development Institute, May 2022.

Maier, Peter, *The rise of digital humanitarianism*, CRC Press, Taylor & Francis Group, 2015.

Metcalfe-Hough, Victoria, Fenton, Wendy, Willitts-King, Barnaby and Spencer, Alexandra, *The grand bargain at five years: An independent review*, Overseas Development Institute, June 2021, https://odi.org/en/publications/the-grand-bargain-at-five-years-an-independent-review

Micklethwait, John and Woolridge, Adrian, *The wake-up call: Why the pandemic has exposed the weakness of the west, and how to fix it*, Short Books, 2020.

Moreland, Will, 'The purpose of multilateralism: A framework for democracies in a geopolitically competitive world', *Foreign Policy at Brookings*, September 2019.

Mulgan, Geoff, *Thinking systems: How the systems we depend on can be helped to think and serve us better*, Department of Science, Technology, Engineering and Public Policy, University College, 2021.

Nauck, Fritz, Poppensieke, Thomas and White, Olivia, *Meeting the future: Dynamic risk management for uncertain times*, McKinsey & Co., 17 November 2020.

OECD, *Covid-19 and policy for science*, OECD Science, Technology and Industry Policy Papers, No. 152, pp.13–14, July 2023.

Peach, Kathy, Berditchexskaia, Aleks, Whittington, Oli, Malliaraki, Erin and Gill, Issy, *Collective crisis intelligence for frontline humanitarian response,* NESTA, 15 September 2021, www.nesta.org.uk › report › collective-crisis-intelligence

Ramalingam, Ben, Jones, Harry with Reba, Toussaint and Young, John, *Exploring the science of complexity: Ideas and implications for development and humanitarian efforts*, Working Group Paper 285, Overseas Development Institute, 2008.

Ramalingam, Ben, Rush, Howard, Bessant, John, and Marshall, Nick, *Strengthening the humanitarian innovation ecosystem*, Ecosystem Research Project. Final Report, May 2015.

Rees, Martin, *Our final century: Will the human race survive the twenty-first century?*, Basic Books, 2003.

Schmidt, Eric and Cohen, Jared, *The new digital age: Reshaping the future of people, nations and business*, John Murray Publishers, 2013.

Skinner, Paul, *Collaborative Advantage: How collaboration beats competition as a strategy for success*, Little Brown Book Group, 2018.

Stevance, Anne-Sophie et al., *The 2019 review of IPBES and future priorities: Reaching beyond assessment to enhance policy impact*, December 2019, https//doi.org/10.1080/25395916.2019.1702590

Taleb, Nassim Nicholas, *The black swan: The impact of the highly improbable*, Penguin Books, 2008.

Twigg, John, *Corporate social responsibility and dssisaster reduction: A global overview,* Benfield Greig Hazard Research Centre, University College, London. Funded by what was then the UK Department for international Development (DFID): ERSCOR award No. R7893.

Vigna, Paula and Casey, Michael, *Crypto currency: The future of money?* Vintage, 2016.

Von Hippel, Karin and Kent, Randolph, 'In a world of pandemics and "Black Sky Hazards," can the UN be rendered fit for the 21st century?' *Commentary*, Royal United Services Institute, 25 March 2020.

Walker, Peter and Maxwell, Daniel G., *Shaping the humanitarian world*, Routledge, 2009.

Weiss, Thomas G. and Campbell, Kurt, Military humanitarianism, *Survival*, 3 March 2008, https://doi.org/10.1080/00396339108442612

2 The Changing Dimensions of Human Agency

I'm delighted. You have given birth to such a very healthy, handsome little boy. As you know, we've adjusted his DNA to ensure that he will not pass on any genetic anomalies, and as we agreed we also inserted a cyber system to strengthen his information intake, decision-making and haptic communications capacities. Clearly all these interventions are consistent with international legal requirements. Now, as you also know, we have inserted the officially required universal implant which will ensure that his health and well-being will always be monitored whether on Earth or elsewhere, and when he arrives at that wonderful age of 120, he will be gently resourced along with his contemporaries.

She leaned back on her pillow, smiled warmly and thanked her life provider. This is exactly what she had hoped for. She didn't quite understand what everything meant, but she did know that this was what everyone else seemed to do.

Human Agency in Context

A restructured DNA, enhanced brain capacities, an implanted monitor both for health and human recycling – what might it mean to be human by the middle of the 21st century, and what will the environment and the contexts be in which human beings exist and engage? In other words, what do we mean by *'human agency'*, and, for the purposes of this book, what might it suggest about future vulnerabilities and ways to mitigate them?

It is important to note from the outset that the term, *human agency*, is not used here to explore the evolving nature of *humanness* based on past or present socio-economic and geo-political distinctions. Rather, the term is used to suggest how the very nature of being human – on planet Earth and beyond – might evolve, and to consider their plausible negative and positive consequences for humans as a species? Readers, therefore, should recognise that what follows are not intended to be predictions. Instead they offer another step to test how anticipatory and adaptive are their approaches for dealing with uncertainty and profound change.

That said, to all of this, there is one certainty. Whoever we might be, wherever we are, whatever we may do, we as human beings will be dramatically transformed

DOI: 10.4324/9781003471004-3

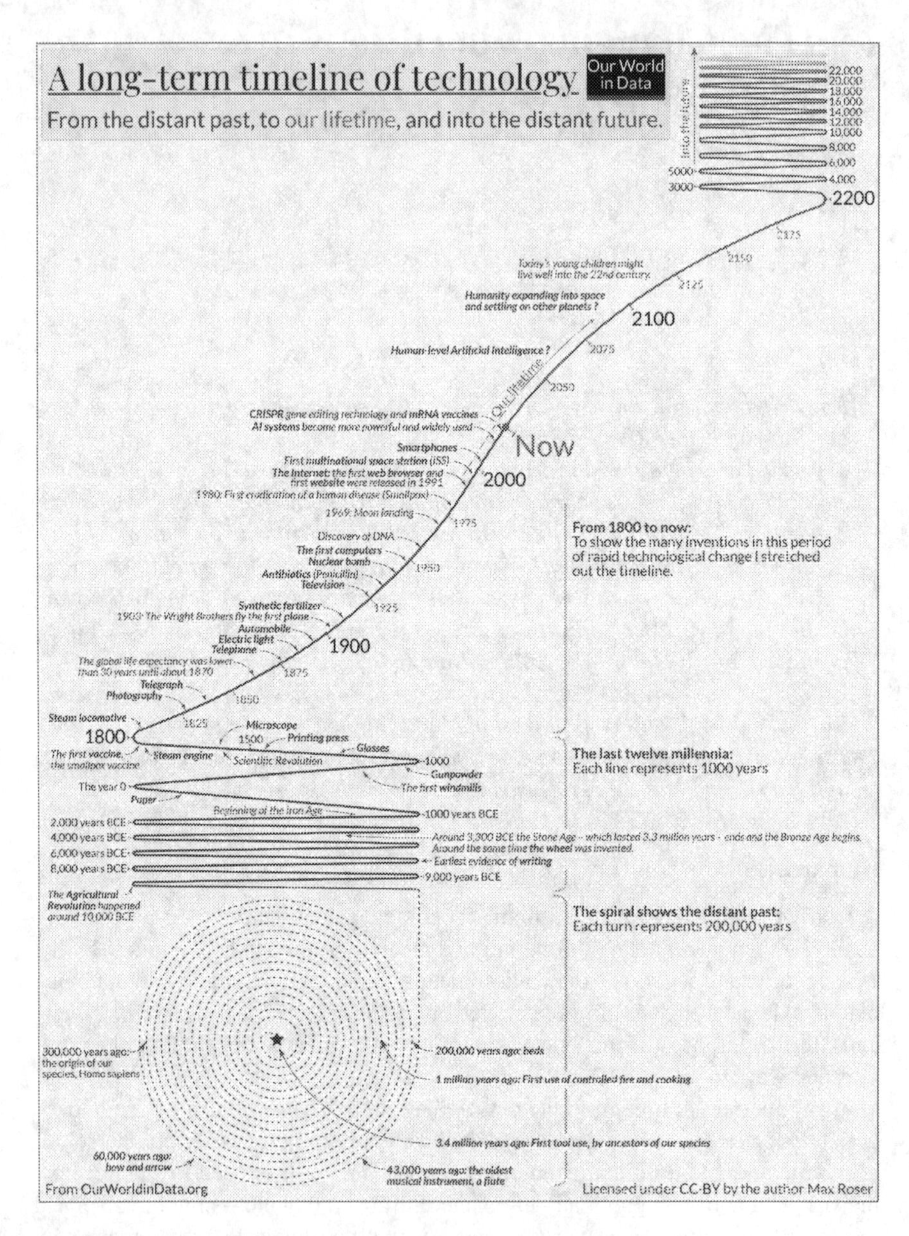

Figure 2.1 A Long-term Timeline of Technology

Source: Max Roser (2023) 'Technology over the long run: zoom out to see how dramatically the world can change within a lifetime.' Published online at OurWorldInData.org. Retrieved from: 'https://ourworldindata.org/technology-long-run' [Online Resource]

over the next three decades. And, as these transformations intensify, our human agency – our sense of who we are within ourselves and our capacities for interacting beyond ourselves – will also change dramatically.[1]

Beyond this certainty, what such transformative drivers could be remain elusive in myriad ways. It is all too evident, for example, that truly transformative technologies – those that result in paradigmatic changes affecting human agency – are frequently the product of happenstance and unanticipated effects. As was too evident in what has been described as the 'chemical age', more often than not, the full consequences of even well-intentioned innovations are not necessarily anticipated, understood or are ignored.[2]

Hence, while acknowledging the uncertainties that underpin change processes in general, the entangled relationship between societal change and transformative technologies clearly offer a compelling launchpad for exploring how human agency could change in the longer term, both on this planet and beyond.

The Weird and the Wonderful: Upsides and Downsides

There can be little doubt that the sciences and related technologies will continue to trigger profound changes in the very nature of 'humanness', only at a faster pace. Similarly, the ways that physical space will be defined and used will undergo significant transformations as will the ways that human beings will engage, communicate, travel and transport themselves. Linked to these are the very requirements that human beings will need to survive and in a related vein the ways that they use time.

From the perspective of the early 21st century, many of the transformations that are suggested here may seem by many unlikely to occur in a mere generation's time, and certainly there may be others who feel that much of the ensuing discussion should be consigned to science fiction. Nevertheless, the social and natural science literature clearly suggests that the sorts of transformations referenced here are by no means implausible.

It is not implausible, for example, 'that machines could one day surpass most distinctively human capabilities; the disagreements are about the rate of travel, not the direction', so suggested the eminent British cosmologist, Martin Rees.[3] And, as a US National Intelligence Director predicted in early 2020,

> Technologies are being invented, used, spread and then discarded at ever increasing speeds around the world and new centers of innovation are emerging.
>
> During the next two decades, the pace and reach of technological developments are likely to increase ever faster, transforming a range of human experiences and capabilities while also creating new tensions and disruptions within and between societies, industries and states. State and non-state rivals will vie for leadership and dominance in science and technology with potentially cascading risks and implications for economic, military, and societal security.[4]

In that context the emerging prospect of Artificial Super Intelligence (ASI), enhanced by breakthroughs in quantum computing, is a step in that direction. ASI systems will possess a reasonable degree of self-understanding and autonomous self-control, and have the ability to solve a variety of complex problems in a variety of contexts, and to learn to solve new problems that they did not know about at the time of their creation.[5]

The exponential growth of AI, possibly leading to the all-encompassing 'Singularity', could eventually result in uncontrollable and irreversible change, according to many experts.[6] Many also forecast that the Singularity might lead to a versatile super-intelligent robot, which 'could be the last invention that humans need to make. Once machines surpass human intelligence, they could design and assemble a new generation of even more intelligent machines.'[7] Some anticipate that prospect in terms of two decades, others suggest that it might take centuries.

A growing number in the ASI field regard the transition from human to the Singularity as not necessarily dystopic. It could be a cause for optimism, say some. 'The civilization that supplants us could accomplish unimaginable advances – feats, perhaps, that we cannot even understand.'[8]

There, too, are counterarguments that do not accept that human beings will be so radically transformed that they will lose the capacity to control, for example, technological transformations. While recognising both the positive and negative consequences of technological developments, human beings by the very uniqueness of their brain capacities will always, so goes the alternative case, be able to be steps ahead of the very systems which human beings create.

In either case, there is an equally relevant debate when considering human agency from a longer-term perspective. That debate centres on the question of whether the Anthropocene age in which human beings dominate the Earth will continue or whether a Novacene age will replace it? The latter would consist of cybernetic organisms that are self-sufficient, though made of engineered materials that will exist alongside humans.[9] The former will reflect the impact on Earth's geology and ecosystems by human beings in essentially their present form.

For the purposes of this book, however, the consequences of such things as ASI, the Singularity and related technological impacts are *not* about predicting whether they will be determinants of human agency. Rather they offer ways to look at the future that might take decision-makers and policy planners well beyond their comfort zones.

The weird and the wonderful – their upsides and downsides – should serve as starting points for challenging assumptions and attitudes about factors that could determine human resilience as well as vulnerabilities in an uncertain future.

R-Evolutionary Dynamics

Analysts foresee that a shift is occurring that is uniting our digital and physical worlds at the deepest architectural and operational levels, on this planet and eventually beyond.[10] In the foreseeable future, nano-scale robots inside the human body could construct sensors and other devices that would help dissolve blood clots, fight cancer and deliver precisely targeted drugs. Cellular programming will have been able to 'rewind the clock' by generating a handful of genes which can make cells young again and rejuvenate organs. All the while advanced robotics and ASI will have provided personalised medical stations which will design and optimise metabolism and microbiome for any single day.[11]

Similar to the prospects for ASI-related transformations will have been those bioengineered innovations that within a three-decade timeframe may have transmuted some of the most fundamental human characteristics. Already during the 2020s, there has been significant progress in growing spare parts for worn-out or diseased bodies, including blood vessels, vaginas, brain parts[12] – all reflecting what has been called 'the evolution machine', designed to evolve new organisms and rewrite whole genomes with ease.[13] Eventually, what might well be emerging is a mix between robotics and human parts, where the former would supplement the mental as well as physical components of the latter.[14] These sorts of admixes would define the *cyborg*.

Such technological shifts would alter global business, government, military and intelligence ecosystems. It is nothing less than a technological singularity and this technology could forever change the ways that humans defined the world. One example is Cyber Physical Systems (CPS), the neuro-science of decision-making, that would enable the human brain to utilise new senses and create new neural pathways to interpret and prioritise vast amounts of data. For the next generation analytics, 'It will not be [about] better data or colours on a dashboard; but rather it will be augmented sensory sensation and individually centric Artificial Intelligence.'[15]

In a related vein, the UK's Ministry of Defence, while acknowledging that the technical barriers were formidable, foresaw that by 2050, 'brain-to-computer interfaces may allow people to augment their mental abilities with automatic access to the memory and processing power of computers'.[16] A plethora of initiatives related to this vision, including the prospect that well before 2030, there will have been brain chips that would enable people to have cognitive boosts as they go about their daily lives. In that regard, a group of analysts suggested that a 'special point will arrive in neuroscience [when] human intelligence will be one of the largest industries, if not the largest industry, to ever emerge'.[17]

Such forms of human agency will certainly have relevance when human beings begin to leave the confines of the Earth to settle elsewhere. However, even beyond these probable changes, there are others which also will most likely occur, and these have to do with the different forms of humanness that might be determined by the locations and environment where humans decide to settle.

In that context, cyborg transformations would reflect where in the cosmos individual settlements might be. Earth provides one set of atmospheric and gravitational characteristics that has determined human evolution over approximately 6 million years. Different planets, moons and space habitats will each in various ways have their own, and human beings will have to adjust accordingly. In that sense, what is human – that relationship between the technological and the organic – will depend as never before upon where one lives. To that extent, human beings will have different biological requirements and capacities that depend upon the habitats which they occupy.

> ...Pioneer explorers will have a more compelling incentive than those of us on Earth to redesign themselves. They'll harness the super powerful genetic and cyborg technologies that will be developed in coming decades. These techniques will be, one hopes, heavily regulated on Earth, but settlers on Mars will be far beyond the clutches of the regulators. We should wish them good luck in modifying their progeny to adapt to alien environments.[18]

The potential settlement-determined changes in the nature of humanness may well in turn relate to the ways that those in different settlements interact. For this reason, what has been called 'astrosociology' will become increasingly important.[19] Clearly, the physical and natural sciences and all the disciplines that relate to STEM fields (Science, Technology, Energy and Mathematics) will be fundamental for the survival of those who inhabit settlements beyond the Earth. Transportation and physical infrastructures and construction will be of fundamental importance, but, so, too, will a deep understanding of emerging social, social psychological and psychological behaviour.

This astrosociological admix may suggest and possibly confirm that who are we really may depend in various ways on where we really are. It will determine how humans see themselves and others – their strengths, weaknesses and vulnerabilities.

All of these changes in the nature of 'humanness' are highly probable. What, however, is far less certain are their possible consequences. To what extent will such transformations, as had been suggested by Hayles, make what might be described as 'the post-humanist' individual more rationale than his or her predecessors, less encumbered with perceptions hitherto determined by upbringing, a range of socio-economic and geographical factors and educational opportunities and physical attributes?[20]

Alternatively, might AGI-determined intelligence and bioengineered improvements create an unparalleled social divide, where the barriers between haves and have nots become seemingly impenetrable?

This clearly raises the issue of ethics. Genome editing such as CRISPR has by the mid-2020s already begun to eliminate a plethora of mutations that result in everything from heart attacks and cancer to Alzheimer and schizophrenia. Indeed, with such increasingly sophisticated interventions the very nature of ageing might be fundamentally transformed – an issue perceived as of growing importance when considering that one in six people in the world will be over 65 by 2050, up from 11 in 2019, and that centurions (those 100 or over) will increase eightfold.

And, what would happen should aging be cancelled? According to *The Genesis Machine*, when Generation Z would become grandparents

> they redefined stereotypes of what elders looked like... . All of the tiny mutations and metabolic failings that had affected every previous generation were no longer causing problems. Zoomers were getting older—but not old.[21]

On the other hand, as one observer commented, Some see it very differently. Gene editing could be a way of 'disappearing' certain types of people... .The issue is whether some states we regard as disabilities are just differences that are only a problem [ed., e.g. dwarfism] because the rest of society treats them as such.

> These are questions our descendants may grapple with for millennia to come. Barring scenarios in which we merge with machines to become superhuman cyborgs, it seems certain we will increasingly shape the genomes of our children. The only question is how.[22]

Human Agency and Human Space

When it comes to *r-evolutionary* change and their impacts on human agency, whether believers or sceptics, most generally focus on what will occur on planet Earth. However, human agency – who we are and the societies of which we are a part – will no longer be confined to a single planet by mid-century.

There can be little doubt that human beings by 2050 will have ventured well beyond the solar system of which the Earth is but one middle-sized component. The dimensions of human agency will have increasingly become intertwined with the oceans beyond planet Earth. 'The moon may just be another country.'[23]

Space aliens are more than a possibility, suggested Avi Loeb, Chair of Astronomy at Harvard University, in 2020. It could be quite likely, he wrote, that the first known interstellar object – referred to as *Oumuamua*, a Hawaiian term for 'scout' – may house aliens beyond our solar system that are monitoring activities on planet Earth.[24] Whether they are or not, the James Webb Space Telescope, launched on Christmas day in 2021, was seen as giving astronomers on Earth a real shot at seeing the details of planets' atmospheres beyond the solar system – *exoplanets* – considered the best bet for finding potential signs of life.[25]

In speculating about the future, it can be assumed that human beings will have become increasingly dependent upon not only the resources which outer space offers but also the opportunities which it provides for global systems on Earth. As one internationally renowned Cambridge physicist had stressed, human survival over the next hundred years would depend in no small part on human beings' willingness to settle in outer space.[26]

It was apparent that early in the 21st century, the transformative consequences of outer space were being recognised across the globe.[27] China's president in 2016 spoke of his country's 'space dream… to take bigger strides to explore further into space'.[28] Six years later, more than 70 countries had established state-funded agencies to facilitate space exploration and research, deployment of artificial satellites and in some instances means to gather space resources. Those 70 included not only those deemed to be major powers, but also countries such as the Philippines (2019), Costa Rica (2021) and Rwanda (2021), and by that time every region across the world was in on the action.[29]

At the same time, according to the United Nations Office for Outer Space Affairs, 31 UN organisations also regularly meet to discuss the use of space technologies for their respective interests, and regional organisations such as the Asian Pacific Space Cooperation Organisation (APSCO), the European Space Agency (ESA) and the Latin American and Caribbean Space Agency (ALCE) have emerged as major players and increasingly shared their assets across regions.[30]

The 'space economy', covering goods and services produced in space for the use in space such as mining the moon or asteroids for material, was worth $469 billion in 2021. It was forecast that by 2040, that figure would increase to $1.1 trillion[31] with the likelihood that by mid-century that amount would triple.[32] Along with a burgeoning space economy, it was forecast that by 2050, Mars and the Moon will have established colonies and that by then there would be means for residing permanently not only on Mars and the Moon but also on other planets within the solar system and possibly beyond.[33]

The numbers of human beings who will have left the Earth to live elsewhere is uncertain. Some suggest that there may well be more than 1 million living on Mars, alone, by mid-century.[34] Others suggest anywhere between '5, 5000 or 50,000'. In any event, whatever the eventual figure, it is generally assumed that space colonialisation will take place over the next three decades. 'The name of the game is sustainability and self-sufficiency,'[35] but in any case, the dimensions of physical space accessible to human beings will have changed exponentially.

While outer space will have emerged as an increasing reality, significant transformations affecting the concept of human space would also be happening at the same time but closer to Earth. By 2050, 'orbital rings', for example, could provide two train tracks approximately 80 km above the Earth that will enable travellers to cross the world in 45 minutes.[36]

Around that same time drone technology resulting in Unmanned Aviation Vehicles (UAVs) will have become an integral part of urban and supra-urban mobility. Something like 100 cities worldwide will have implemented drone services ranging from 60 drones for the smallest metropolitan areas to more than 6,000 in the largest. Of course, drones will by then have also become the basic system for delivery of goods as well as assuming various defence and security functions.[37]

When it comes to Earth-based access, it is also worth considering the likelihood that by mid-century long-distance aircraft will have been able to fly at approximately 3800 miles per hour, and would take approximately one hour to go between London and New York. Based on future ambitions for military aircraft, the United States as well as China, India, Russia and several European nations also are focusing on hypersonic aircraft that would be able to fly anywhere on Earth in under three hours. All of these might be made more comfortable by airlines providing virtual reality cabins, where cabin space could be transformed into golf courses and offices.[38]

Of all those factors that could in the longer term affect travel dynamics, perhaps the most transformative and controversial is *teleportation*. Boiling down this highly complex and, at this stage, very hypothetical phenomenon to its simplest definition, teleportation involves disassembling objects – matter or energy – at the subatomic level from a point A and forwarding that scanned data within a fraction of a second to a point B. At point B, a computer would build back the object, even though it would not have traversed physical space, *per se*.

The concept, let alone its feasibility, has generated persistent criticisms, including the sort suggested by one journalist that it was a Star Wars 'tease'.[39] And, without ignoring its science-fiction connection, the fact of the matter is that teleportation's conceptual underpinnings and a growing number of micro-experiments have indicated that human beings might be at the edge of a realistic mode of travel hitherto unimaginable.[40] One example that had been suggested was teleporting a baseball:

> [A baseball] 'couldn't be sent by radio waves, but all the information about it could. If you can read what the quantum state of a baseball is in London, you could send that information around the world and imprint atoms with the same chemical elements in India, where they would be assembled to become the exact same ball.[41]

There are those who indeed support teleportation as feasible in terms of decades rather than centuries, and if they are right, how and where humans appear physically – on and beyond Earth – will clearly have extraordinary consequences when it comes to human access.

As with all emerging transformative change, those affecting *human space* are replete with downsides. Overreliance upon transformative innovations such as orbital rings, drone technologies and interplanetary transportation might mean that systems failures could leave large swathes of communities on Earth and beyond in deep physical isolation. It, too, could result in the breakdown of supply chains where time and not proximity is the principal determinant, and should monitoring technologies such as the Space-based Positioning, Navigation and Timing services go down, the force multiplier would have been reflected in the collapse of a vast range of systems upon which human engagement depended. That would include land, air and sea navigation, precision agriculture, water source monitoring, security analyses, energy requirements and population movements.

Yet, whatever the upsides and downsides of these transformative factors might prove to be, a far more fundamental and enduring transformation will have been that human beings' perceptions of who they are, the nature of time, place and space will have altered paradigmatically.

Human Engagement

Issues of *human space* flow naturally into how humans in a possible future will have begun to engage, virtually and physically. Like the fundamental transformations that will have been witnessed in human space, *human engagement*, too, will have been transformed by paradigm shifting technologies. Of course, new forms and approaches to engagement are not always received well, as was all too evident when one author complained that

> in the age of digital distractions, we've been fooled into believing we're more connected, informed, productive and happy. But in reality, this kind of social

> reciprocity eats away at our norms and values and rebuilds them in harmful ways. As a former Facebook executive put it, "The short-term, dopamine-driven feedback loops that we have created are destroying how society works".[42]

It is more than likely that there will be disparities when it comes to availability and access. When, for example, data and cross-border data flows were assessed by the UN in 2021, only 20 per cent of people in least developed countries (LDCs) used the internet, and 'when they did so, it was typically at relatively low download speeds and with a relatively high price tag attached'.[43] Indeed, the UN Secretary General had expressed one year before his belief of the existential importance of 'connecting the unconnected'.[44]

However, from a global perspective, myriad economic, social, political and personal boundaries will have been crossed as digital services continue to expand. The rate of uptake for digital services had already doubled between 2009 and 2019 to 53.6 per cent, or, 4.1 billion people.[45] Traditional and virtual communities have begun to mesh through virtual reality and already have begun to create virtual communities across the planet and most likely will eventually do so in outer space. While access to such communication opportunities has not been available to all at this stage, the likelihood as suggested by those who should know was there.[46] Towards that end, transmitters in the stratosphere and 'loitering' solar-powered drones rather than land-based fibre-optic cables could well open up the world of the internet for virtually all.

Such innovative technologies – possibly based on the Artificial Super Intelligence – could well result in fundamental changes in the ways that human beings engage, and perhaps one of the most transformative would be the Tactile Internet (TI).[47] Based on 'haptic' technology, TI may enable users to engage with humans and cyber-physical systems as if they were close but in reality vast distances away. 'Haptic feedback', using sensations generated through virtual systems, could produce real capacities and feelings in real time. This would include not only control of highly dynamic processes, but even hugging and handshaking.

For all intents and purposes, these may well have replaced in many instances the need to be physically present for surgeons, drivers, pilots, hairdressers and virtually all other professions. It is by no means improbable that delivering or indeed creating hospitals in times of emergencies is one. Another would be the ability of doctors and surgeons to remotely undertake diagnostics and even surgery using connected, tactile technologies.[48] Similarly, identifying pandemics such as Covid-19 and providing essential vaccines could all be facilitated through 'haptic feedback'. Even medicine transferred virtually into outer space, e.g. to the International Space Station, is a serious prospect being actively explored.[49]

The forms and types of human engagement that will have emerged out of the technologies of the early 21st century might well be regarded as first steps in an ever more adventurous and uncertain future. Beyond the sorts of haptic examples already noted, there are prospects such as very small (e.g. 2 cm) robots that could navigate across a user's clothing, choosing the best location to perform a task, ranging from a medical measurement to a dynamic display.

The prospect that human engagement will have also included physical and virtual meetings across planets has become ever more plausible. So, too, is the possibility that the more outer space became a norm, the more likely that human engagement would by necessity involve cyborgs. Brain implants would become normal means of engagement. And, of course, as noted in the next chapter dealing with governance, the all-pervasive nature of the internet would mean that authorities would be able to monitor the needs of society with unparalleled sensitivity to the individual, and learning and education would be an accessible process any time.

Transformative technologies leading to enhanced human engagement might also address what has been a persistent concern of observers dealing with crisis threats, namely, that earlier technologies had reflected unintended biases of relief workers 'either through a shift to digital registration unintentionally excluding those most in need, or humanitarian independence being compromised'.[50] This concern could clearly be addressed through technologies which will preprogramme themselves to recognise individual needs without depending upon pre-programmed categories such as gender or race. Technological developments, including distributed technology, 5G supercomputing and quantum computing could continue to improve the efficiency and targeting of crisis assistance operations, including the swift diagnoses of infectious diseases.[51]

Yet, as with all advances in technology and their societal impacts, those involving human engagement would also pose serious and on occasion existential challenges. The positive dimensions of human engagement could also feed in various ways into large-scale threats. For example, what might be the consequences of IoT dependent systems being severely damaged by attacks on cyber systems in outer space? It is quite likely that large portions of global infrastructures would be destroyed, resulting in unprecedented types of interactive crises and new dimensions of human vulnerability.

Certainly since 1988, when a computer at the Massachusetts Institute of Technology unleashed a malicious programme on the internet, cyber security had increased exponentially as a threat of global consequence. Issues of defence, finance and economics, and health would be just some of the potential victims to the cyber disrupters. Thirty-three years after that MIT malware attack, one hacker was reported to have leaked 8.4 billion passwords.[52] Cybercriminality and state-sponsored cyber-attacks, all had been indicative of the ways that the instruments of human engagement paradoxically could have undermined all their positive benefits. Maybe the downside of such plausible futures had been captured in the following reflection:

> Suppose…that COP36 asks for help in deacidifying the oceans; they know the pitfalls of specifying objectives incorrectly, so they insist that all the by-products must be non-toxic, and no fish can be harmed. The AI system comes up with a new self-multiplying catalyst that will do the trick with a very rapid chemical reaction. Great! But the reaction uses up a quarter of all the oxygen in the atmosphere and we all die slowly and painfully. From the AI system's point

of view, eliminating humans is a feature, not a bug, because it ensures that the oceans stay in their now-pristine state.[53]

Human Needs

The changing nature of humanness, human space and human engagement are clearly intertwined with all things essential for human well-being. Here, the principal areas of interest would be of no surprise to the reader: food and nutrition, water, energy and healthcare. For each, transformative technologies will be of considerable importance and will inevitably impact upon issues essential for the survival of a population forecast to be almost 9.7 billion by 2050.[54]

In speculating about how human needs might be fulfilled in a generation's time, it is difficult to embark on a discussion about them without recognising the potential consequences of climate change. Climate change might well continue to expose existential threats across planet Earth; and, while at the time of writing, it is difficult for this author to predict with any accuracy the extent to which the global community will have responded adequately to such threats, the following assumption underpins the discussion that follows.

The 1.5 centigrade target might be met by 2050, and in so doing as much emissions as had been placed into the atmosphere would have been removed.[55] No doubt carbon capture technologies, geo-engineering, nuclear energy, space-based solar systems and solar and wind-energy will have positive impacts as would related changes in manufacturing processes and forest preservation. However, to overcome the existential threat posed by climate change will also require fundamental changes in the nature of human needs.

Transformations affecting available land mass, air quality, new sources of water, food and energy as well as innovations dramatically affecting human well-being could offset changing climate's worst effects by 2050. Nevertheless, the ways that such transformation might be adopted will determine whether or not much of humanity will find itself on the brink of extinction.

Take food, for example. A positive perspective might begin with the prospect that the very nature of food might change. More bio-engineered foods could well begin to play an increasingly important and positive nutritional role across the globe.[56] For example, Solein consists of 50 to 60 per cent protein and the remainder carbohydrate and fats,[57] and is produced using hydrogen-oxidising bacteria, electricity from solar panels, a small amount of water, carbon dioxide drawn from the air, nitrogen and traces of minerals such as calcium, sodium, potassium and zinc.

NovoNutrients, Air Protein and Solar Foods follow similar paths – all using 'constituents of air, waste CO2, and water to make plentiful amounts of nutritious protein'.[58]

Thirty-metre-tall vertical 'farms', robotically managed, are already becoming features in urban and semi-urban areas. Some even specialise in what are described as 'delectable' flour beetles and black soldier flies as part of changes that could significantly contribute to human nutrition.[59] Then, too, others suggest the creation of whale farms, where vast 'ranches' and underwater electric fences could keep giant, vegetarian baleen whales herded, and like cattle, eventually eaten.[60] Urban farming,[61] under-water farming[62] and 3D Ocean Farming[63] are all foreseen as ways that the human species might feed itself in the future, certainly by 2050.

Beyond Earth, it is also assumed by many experts that once space technology has advanced to the point where self-sustaining space settlements of perhaps millions of people were possible, the vastly larger resources of space could be used to grow food for people on Earth as well. Indeed, it can be argued that tensions about the uses of land on Earth for human habitation, agriculture, industrial activities and preservation of nature could in various ways be resolved directly and indirectly by going beyond the planet. While initially only small amounts of food or specialty items deemed too expensive or taxing on Earth's ecosystems would be shipped to Earth, eventually portions of the world might be fed from space.[64]

Countering these more positive perspectives are other concerns about the nature of land and the consequences of growing urbanisation. As for the former, it is more than likely that despite a range of positive innovations, agricultural land still would remain of fundamental importance in a generation's time. Therefore, findings that availability of sufficient landmass could not be assumed is disconcerting.[65]

Of the 1,500 million hectares of arable land worldwide, approximately 1/3rd is likely to increasingly suffer from soil erosion, lack of biodiversity and pollutants which would impact on soil health and biological productivity. At the same time, from a 2022 perspective, wildfires will have reached as far as the Arctic and by 2050 could have increased by 50 per cent, with severely negative impacts on land usage.[66]

When it comes to the nutritional consequences of growing urbanisation, it is forecast that 70 per cent of the world's population will be living in urban areas and that term, *urban*, would include *megalopolises*, defined as densely clustered groups of metropolitan centres tied together by varying degrees of common infrastructures.[67] And, while vertical farms in urban areas and artificially produced foods on planet Earth and beyond might address varying degrees of nutritional requirements for such bourgeoning populations, it is more than likely that from a global perspective the mainstay of food production will remain agricultural land. Hence, it is clearly disturbing to anticipate that agricultural lands will continue to deteriorate and competition for remaining lands will intensify.

Linked to issues of land and food availability is that of water. Certainly up though the mid to late 2030s, water availability from a planetary perspective will have become an issue of major concern. Water use increased sixfold over this century and continues to rise by at least 1 per cent a year. The paradox, if not irony, is that the issue will not be the amount of water but access to drinkable water. According to the Commission on the Economics of Water, demand is expected to outstrip supply by 40 per cent in the 2030s.[68] However, due to climate change, resulting in the increasing frequency and intensity of extreme events – storms, floods and droughts – countries that already had been experiencing 'water stress' now were most likely to be joined by other areas that had not previously been so severely affected.

Some of the most severely affected will result from the consequences of steadily rising temperatures affecting some of the world's largest ice sheets and mountain glaciers. The Greenland and Antarctic ice sheets and the Alaskan, Patagonian and other mountain glacier systems will most likely continue to disintegrate at alarming rates, pouring billions of tonnes of water into the oceans each year, driving sea levels to dangerous new heights. Areas of unprecedented flooding would include the upper Midwest in the United States, southern Albert in Canada, Amazon and Orinoco River basins in South America and the Okavango Delta in southern Africa.[69]

Already by the early 2020s, more and more megalopolises and more conventional urban conurbations, found themselves 'underwater'. In the case of West Africa, for example, whatever type of conurbation, all countries have urban areas where at least 23 per cent of populations are exposed to serious flooding, and as a series of climate change conferences (viz, Conferences of the Parties, or CoPs) recognised, growing proportions of island landmass are underwater as are coastal cities elsewhere, for example, in North and South America, and East and South East Asia, including two of the most populous countries, China and India.

At the same time, over half of the world's major aquifers – the basis of ground water – would be consumed at far greater rates than they were being replenished. The Central Valley and Ogallala aquifers in the US, the Northwest Sahara aquifer system, across the Middle East, north-western India, northern Bangladesh, the North China Plain aquifer in Beijing, the Pilbara basin in north-western Australia and the Guarani aquifer in southern South America would most likely be over exploited. These great aquifer systems would continue to be mined, primarily for irrigation in the overlying, mega-food-producing regions of the world. This disappearance of groundwater would continue to place regional and global water and food security at ever increasing risk.[70]

Some of these dystopic visions about land, food, water and energy may be offset overtime in various ways.

Looking across the decade, there were and will continue to be emerging technologies beginning to address the consequences not only of lack of potable water but lack of sufficient water at all. At the local levels, desalination will continue to have significant impact on municipal water supplies in urban coastal centres in some instances accounting for an estimated 10 per cent of water needs. By 2030 that figure could well have increased to approximately 25 per cent of municipal water supply of urban coastal centres worldwide.

Regarding water, Nigeria's use of space-based sensors already has begun to identify how much water is needed for agricultural production by providing information about what each square inch of ground requires, including customised fertiliser and water.[71]

In the Sidi Ifni region of Morocco, where entire villages had suffered from severe water shortages, innovators decided to use the one thing that the region had in abundance to offset the looming water crisis, namely, fog, by using fog-harvesting to create water.[72] In India, during this same period, over 181,000 solar power pumps were being used to harvest water, which, ironically, resulted in many instances in over-irrigation.[73]

In a related vein, China had proposed to turn 16 flood-prone urban areas into 'sponge cities', absorbing and reusing at least 70 per cent of rainwater in the 2020s. And, as another example, Israel – a country consisting of 50 percent desert – during this same period got 60 per cent of domestic water supply from 5 large and 34 small desalinisation plants around the country. It also had been a world leader in the development and operation of desalination plants, including 400 plants in 40 countries such as China, India, Australia and the US.

Added to these innovations have been at least three others. Remote sensors, drones and blockchain that can provide precise, real-time information about sources and availability of water throughout the world.[74] This would include linking water infrastructures to the internet and enabling real-time monitoring via sensors. In other words, 'pipes, wells, treatment plants, just about anything can become smarter once they are hooked up to the internet. Loss management and loss detection then becomes much easier'.[75]

'Evapotranspiration' is another example, consisting of outer space monitoring systems which can measure the amount of water being expelled by plants, crops and surface areas more generally. This sort of information should enable farmers, for example, to better calculate crop water requirements, helping them use water more efficiently and better plan irrigation.[76]

A second transformative factor involves the use of nanotechnology (nanocellulose) materials to provide a stable and long-lasting methods for removing impurities such as bacterial and chemical contaminants, including dyes, oils and pesticides from polluted water. Closely linked to this nanocellulose method of water purification is a third factor, namely, the likelihood that increased access to graphene, which enhanced desalination membranes to produce potable water for an estimated 140 countries.[77]

Whether it comes to food production or access to water, the energy factor is fundamental to both. And, as with both, technological transformations will affect the use and access to energy, negatively as well as positively, over the next three decades. Some analysts forecast that energy usage would increase in relation to Gross Domestic Product, but that growth would be slower – an average of about 0.7 per cent a year through 2050 (versus an average of more than 2 per cent from 2000 to 2015). The decline in the rate of growth would be due to digitisation, slower population and economic growth, greater efficiency, a decline in European and North American demand, and the global economic shift towards services, which would use less energy than the production of goods.[78]

Nevertheless, it can be assumed that by 2050 electricity will account for a quarter of all energy demands, compared with 18 per cent in the 2020s. China and India may have generated 71 per cent of such outputs. How will that additional power be generated? In 2016, a leading consultancy firm had estimated that by 2050 more than three-quarters of new capacity (77 per cent) would have come from wind and solar, 13 per cent from natural gas, and the rest from everything else. The share of nuclear and hydropower are also expected to grow, albeit modestly.[79]

What that analysis had not taken into account was the creation of means to capture a new energy source, namely, geothermal energy derived from magma, or hot molten rock (mixed with gases and mineral crystals) that collects in chambers normally around 3 kilometres below the Earth's crust. The energy technology called 'near-magna geothermal' (NMG) would be able to capture geothermal fluids, with temperatures of about 900 degrees centigrade, which could produce pressure roughly 500 times that of the atmosphere. The results would be energy outputs that would be about 1/6th of the cost of electricity available in 2024, the source of which would be limitless. Many places on Earth have the potential to exploit this near-magma geothermal method, including Kenya, the United States, the mid-Atlantic ridge and 'all the rift zones in the oceans'.[80]

In parallel with the development of NMG would be giant space-based solar farms, which could offer another completely environmentally friendly answer to longer-term energy crises. 'Sun-powered chemistry' would enable the manufacturing of chemicals important to human life not to be fossil fuel dependent. Instead, it would use sunlight to convert waste carbon dioxide into needed chemicals. In so doing, it would use unwanted gas as a raw material and sunlight – not fossil fuels – as the source of energy for production.[81]

A second example would be the benefits arising from *space-based solar power* (SBSP). In this instance, solar energy would be transmitted from outer space through a number of large platforms positioned in high earth orbit where they can collect and convert solar energy into energy on earth on a global scale. According to one analyst, power captured in outer space through such platforms could 'provide an energy source that would be continuous, clean and unlimited.'[82] To a very significant extent, SBSP could eliminate the need for any type of fossil fuels, recycled or otherwise, and pose far fewer hazards than nuclear and far greater certitude and continuity than tidal or wind generated energy sources.

Since the 1970s there have been many such proposals concerned with solar panels in outer space, which would orbit about 22,000 miles above the Earth, and gather sunlight and 'beam' the energy back down to the surface. The photovoltaic array of solar satellites could 'harvest' sunlight, and through that array convert sunlight into electricity. This electricity would be converted into radio frequency electrical power (microwaves) beamed wirelessly to ground-based receivers. They would not be affected by the Earth's atmosphere, including clouds and weather.

The receivers that would capture the energy would take the form of giant wire nets measuring up to four miles across that could be installed across deserts or farmland or even over lakes. Its potential, even at an early stage of development, has been compared to the largest earth-based solar facility, namely, in Aswan, southern Egypt. The latter produces a maximum of 1.8 gigawatts, the former could produce 2000 gigawatts. And, industrial giants such as Northrup Grumman had as far back as 2015 committed themselves to the project, and similarly so had the governments of China and Japan.[83]

Less than a decade after the Northrup Grumman announcement, the Co-Chair of the multi-institutional Space Energy Initiative (SEI) said that the power that could be generated by harvesting solar energy could be almost limitless. 'In theory it could supply all of the world's energy in 2050.'[84]

At the same time, what also has to be taken into account are the downsides of over dependence on SBSP. One certainly is that space debris and dust, asteroids, and extreme solar radiation could significantly destroy these major power providers or at least disrupt them for extensive periods. Another is the prospect that they could be weaponised, with microwaves aimed at specific targets. And, inevitably there is the issue of control. Who in the final analysis will determine when and whom will be the beneficiaries, and who will ultimately determine how and when they will be used?

The Use of Time. How in the longer term technologies might affect ways that humans might use time are also replete with uncertainties. Employment, work, personal life and leisure will all be affected, and from a 2050 perspective, there is a wide range of possibilities.

Employment and work already began to undergo major transformations by the early 2000s due to rapid technological, political and social change. Except in a decreasing number of circumstances such as small hold farming, the ways that human beings will seek to ensure their livelihoods will most likely undergo exponential change. ASI and robotics could prove to be positive factors in that regard. *Assisted Intelligence* (e.g. GPS navigation systems) and *Augmented Intelligence* enabling human beings to do things that they otherwise could not do are but two examples.

By 2050 and indeed well before, these sorts of innovations may well have changed the nature of employment quite fundamentally. Generally speaking, employment might be less geared to long-term contracts and more based upon individual talents and capacities that different employers could use for defined periods of time.

It is quite likely that by mid-century, at least 40 per cent of workers worldwide would be employed in more 'gig' type economies, where freelancers would work on as many as 20 projects at once with as many teams or companies. Their boss *per* project might be pieces of software, or, supercharged brainpower, in organisations where interacting systems predominated and hierarchical structures far less so.

There, too, might be elite groups of professionals who would rely on 'genius apps' to augment their intelligence in order to carry out knowledge-specific roles. Theoretical physics is a case in point, or 'lawbots' that churned through legal cases in microseconds. Here, too, professional networks rather than hierarchical management chains would advance their careers.[85]

ASI could assist with 'people processing', resulting in expanded and reshaped skills. In that sense, few analysts would disagree that technology has and will continue to reshape skills defined as work and employment and would do so exponentially. But, to do what?

One answer is that employers would not think in terms of employees – but rather in terms of specialisms. 'Who do I need? And for how long?' Future work would also be focused around making complex decisions – using creativity, leadership and high degrees of self-management.'[86] Most of all, it would be based on ensuring that capacities to deal with rapidly transforming products would, when and where necessary be available.

At the same time, others believed that the demand for advanced cognitive skills, socio-behavioural skills and skill combinations associated with greater adaptability was rising.[87] In other words, some anticipated a growing tension between high-level, leadership roles and then less highly-specialised jobs that could be automated.

Whether in what had been called the developed or developing worlds, technology would witness general *disruption*. Disruption, regarded as inherent in any dynamic economy, would result in the upshot of markets responding to changing conditions. While such disruptors could be devastating for any particular individual or community, their effects for workers as a whole could be positive if old jobs were replaced with new ones that would be safer, less physically arduous, more stimulating and providing greater autonomy.

That perspective globally speaking hinged for many on whether, for example, ASI might develop beyond human control or not, and whether other related technologies such as synthetic biology, computational science, nanotechnology, quantum computing, 3D and 4D printing and robotics would result in exponentially increasing long-term structural unemployment.

The increasing ubiquity of ASI no doubt could result in profound societal upheavals, including unparalleled levels of displacement, as traditional work and skills and limited education might become substantively irrelevant.[88] They might offer little societal purpose. That agricultural worker, who had followed in the footsteps of previous agriculturally-dependent generations, now found that he or she has been replaced by robotic systems. Those with mental or physical disorders who had hitherto survived on the fringes of society may be even further side-lined.

On the other hand, this dystopic proposition might well be countered by those who feel that, despite these perceived 'exceptions', the positive consequences that resulted from the 19th century Industrial Revolution offer examples that bode well. That 19th century period of unprecedented phenomena, so they would argue, eventually opened up new opportunities for a spectrum of people never previously considered in any positive way.[89]

In other words, human beings might have opportunities in a world in which the nature of work might have been changed significantly but by no means to the detriment of the many.

From a 2050 perspective, technology would have allowed jobs to become customisable, with individuals able to choose who they worked for, where they worked, how much they worked and the pace at which they worked. Instead of creating vulnerabilities, technology and its consequences would have enhanced resilience throughout society. This perspective, of course, would depend upon the assumptions one made about levels and types of 'non-employment'.[90]

As jobs became increasingly automated and fluid, people may frequently become redundant, but opportunities to be retrained become a norm. A 'job for life' would be well and truly passé, and instead

> there will be constant new areas of work for people to stay on top of. In 2050 people will continually need to update their skills for jobs of the moment, but

> I have an optimistic view that there will continue to be employment if these skills are honed.[91]

Private sector companies as well as governments might begin to undertake measures to reduce the social costs of automation – avoiding factors that could even weaken national economies more generally. Either on their own or with government incentives, workers could be trained in new skills before their jobs became completely automated, and governments provided them with a basic income during such transitions.

For those in the workplace, collaboration and co-creation of ideas and tasks would open up new opportunities for work, one which it had been argued would also lead to better natural resource management. Globalisation, too, could maximise workers' potentials since, though dispersed around the world in a physical sense, they would collaborate and co-create via computational tools such as augmented and virtual reality. Such ASI-mediated work will have redefined the nature of the workplace.

It has been suggested that these sorts of transitions could ensure consistent continuous patterns of product consumption and exchange, which would stabilise rather than damage society.[92]

The ways that time might be used for work also relates to how time might be used in non-work situations, e.g. homes and families. Home, for example, could become an accepted alternative to the office, the factory or the farm. However, unlike the post-Covid period of the 2020s, haptic connections by mid-century would mean that 'real' space and 'virtual' space from a productivity and collaboration point of view could become indistinguishable. This would apply as much to agriculture as it would to medical care, energy systems production, legal and political processes and even to construction.

Such virtual space, it has been proposed, could bring workers closer to their families in terms of real space. The boundaries between work and personal life would become increasingly blurred and there would be a gradual move away from individuals trying to achieve a better 'work-life balance' towards a greater 'work-life integration'.

However, the 'Orwellians' would be less optimistic. Societies might have to face the fact that technological unemployment could mean that many careers would cease to exist. More and more individuals would rely solely on governments to prepare them for new jobs. Yet, the emerging reality might be that many governments lacked the resources or were unable to keep up with the momentum of employment changes. At the same time, there could well be divides between government and those bodies outside governments about required and acceptable types of employment. Hence, large swathes of populations would be unable to gain adequate sources for survival.[93]

This could well lead to a class of citizens that were economically irrelevant to society. They neither worked nor consumed. It was those that had control over 'the machines' – that super elite – that produced most of the wealth in the world, and they would form a super elite, even richer and more powerful than the top 1 per cent as we know it. The super elite might reap the benefits of automation and jobless growth making inequality even greater. This will lead to the rise of two highly divided classes – an elite and an ever-increasing 'under class'.

As urbanisation grew, those in rural areas would have streamed into cities, including megalopolises, looking for employment which was not readily available. As a result, unemployment would have increased significantly. And, in a related vein, such realities reflected governments' own deficiencies in dealing effectively and consistently with the interrelationships between technological change, employment and societal needs. Inevitably, these failings and their consequences might well result in spillovers affecting societies as a whole such as decline in air and water quality and ultimately health.

Contextualising Human Agency

There can be little doubt that human agency by mid-century will have changed in myriad ways. The nature of humanness – whether the result of gene modification or brain implants or a host of other factors that are foreseen by social and natural scientists – will have rapidly changed and would continue to do so. Perhaps the Novacene age by then would have been recognised as an alternative to the Anthropocene.

More than likely, the conventional distinctions between real, physical and virtual would have decreasing relevance when it came to the ways that human beings connected and interacted, and certainly when it came to human access, human beings will have been able to move locations on this planet and perhaps others in ways and at speeds that hitherto had been relegated to the realm of science fiction.

Where and how humans might live and engage and how they will and will need to use time are all questions the answers to which are at best speculative. In that sense, no one can predict the longer term with any assurance that such speculations will become reality, let alone what their consequences might be.

Nevertheless, whatever their consequences, they will mirror ways that societies may be structured and resources distributed – and these will be reflected in the dynamics of governance and resource distribution.

Notes

1 'Blurring the lines of what it means to be human', *New Scientist*, 22 February 2020, pp. 18–19.
2 See, for example, Frank A. Von Hippel, *The chemical age: How chemists fought famines and disease, killed millions and changed our relationship with earth*, University of Chicago Press, 2020.
3 Martin Rees, *On the future: Prospects for humanity*, Princeton Press, p. 108.
4 Office of the Director of National Intelligence, Global Trends, www.dni.gov/index.php/gt2040-home/summary

5 Ben Goertzel and Cassio Pennachin (Eds), *Artificial general intelligence*, Springer-Verlag Berlin Heidelberg, 2007, p.vi.
6 The Singularity is a hypothetical future point in time at which technological growth becomes uncontrollable and irreversible, resulting in unforeseeable changes to human civilisation. See, for example, Ray Kurzweil, *The Singularity is near: When Humans transcend biology*, Viking, 2005.
7 Op. cit., #3, Rees, p. 136.
8 Op. cit., #3, p. 108.
9 James Lovelock, *Novacene: The coming age of hyperintelligence*, Penguin/Random House UK, 2019.
10 BBVA's *Next Step: Exponential Life* views transformative technologies as the basis of 'exponential life', having environmental, ethical, and even ontological implications. From the perspective of the Chairman of the BBVA, Francisco González, 'Humanity is at the beginning of a technological revolution that is evolving at a much faster pace than earlier ones, and that is so far reaching itis destined to generate transformations we can only begin to imagine.'
11 Nicholas St Fleur, Chloe Williams and Charlie Wood, 'How long can we live: In the last century, the average human life expectancy doubled. Here's a roadmap to the innovations that could help us do it again—maybe', *New York Times*, 27 April 2021. See, also, Antonio Regalado, 'Meet Alto Labs, Silicon Valley's latest wild best on living forever', *MIT Technology Review*, 4 September 2021.
12 See, for example, R. D. Kirkton et al., 'A bioengineered blood vessel', *Science Translational Medicine* (2019), 27 March 2019.
13 Jo Marchant, 'Evolution machine: Genetic engineering on fast forward', *New Scientist*, 22 June 2011.
14 See, for example, 'E-Skin: From humanoids to humans (Point of View)', *IEEE Journal*, 107 (2), February 2019.
15 Marty Travino, 'Cyber physical systems: The coming singularity', *Prism*, National Defense University, 8 (3), 2019.
16 Ministry of Defence, *Global strategic trends: The future starts today*, Sixth Edition, 2018.
17 Jessica Hamzelou, '$100 million project to make intelligence-boosting brain implant', *New Scientist*, 20 October 2016. This assumption stems from the driver of the brain chip initiative, the entrepreneur Bryon Johnson who invested $100 million into the project, and who continues to work with scientists from the Massachusetts Institute of Technology and the University of Southern California.
18 Martin Rees, *On the future: Prospects for humanity*, Princeton Press, 2018, p. 151.
19 Jim Pass, 'Astrosociology on Mars' in Giuseppe Pezzella (Ed.), *Mars exploration: A step*, Interchange Publisher, 2020 [Available in the Virtual Library at https://lnkd.in/gY2eA5j] .
20 N. Katherine Hayles, *How we became posthuman: Virtual bodies in cybernetics literature and informatics*, University of Chicago Press, 1999. 'In this age of DNA computers and artificial intelligence, information is becoming disembodied even as the "bodies" that once carried it vanish into virtuality.'
21 Amy Webb and Andrew Hessel, *The Genesis Machine: Our Quest to Rewrite Life in the Age of Synthetic Biology*, Public Affairs, Hatchett Book Group, Inc., Kindle Edition, 2022, pp. 193 ff.

22 Michael LePage, 'The ethics issue: Should we edit our children's genomes?', *New Scientist*, 5 July 2017, www.newscientist.com/article/mg23531330-700-the-ethics-issue-should-we-edit-our-childrens-genomes/#ixzz5wIlLPdni.
23 Comment made by Laura Sandys, Founder and Director of Challenging Ideas, a UK-based consultancy, 11 October 2021
24 Avi Loeb, *Extraterrestrial: The first sign of intelligent life beyond earth*, Houghton Mifflin Harcourt, 2021.
25 Stuart Clark, 'Alien skies', *New Scientist*, 12 November 2022, pp. 36 ff.
26 Stephen Hawking, *Brief answers to the big questions*, John Murray Publishers, 2018, pp. 165 ff.
27 It is interesting to note that, according to the *New Scientist* ('From Ethiopia to the stars', 23 January 2016, p. 27), the Ethiopian director of Ethiopia's Entoto Observatory and Research Center, Solomon Belay Tessema, believed that 'a space programme is not a luxury, but a key to securing food, increasing the productivity of agriculture and developing scientific thinking. Space technology is important for many things: satellites for are used for environmental and water management, soil assessment. We use them for disaster planning to gather meteorological data and to improve communications.'
28 Namrata Goswami, 'China's get-rich space program', *The Diplomat*, 28 February 2019.
29 Ryan Brukardt, Jesse Klempner, Brooke Stokes and Mary Kate Vaughn, *Space around the globe*, McKinsey & Co., 20 April 2022.
30 During this same period, citizens from 41 counties – ranging from Afghanistan to Iran, from South Africa to Mongolia – had travelled to outer space, and of those countries, 11 had their own capacities to send objects into orbit using their own launch vehicles.
31 Morgan Stanley Research expects the global space industry to grow into a $1.1 trillion dollar market by 2040, from about $350 billion in 2016. *Morgan Stanley Research*, 25 October 2022.
32 Op. cit., #26, Hawking.
33 In this context, Christer Fuglesang, a Swedish astronaut, noted in 2021 in an interview, that 'the key space exploration issue we will need to solve by 2050 is how to live outside Earth'. But, in spite of the urgent challenges posed by climate change, the Swedish astronaut did not mean that humans 'will have to leave our own planet behind, but that there will be life on Mars by 2050 and a greater human presence in space generally. By 2050, there will be an established research base on the moon with a permanent population and we'll be able to find resources on the Moon that will help people stay there... . I also think that there will be people living on Mars, perhaps starting some colonies... .' www.saab.com/newsroom/stories/2021/may/what-will-space-exploration-look-like-in-2050
34 'Mars settlement likely by 2050 says expert – but not at levels predicted by Elon Musk', *SciTechDaily*, University of New South Wales, 19 March 2021.
35 Matthew S. Williams, 'Making a greenhouse on another world: Where can we paraterraform in our solar system?' *Interesting Engineering*, April 2019.
36 In addition, steel cables will be held in place by Earth-based cables which will also serve as elevator links that will enable travellers to move to and from the rings in approximately 1 hour. John Grant and Keith Baker, 'How we shall travel the world in 2050, from electric planes to helium airships', *The Independent*, 21 August 2019. John Grant is a Senior Lecturer in natural and built environments at Sheffield Hallam University, and Keith Baker is a Research Associate in sustainable urban environments at Glasgow Caledonian University.

37 Roland Berger, *Urban air mobility; The rise of a new mode of transportation*, 23 November 2018,
www.rolandberger.com/en/Publications/Passenger-drones-ready-for-take-off.html
38 BBC with *Lonely Planet Magazine*, 'What will travel look like in 2050?', 23 April 2013.
39 'Not content to tease us with unreasonable expectations of phasers and warp drive, it also thrust into the popular imagination the idea of teleportation, in which we step into a giant scanner of some sort and instantaneously find ourselves somewhere else, mind, body and soul intact.' Dave Hall, 'Teleportation: Will it ever be a possibility?', *The Guardian*,12 June 2018. The article also notes that 'according to a highly entertaining University of Leicester study into the computing power required to teleport a human being, your cells, broken down into data, equates around 2.6 x 10^{42} bits, which is 2.6 followed by 42 zeroes'.
40 For example, Canadian scientists in 2016 successfully teleported tiny atoms faster than the speed of light. One year later, Chinese scientists reported that they had teleported a photon particle from the ground to a satellite orbiting approximately 870 miles away. To teleport a human being, however, would require 'billions of billions of billions of particles that form a person', explained Professor Sandu Popescu from Bristol University. No one is denying the complexity of the task nor the staggering number of atoms that would be required to teleport a human being – 2.6×10^{42} bits of data in the human body, or 26 followed by 42 zeros.
41 Sajan Sani, 'Will we ever be able to teleport?' TED Talk, 18 July 2017.
42 Brian Sollis, *Lifescale: How to live a more creative, productive, creative, and happy life*, Wiley, 12 April 2019.
43 UNCTAD, *Digital economy report 2021: Cross border data flows and development: For whom the data flows*, p. xv. The report noted that within LDCs, 'There are significant divides between rural and urban areas as well as between men and women.'
44 'Exploring space technologies for sustainable development and the benefits of international research collaboration in this context: Report of the Secretary-General', Commission on Science and Technology for Development, 23rd session, Geneva, 23–27 March 2020
45 *New and emerging technologies are improving humanitarian action*, https://gho.unocha.org/globaltrends/new-ArticleI.and-emerging-technologies-are-improving humanitarian-action
46 The vision as outlined by Facebook's founder is a world in which social media will be able to help people build an inclusive community that reflects collective values and common humanity from local to global levels, spanning cultures, nations and regions in a world with few examples of global communities. Greg Sterling, Mark Zuckerberg's manifesto: How Facebook will connect the world, beat fake news and pop the filter bubble. The CEO describes the next phase of Facebook in a nearly 6,000-word missive, MarketingLand, 20 February 2017.
47 'The Tactile Internet will enable haptic interaction with visual feedback. The term haptic relates to the sense of touch, in particular the perception and manipulation of objects using touch and proprioception. Proprioception is the sense of the relative positioning of the parts of one's body and the strength of effort used in movement.' Sacha Kavanagh and Jon Mundy, 5G Comparison Site, 17 November 2021.
48 'What's after the Internet of Things? The tactile internet!', *World Sensing: Connected Operational Intelligence*, January 2015.

49 Panellria Seoane-Viano, Jun Jie Ong, Abdul W. Basit, Alvaro Goyanes, 'To infinity and beyond: Strategies for fabricating medicines in outer space', *International Journal of Pharmaceutics*, X Volume 4, December 2022.
50 John Bryant, *New technologies are changing humanitarian action, but don't assume their inclusive: Comment*, Overseas Development Institute, 29 November 2019.
51 'Six trends that will shape the future of humanitarian action', https://medium.com/humanitarian dispatches/six-trends-that-twill-shape-the future-of-humanitarian-action-a47d19f6ac61
52 Sylvia Pellegrino, 'The six biggest cyberattacks in history', *TECHMONITOR*, 5 August 2022.
53 Stuart Russell, Professor of Computer Science and founder of the Center for Human-Compatible Artificial Intelligence at the University of California, Berkeley. BBC Reith Lecture, *The biggest event in human history*, 2021.
54 In 2019, the United Nations confirmed that the world's population was growing older due to increasing life expectancy and falling fertility levels, and that the number of countries experiencing a reduction in population size was growing. The new population projections indicate that nine countries will make up more than half the projected growth of the global population between now and 2050: India, Nigeria, Pakistan, the Democratic Republic of the Congo, Ethiopia, the United Republic of Tanzania, Indonesia, Egypt and the United States of America (in descending order of the expected increase). Around 2027, India is projected to overtake China as the world's most populous country. While growth rates will continue to decline by 2050, predictions suggest that world population will continue to grow – arriving at 11 billion by 2100. Department of Economic and Social Affairs, United Nations, *World Population Prospects 2019.*
55 Jennifer Chu, 'Explained: The 1.5 C climate benchmark', *MIT News*, 27 August 2023.
56 The 2016 US National Bioengineered Food Disclosure Law defines 'bioengineered' to mean any food '(a) that contains genetic material that has been modified through in vitro recombinant DNA techniques; and (b) for which the modification could not otherwise be obtained through conventional breeding or not found in nature'.
57 Solein had by 2019 already been selected an incubation project by the European Space Agency.
58 John Cumbers, 'Food from thin air: The forgotten space tech that could feed planet Earth', *Forbes*, 6 March 2020. It is worth noting that the technology used for creating these foods were the result of NASA's initial experiments for feeding astronauts in outer space.
59 'Farming insects: Grub's up', *The Economist*, 6 July 2019, p. 71.
60 Adrian Berry, *The next 500 years: Life in the coming millennium*, Headline Book Publishing, 1996, p. 157.
61 While the degree to which urban farming could significantly reduce the need for rural space is very uncertain, it is worth noting that the US Department of Agriculture had been promoting the idea, and noted in its 2016 Urban Agriculture Toolkit that, 'while a large-scale aquaponic facility located in a warehouse-type building may be a multi-dollar investment, a small aquaponics system housed in a greenhouse could be built for a few thousand dollars, or even less if you are able to use salvaged material.' US Department of Agriculture, *Urban Farming Toolkit*, item #1, 2016.
62 Through the work of the Italian Ocean Reef Group, crops such as strawberries, red cabbage, lettuce, beans and basil emanate from a cluster of balloon-like pods pegged to the seabed by ropes half a dozen or so metres long. Rich McEachran, 'Under the

sea: The underwater farms growing basil, strawberries and lettuce', *The Guardian*, 13 August 2015.

63 3D ocean farming is a system that grows a mix of seaweed crops and shellfish – including mussels and oysters – under the water's surface. This polyculture vertical farming system requires zero input because the sea plants filter and sequester carbon, making it, at this moment, the most sustainable means of food production on the planet.

64 Jeff Greenblatt and Al Anzaldua 'How space technology benefits the Earth', *The Space Review* in association with *Space News*, 29 July 2019.

65 While around half of the world's land currently held around 2 per cent of the planet's population, only about 3 per cent of total land supports more than half of humanity. Rachel Nuwer, In an increasingly crowded world, will we still be able to find respite from one another?, BBC Future, 1 September 2015. And, yet, human use directly affected more than 70 per cent of the global, ice- free land surface. IPCC, Special Report on Climate Change, Desertification, Land Degradation, Sustainable Land Management, Food Security, and Greenhouse gas fluxes in Terrestrial Ecosystems, A1, p. 2, 7 August 2019.

66 United Nations Environment Programme *Spreading like Wildfire – The Rising Threat of Extraordinary Landscape Fires*. A UNEP Rapid Response, 2022.

67 Examples of *megalopolises* are coastal areas in West Africa that began with Abidjan, the economic capital of Ivory Coast, and extends 600 miles east – passing through the countries of Ghana, Togo and Benin – before finally arriving at Lagos in Nigeria. In the United States, the term 'Bowash' reflects a tightly integrated metropolis that extends from Boston, Massachusetts to the nation's capital, Washington, DC; and, already, by 2018, the Chinese government had officially approved nine megalopolises.

68 Global Commission on the Economics of Water, *Turning the tide: A call to collective action*, March 2023.

69 Pew Charitable Trusts, *A map of the future*, 8 February 2022.

70 Pew Charitable Trusts, op. cit., #59, 'We know this thanks to 14 years' worth of satellite data collected by a unique NASA Earth-observing mission called the Gravity Recovery and Climate Experiment—which has the gratifying acronym GRACE. Unlike some satellite missions that rely on images, GRACE, which was launched in 2002 and decommissioned at the end of 2017, was more a "scale in the sky." It measured the very tiny space-time variations in Earth's gravity field, effectively weighing changes in water mass over large river basins and groundwater aquifers—those porous, subterranean rock and soil layers that store water that must be pumped to the surface.'

71 Alec Ross, *The industries of the future: How the next ten years will transform our lives at work and home*, Simon & Schuster, 2016, p. 163.

72 Fog collector panels were mounted on the slopes of the region's Mount Boutmezguida, and these fed into 6,460 square feet of netting and 8 km of pipes and solar water pumps which began to address some of the water woes of at least 400 people. Though only harvesting 6,300 litres of water daily, it was nevertheless a demonstration of yet another way that looming water crises might be offset.

73 The International Water Management Institute therefore recommended that one way of dealing with this was to incentivise farmers to return excess power back to the grid, https://energy.economictimes.indiatimes.com/news/renewable/india-installed-181000-solar-power-pumps-for-irrigation-in-three-years-under-pm-kusum-scheme/73030827?redirect=1

74 In 2021, the Surface Water Ocean Topography mission, a joint satellite mission between Nasa and France, will have used radar technology to provide the first global survey of Earth's water, measuring how bodies of water change over time. The satellite will survey at least 90 per cent of the planet, studying lakes, rivers, reservoirs and oceans roughly twice every 21 days.

75 Dominic Basulto, '6 innovations to cope with the threat of a megadrought', *Washington Post*, 19 February 2015.

76 Aries Keck, NASA Earth Science, 'Evapotranspiration: Watching over water use', 19 August 2021; Anita Gibson, OECD Directorate for Science, Technology and Innovation, E-mail: anita.gibson@oecd.org, August 2020, 'Keeping track of the world's water supplies: satellites contribute to the understanding of the global water cycle and to improved fresh water management. Clouds, water vapours, precipitation and sea-levels are all measured from space, in co- ordination with in-situ systems. Already in many OECD countries, satellite data are used to monitor daily the quality of water bodies, detecting in particular natural and man-made pollutants (e.g. harmful algal blooms, oil spills).' See: http://oe.cd/spaceforum

77 Thomas Sumner, 'New desalination tech could help quench global thirst: Scientists seek cheaper strategies for producing freshwater', *Science News*, 9 August 2016. also see Hilla Shemer, Shlomo Wald and Raphael Semiat, Challenges and Solutions for Global Water Scarcity, National Library of Medicine, June 2023, 13 (6), p. 612. doi: 10.3390/membranes13060612

78 Scott Nyquist, *Energy 2050 from the ground up*, McKinsey & Co., November 2016 mckinsey.com

79 Ibid.

80 Graham Lawton, 'Fire in the hole', *New Scientist*, 261 (3472), 6 January 2024, pp. 33 ff.

81 Javier Garcia Martinez, 'Sun-powered chemistry', *Scientific American*, December 2020.

82 'Space-based solar panels beam unlimited energy to Earth', *Business Insider*, p. 1, http://uk.businessinsider.com/space-based-solar-panels-beam-unlimited-energy-to-earth-2015-9/R=US&IR=T

83 Space Solar Power Project, CalTech spacesolar.caltech.edu

84 'How solar farms in space might beam energy to Earth', World Economic Forum in collaboration with EcoWatch, 9 November 2022.

85 Lyndsey Jones, 'In 2050, will gig economy workers answer to robo-bosses?

Futurologists present their vision of the workplace and how to succeed in it', *Financial Times*, 5 November 2019. This article was a consolidation of views of Jerome Glenn of the Millennium Project, Shivvy Jervis, a UK-based futurologist. Amy Fletcher, associate professor of political science and international relations at Canterbury University in Christchurch, Rob Cross, the Edward A Madden professor of global business at Babson College, Massachusetts, Emily He, senior vice-president of marketing at Oracle, Eli Sutton, vice-president of global operations at Teramind.

86 Charlotte Seager, 'Will jobs exist in 2050?', Guardian Careers, *The Guardian*, 13 October 2016.

87 World Bank, *The changing nature of work*, 2019.

88 Keith Dear and Ali Hossaini, The AI Special Issue, *RUSI Journal*, 164 (5/6), July/August 2019. See also, Beazley, *Risk and resilience: Spotlight on technology risk*, 21 September 2021.

89 According to Daron Acemoglu in 'Technical change, inequality and the labour market', *Journal of Economic Literature* 40 (1), 2002 as referenced by Daniel Susskind, *A world without work: Technology, automation and how we should respond*, Metropolitan

Books, 2020, p. 34, 'When the industrial Revolution got underway in Britain, new machines were introduced to the workplace, new production processes were set up, and so new tasks had to be done. But it turned out that those without the skills of the day were often placed to perform these tasks. Technology, rather than being skill-biased, was "unskilled-biased" instead.'

90 Carl Benedikt Frey and Michael A. Osborne, *The future of employment: How susceptible are jobs to computerisation*, oxfordmartin.ox.uk, 17 September 2013.

91 Carl Benedikt Frey's comments at the Deloitte-Guardian Newspaper roundtable on the Future of Work, 13 October 2016.

92 Carlos Eduardo Barbosa et al., *Working in 2050: A view of how changes on the work will affect society*, December 2017, 10.13140/RG 2.217314.0736.

93 Ibid.

Bibliography

Acemoglu, Daron, 'Technical change, inequality and the labour market', *Journal of Economic Literature* 40 (1), 2002.

Barbosa, Carlos Eduardo, Lima, Y., Souza, J., Santos, E., Costa, L., Carmo, A. and Kritz, J., 'Working in 2050: A view of how changes on the work will affect society', *European Journal of Futures Research,* December 2017, 10.13140/RG 2.217314.0736.

Berger, Roland, *Urban air mobility; The rise of a new mode of transportation*, 23 November 2018, www.rolandberger.com/en/Publications/Passenger-drones-ready-for-take-off.html

Berry, Adrian, *The next 500 years: Life in the coming millennium*, Headline Book Publishing, 1996.

Brukardt, Ryan, Klempner, Stokes, Jesse Brooke, and Vaughn, Mary Kate, *Space around the globe,* McKinsey & Co., 20 April 2022.

Bryant, John, *New technologies are changing humanitarian action, but don't assume their inclusive: Comment*, Overseas Development Institute, 29 November 2019.

Clark, Stuart, 'Alien skies', *New Scientist*, 12 November 2022.

Cumbers, John, 'Food from thin air: The forgotten space tech that could feed planet Earth', *Forbes*, 6 March 2020.

Dear, Keith and Hossaini, Ali, The AI Special Issue, *RUSI Journal*, 164 (5/6), July/August 2019.

Frey, Carl Benedikt and Osborne, Michael A., *The future of employment: How susceptible are jobs to computerisation*, oxfordmartin.ox.uk, 17 September 2013.

Global Commission on the Economics of Water, *Turning the tide: A call to collective action*, March 2023.

Goertzel, Ben and Pennachin, Cassio (Eds), *Artificial general intelligence*, Springer-Verlag Berlin Heidelberg, 2007.

Goswami, Namrata, 'China's get-rich space program', *The Diplomat*, February 28, 2019.

Greenblatt, Jeff and Anzaldua, Al, 'How space technology benefits the Earth', *The Space Review* in association with Space News, 29 July 2019.

Hamzelou, Jessica, '$100 million project to make intelligence-boosting brain implant', *New Scientist*, 20 October 2016.

Hawking, Stephen, *Brief answers to the big questions*, John Murray Publishers, 2018.

Hayles, N. Katherine, *How we became posthuman: Virtual bodies in cybernetics, literature and Informatics*, University of Chicago Press, 1999.

IPCC, *Special report on climate change, desertification, land degradation, sustainable land management, food security, and greenhouse gas fluxes in terrestrial ecosystems*, A1, August 2019.

Jones, Lyndsey, 'In 2050, will gig economy workers answer to robo-bosses? Futurologists present their vision of the workplace and how to succeed in it', *Financial Times*, 5 November 2019.

Kavanagh, Sacha and Mundy, Jon, *5G Comparison Site,* 17 November 2021.

Keck, Aries, NASA Earth Science, 'Evapotranspiration: Watching over water use', 19 August 2021. www.nasa.gov › missions › landsat › evapotranspiration

Kirkton, R. D., 'A bioengineered blood vessel' *Science Translational Medicine* (2019), 27 March 2019.

Kurzweil, Ray, *The singularity is near: When humans transcend biology*, Viking, 2005.

Lawton, Graham, 'Fire in the hole', *New Scientist*, 261 (3472), 6 January 2024.

LePage, Michael, 'The ethics issue: Should we edit our children's genomes?', *New Scientist,* 5 July 2017. www.newscientist.com/article/mg23531330-700-the-ethics-issue-should-we-edit-our-childrens-genomes/#ixzz5wIlLPdni

Loeb, Avi, *Extraterrestrial: The first sign of intelligent life beyond earth*, Houghton Mifflin Harcourt, 2021.

Lovelock, James, *Novacene: The coming age of hyperintelligence*, Penguin/Random House UK, 2019.

McEachran, Rich, 'Under the sea: The underwater farms growing basil, strawberries and lettuce', *The Guardian,* 13 August 2015.

Marchant, Jo, 'Evolution machine: Genetic engineering on fast forward', *New Scientist*, 22 June 2011.

Martinez, Javier Garcia, 'Sun-powered chemistry,' *Scientific American*, December 2020.

Ministry of Defence, *Global strategic trends: The future starts today*, Sixth Edition, 2018.

Nuwer, Rachel, *In an increasingly crowded world, will we still be able to find respite from one another?*, BBC Future, 1 September 2015.

Nyquist, Scott, *Energy 2050 from the ground up,* McKinsey & Co., November 2016. mckinsey.com

Office of the Director of National Intelligence, *Global trends*, www.dni.gov/index.php/gt2040-home/summary

Pass, Jim, 'Astrosociology on Mars', in Giuseppe Pezzella (Ed.) *Mars exploration: A step*, Interchange Publisher, 2020 [Available in the Virtual Library at https://lnkd.in/gY2eA5j].

Pellegrino, Sylvia, 'The six biggest cyberattacks in history', *TECHMONITOR*, 5 August 2022.

Pew Charitable Trusts, *A map of the future*, 8 February 2022.

Rees, Martin, *On the future: Prospects for humanity*, Princeton Press, 2018.

Ross, Alec, *The industries of the future: How the next ten years will transform our lives at work and home*, Simon & Schuster, 2016.

Seager, Charlotte, 'Will jobs exist in 2050?', *Guardian Careers, The Guardian,* 13 October 2016.

Seoane-Viano, Panellria, Jun Jie Ong, Basit, Abdul W., and Goyanes, Alvaro, 'To infinity and beyond: Strategies for fabricating medicines in outer space', *International Journal of Pharmaceutics,* X Volume 4, December 2022.

Shemer, Hilla, Wald, Shlomo and Semiat, Raphael, 'Challenges and solutions for global water scarcity', *National Library of Medicine*, 13 (6), 612, June 2023. doi: 10.3390/membranes13060612

Sollis, Brian, *Lifescale: How to live a more creative, productive, creative, and happy life*, Wiley, 12 April 2019.

Sumner, Thomas, 'New desalination tech could help quench global thirst: Scientists seek cheaper strategies for producing freshwater', *Science News,* 9 August 2016.

Susskind, Daniel, *A world without work: Technology, automation and how we should respond*, Metropolitan Books, 2020.

Travino, Marty, 'Cyber physical systems: The coming singularity,' *Prism,* National Defense University, 8 (3), 2019.

United Nations Department of Economic and Social Affairs, *World population prospects,* 2019.

United Nations Environment Programme *Spreading like wildfire: The rising threat of extra-ordinary landscape fires*, A UNEP Rapid Response, 2022.

United Nations Report of the Secretary-General, Commission on Science and Technology for Development, 23rd session, Geneva, 23–27 March 2020.

US Department of Agriculture, *Urban farming toolkit*, item #1, 2016.

Von Hippel, Frank A., *The chemical age: How chemists fought famines and disease, killed millions and changed our relationship with earth*, University of Chicago Press, 2020.

Webb, V. and Hessel, Andrew, *The genesis machine: Our quest to rewrite life in the age of synthetic biology*, Public Affairs, Hatchett Book Group, Inc., Kindle Edition, 2022.

Williams, Matthew S., 'Making a greenhouse on another world: Where can we paraterraform in our solar system?' *Interesting Engineering*, April 2019.

World Bank, *The changing nature of work [World Development Report 2019: The Changing Nature of Work],* World Bank, 2019. doi:10.1596/978-1-4648-1328-3. License: Creative Commons Attribution CC BY 3.0 IGO

World Economic Forum in collaboration with EcoWatch, 'How solar farms in space might beam energy to Earth', 9 November 2022.

3 Governance and Resource Prioritisation

From a Futures Perspective

Amid fears that we were witnessing the creation of a caste system based on genetic differences, the Gene Equality Project (GEP) was a philanthropic effort to bring cognitive enhancements to low-income communities. In May 2059 the results of the project were made public.

According to the New York Times, *the results were largely disappointing. The intentions of the GEP were good and therapeutic interventions well intentioned. It had begun 25 years ago, and enabled 500 pairs of low-income parents to increase the intelligence of their children through a common cognitive-enhancement protocol involving modifications to 80 genes associated with intelligence. Each individual modification had only a small effect on intelligence, but in combination they typically gave a child an IQ of 130, putting the child in the top 5 per cent of the population.*

This GEP has been one of the most popular enhancements generally purchased by affluent parents, and is often referenced in media profiles of the 'New Elite', the genetically engineered young people who are increasingly prevalent in management positions of corporate America today. Yet, the 500 subjects who came from lower-income families are not enjoying career success that is remotely comparable to the success of the New Elite, despite having received the same protocol. The fact of the matter is that those subjects of the GEP experiment could not rise above their social status.[1]

The Boundaries of Governance and the Dynamics of Resource Distribution

The implications of that 2059 *Gene Equality Experiment* reflect the sorts of changes in both human agency and human space discussed in the previous chapter. Beyond the upsides and downsides of transformative biotechnologies, the experiment raised issues, for example, about who permitted and controlled the development of such innovations, and who sanctioned their use and for what purposes? To what extent did they reflect a more global trend, and, if so, were they more positive than negative disrupters? Was the social status reflected in the GEP ultimately fixed

DOI: 10.4324/9781003471004-4

and enduring, or could it have eventually resulted in a more fluid pattern of societal behaviour, or, indeed ultimately, greater cross-societal equality?

These questions in turn open the way for issues about the nature of governance and resource distribution more generally – so important for identifying plausible types of vulnerabilities and ultimately possible types of humanitarian crisis threats.

When it comes to governance, what could be the dominant construct in a generation's time? Will it be 'the state', and what would determine state authority and its enforcement capacities? Will the state be geopolitically defined or perhaps more virtual than geographical? Will its boundaries include outer space, and how might such boundaries be defined? If the state should prove to be merely part of more dispersed governance structures, what else might be relevant components and how would they interact, with whom, how and from where?

And, reflecting back on the assumptions that had underpinned the Gene Equality Project, who were to be the policy planners and decision-makers? Were they those that had enhanced intellectual – perhaps cyborg-like – capacities, or did they reflect a new societal norm based upon equal access to all human-enhancing benefits? And, how were societal resources identified and distributed and by whom?

Once again, it should be borne in mind that the questions and answers posited in this chapter are by no means about predictions. Rather, they are about portraits of a future intended to pose another question to the reader: what would be required to anticipate and adapt to complexities which hitherto have few precedence? What would the answer be?

Evolving Governance Constructs

Consistent with the 'normal life proposition', risks, crises and response are determined in very fundamental ways by the dynamics of governance. Even in the mayhem of anarchy there are assumptions about the ways that humans have and will organise their lives and respond or not to perceived authority. Those assumptions have varying degrees of historical precedence. Yet, the extent to which the past will provide adequate insights into the future of such constructs or whether in the future they might be determined by different paradigmatic assumptions is a fundamental issue when it comes to *planning from the future*.

Governance Paradigms in an Historical Context

The renowned political scientist, Samuel P. Huntington, once noted that civilisations evolve: 'They are dynamic; they rise and fall; they merge and divide; and as any student of history knows, they also disappear and are buried in the sands of time.'[2]

That insight certainly pertains to assumptions about the nature of governance. The vast majority of the governed consciously or unconsciously make or accept certain assumptions about the types of systems and their allocative authority when it comes to the paradigms that underpin governance constructs. They may dislike the ways that such constructs are organised and manipulated, the ways that their boundaries and powers are determined and asserted and ultimately may revolt against them. And, yet, those in each historic period consciously or unconsciously reflect an intersubjective consensus based upon concepts, values and practices that constitute a way of viewing a reality – a paradigm – until it also is buried in the sands of time.

Paradigmatic assumptions about the nature of governance may change dramatically though by no means consistently. Loose knit clanic communities, Italian city states, fluctuating types of empires, nation states – authoritarian, democratic, all suggest that the underpinnings of governance have taken different forms over millennia but not necessarily in a pattern that was consistent, let alone consistently progressive. Over the course of human history, there has been no consistent pattern, and each reflected ways that authority was accepted and that resources were obtained and distributed.

The architecture of governance only changes when existing paradigms are so profoundly challenged by fundamental transformations, including technological transformations, that governance systems lose their relevance. 'Ideas and technology move from civilisation to civilisation, but it often [takes] centuries.'[3]

In 1452, for example, the printing press that resulted in the Guttenberg Bible challenged the Catholic Church's monopoly over biblical interpretation, and eventually led to the breakup of the Catholic church's control over much of Europe, including England. Final authority in doctrinal and legal disputes rested no longer with a universal pope but now with a growing number of monarchs free from the dictates of Rome, as evidenced by the Peace of Westphalia over two hundred years later.[4]

That said, though governance architecture and government systems change over time, they do not necessarily do so in positive or progressive ways. Rather they reflect random and normally unanticipated change where values are unpredictable and patterns of behaviour equally so. The evolution of the Roman Empire suggests the paradigmatic consequences of slow, transformative change:

> A Rome at peace could still offer wealth to its people. But the wealth that was generated by peace was no longer in the gift of the ruler but the result of the trade that flourished in peacetime, created by multiple transactions between thousands of people. Divinity maintained the emperor's position as the source of blessings. But trade provided an alternative source of good fortune and would eventually kill off emperor worship by creating the conditions for a new all-encompassing religion.[5]

Alternatively, transformative consequences of 1421 – the year that China's vast armada discovered the world – points to a governance change that was quick and paradigm shifting. So, it has been suggested, had China's Imperial government continued to establish permanent colonies in Africa, the Americas and Australia, China's approach to governance would have witnessed a radical departure from its isolationist empire. Had the armada not been ordered to return to port, 'Would New York have become the New Beijing?' However, lightning struck the Forbidden City that same year, and therefore

> … had fire not roared down the Imperial Way and turned the Emperor's palaces and throne to cinders. Would the Emperor have kept his nerve? …Would he have ordered Admiral Zeng He's squadrons to continue their voyages…Would Buddhism rather than Christianity have become the religion of the New World? Instead of the cultured Chinese, instructed to 'treat distant people with kindness, it was the cruel, almost barbaric Christians who were the colonisers.[6]

Disintegration, Fragmentation and Reconfiguration

All governance constructs go through patterns of disintegration, fragmentation and reconfiguration. Increasingly, as one approaches the mid-21st century, the impact of *informatised* technology will add exponential speed to that process, simultaneously enhancing and disrupting the fabric of life in every society. The slow-motion collapse of parts of the 20th century's legacy may well have accelerated by the 2050s, resulting in monumental realignments of societal institutions, the nature of resources, methods of production and business and certainly fundamental ideas about national security.[7] And, in the words of a cognitive analyst,

> … the pre-informatized infrastructure has been destroyed, but societal processes—especially those of government, defense, and the law—are still those of the pre-informatized world, a world that is rapidly going out of existence. The world is using digitized, sharable information, transitioning from one-way, single-supplier siloed, one-function stovepipes to interactive ecosystems where software is orchestrating the movement of goods and services, the making of decisions, and impacting the way humans live. In just one generation, every industry has come to depend on interactive real-time decision-making.[8]

In 2016, PWC – one of the world's largest management consultancies – made forecasts about the growth of the global economy and those states that would take the lead in such growth. By 2050, according to PWC, it was more than likely that the world economy will have more than doubled in size, far outstripping population growth due to continued technology-driven productivity arrangements.[9] That growth would be measured based on the economies of conventional, boundary-determined states.

It was anticipated then that six of the seven largest economies in the world would be led by China, then India and Indonesia, and it was likely that the US could be down to third place, and that states such as Nigeria, Vietnam and the Philippines as well as many more economically emerging states would rapidly climb the GDP ladder.

Whether or not that prediction will prove to be accurate, it is worth noting that the focus of the analysis was on 'the state' and that the underpinning assumption was that state-based 'gross domestic product' would be the basic criterion for determining wealth. Of course, that assumes that states will be the main global actors in a generation's time, and that they will maintain that role through a plethora of institutional mechanisms over which in the final analysis they would have control.

However, as one looks to the future, it can be argued that the very definition and construct of 'the state' will change in ways too rarely anticipated. Closely linked to that proposition is that multilateralism, for all its strengths and weaknesses will no longer remain the global paradigm which explains the dynamics of what is normally referred to as 'the international system'.

The durability of the state as concept and reality may be challenged along several lines. As regards the latter, it is very possible that a number of states may have already disintegrated by 2050. Their authority may no longer exist, and a sense of citizenship could disappear, replaced by non-state societal linkages ranging from private companies on some distant planet to virtual communities, to clanic and religious links. In the case of Africa, it is quite plausible that some states based on outdated treaties or 'maps of widely varying quality'[10] would fragment into loosely defined sub-states. Similarly, certain states in Central Asia might also begin to collapse as early as the 2030s, and conventional authority replaced by a combination of clanic and local governance systems.[11] Functional linkages could bring those who had once been deemed to be 'local authorities' into 'cross boundary relationships' which could bring the interests of the private sector, transport, water sources and regional threats into an essentially political network based upon common interests.

In a related vein, there, too, might be active adjustments to various state boundaries which certainly had generally been presumed to be immutable. Several states, for example, in the United States, including California, Oregon and Wyoming, could become – despite considerable federal resistance – far more *confederal* than the US constitution had anticipated. One state, namely, Washington, with more than 13 land border crossings into British Columbia, could well merge with its neighbour. In Europe, the impetus for fragmentation has a long history, and one can foresee that by mid-century more than 1/3rd of EU member states might have witnessed fundamental transformations, including the United Kingdom (i.e. Scotland and Northern Ireland), Spain (i.e. Catalonia) and Eastern Europe's so-called 'authoritarian belt', which includes Poland.[12]

The sorts of disintegration and fragmentation of various states that could occur over a thirty years period clearly have antecedents. As in the past, so, too, now and in the future, the fluctuating patterns of state development, disintegration, fragmentation and reconfiguration might well reflect changing types and dynamics of societal interests, in various ways influenced by technological transformations.

The Evolving Nature of State: From Geographical Boundaries to Virtual

Five hundred years after the Peace of Westphalia, the concept and practical implications of fixed state boundaries might well have evolved in very fundamental ways as will those responsible for guiding governmental processes. The assumption that fixed boundaries, defined populations, ultimate control over assets and currencies are all fundamental characteristics of the state could have been challenged in various ways by 2050. It could well be that the state by then would have increasingly fluid boundaries and state responsibilities for its citizens and resources could have transcended the sorts of geopolitical boundaries assumed for centuries and more often than not may become more virtual.

At the same time, city-to-city collaboration, extra-terrestrial communities, AGI-guided social networks, global corporations based on Earth and beyond and issue-focused coalitions suggest the sorts of actors that not only could impact governance but also determine its construct and direction. To sustain some sort of authority and control, the state may have to be increasingly fluid and dependent upon technology-driven capacities to achieve basic control, prioritisation processes and resource collection and distribution.

If states might often trail behind the contending interests of a burgeoning number of non-state actors that were truly 'multinational' and social networks that were truly global, then governance would increasingly transcend geopolitical boundaries, even to deal with so-called, 'domestic responsibilities'. More and more boundaries could well be determined by those states 'that go virtual' – where authority, influence and responsibilities were framed by AGI and less and less by physical capacities.

Those virtual states can be described in various ways. A virtual nation, a micronation, a bitnation, are all terms that suggest entities that could be capable of sustaining to varying degrees their monopoly of power. That monopoly, though quite likely in decline, might reflect an *informatised* world and all-pervasive data flows might have become major factors determining governance between habitats in outer space and certainly between Earth and those habitats.

That is not to suggest that in outer space, as on Earth, engagement between humans would not be possible, but rather, like those state and non-state actors of which in various ways they might be a part, it, too, could also be virtual.

Box 3.1 Emerging Virtual States

Estonia, one of the smallest states on planet Earth, had by 2015 already become a well-recognised example of an increasing digitally-based virtual state. That year the government had introduced an 'e-Residency' which allowed anyone anywhere in the world to receive a government-issued digital identity. This identity gave people access to digital public services and the ability to register and run online businesses from other countries in exactly the same way as someone born in Estonia. As of November 2017, over 27,000 people had applied to be Estonian e-Residents, and had established over 4,200 companies. By 2025, the government aimed to have somewhere in the region of 10 million Estonians with digital identities.[13]

Less than a decade later, at the 2022 United Nations Climate Change Conference (COP27)min Egypt, Tuvalu's foreign affairs minister, Simon Kofe said,

> *Our land, our ocean, our culture are the most precious assets of our people and to keep them safe from harm, no matter what happens in*

> *the physical world, we will move them to the cloud...Islets like this one won't survive rapid temperature increases, rising sea levels, and drought, so we'll re-create them virtually. Piece by piece, we'll preserve our country, provide solace to our people, and remind our children and our grandchildren what our home once was.*

These examples reflected at the time the inclinations of small nation-states. However, they were increasingly indicative of a more global propensity to go 'virtual' due to growing distrust of the nation-state, regional alliances and intergovernmental bodies.

What was being increasingly recognised was that a virtual state would enable people with shared values to create a digital territory, likely in the metaverse, with its own decentralised governance, powered by blockchain. 'It would resemble a cross between a social network and an "invisible" country layered over our reality. It would be populated by global citizens drawn together across borders by common values and common purpose, and who use the cloud and its technologies to work, rest and play.'[14]

Global Architecture and the Entanglement Nexus

'In less than a generation', noted the former US presidential advisor and Nobel Prize winner, Henry Kissinger,

> the most successful network platforms have brought together user bases larger than the populations of most nations and even some continents. However, large user populations gathered on popular network platforms have more diffuse borders than those of political geography, and network platforms are operated by parties with interests that may differ from those of a nation.[15]

As in the past, so, too, in the future, patterns of governance will reflect the ebbs and flows of contending and common interests and varying types and levels of interconnectedness. Fluctuating patterns of governance will depend more and more upon who controls and over what, and that does not mean that state and its presumed monopoly of power – whether virtual or physical – would automatically hold sway.

In the aftermath of a growing number of state failures in the early years of the 21st century there has been a growing consensus that the 'overloaded state' may lack the capacities for dealing with complex problems.[16]

> Institutions that were designed for one set of problems in another era are now being tasked to come up with solutions to quite different challenges in a different context. Social security systems designed 60 years ago are coping with the rise of flexible, independent work and the gig economy; mental health services designed for a small minority of the population are dealing with widespread anxiety and depression amongst young people.[17]

Even in some of the richest states in the world there are signs that opaque, drawn-out processes combined with contending bureaucratic interests all too often reflect and will increasingly reflect pervasive dysfunctionalities.[18] And, many analysts and practitioners who still regard the state and its multilateral construct as central to global governance, nevertheless recognise that the state and its components need to be more adaptive and agile, 'refreshed'.

As one observer noted when reviewing the US government's 2040 futures report, it had been accepted that there would emerge a coming shortfall in the US's ability to keep up with infrastructural demands. That shortfall, for example, might possibly result in a 'sharing economy' in which business empires would successfully run themselves with little government intervention, and blockchains will have allowed everyone to just get on with their lives without being mired in endless government bureaucracy.[19]

A growing number of critics, too, point to state-based multilateral systems such as the UN as 'constitutionally unfit'. Examples of its failures, so it is asserted, are many. The consequences of unregulated transnational capitalism and related financial flows, radicalised nonstate armed actors, the proliferation of nuclear, biological and autonomous weapons, the seemingly ceaseless flows of displaced peoples across borders, the relatively ineffective handling of the 2020 Covid-19 pandemic and the Palestinian and Ukraine crises and persistent failures to gain operational consensus to deal with climate change and biodiversity are just some of the criticisms launched at the UN, and which underscore growing uncertainties about the capacities of state-based multilateral systems to handle ever more complex threats.[20]

Even the United Nations Secretary General had acknowledged in 2021 that the UN was at an inflection point in history. 'The choices we make, or fail to make, today could result in further breakdown, or a breakthrough to a greener, better, safer future.'[21] Towards that end, he proposed that the conventional multilateral system would have to change. States alone could not determine the direction of the United Nations, and its constituency would have to expand. The sciences, the private sector and communities should come together at the policymaking table. Ironically, however, the greater the UN's institutional and sectoral diversity, the less able it might be to generate consensus on many issues of global consequence.

Emerging out of these uncertainties is a plethora of theories that attempt to capture what appears to be an evolving global governance architecture. States' monopoly of power, however, still remain the abiding paradigm for most analysts for understanding global governance. It is the state, so many argue, that determines not only governance at a national level, but also at intergovernmental and ultimately non-governmental levels as well.

At the same time, there is a growing contingent who believe that the failings of multilateralism has to be recognised and accepted. Instruments influencing global governance increasingly depend less upon global consensus but rather upon *minilateralism*. All too often what some suggest is that small groupings of states, reflecting 'coalitions of the willing' – *minilateralism* – will increasingly bypass intergovernmental institutions and focus on specific issues or engage within a defined geographic region to achieve a specific objective or set of objectives.[22] This does not foretell an end to multilateralism, but rather the perceived reality that states will continue to dominate but less and less through intergovernmental institutions and less and less on a global scale.

That last premise also feeds into what might be a more dystopic view of an emerging global architecture, namely, *atomisation.* Essentially, in a world reflecting ever increasing complexities and exponentially increasing numbers of actors – a substantial number based upon AGI and network defined 'borders' – atomisation again put into question states' supposed monopoly of power. 'Was the world becoming so fragmented,' ask analysts, 'that there were few consistent patterns of behaviour?'

To what extent might the consequences of state and non-state based cyber weapons, blockchain and cyber economies, private sector interests in outer space, exponentially increasing numbers of social networks and growing numbers of settlements on planets beyond Earth be just a few factors to suggest that there will be no overarching system of control, that the architecture of future governance – even more than minilateralism – could be issue-dependent and with no consistent pattern of behaviour. Randomness and fluctuating capacities to assert authority also could be a relevant governance scenario.

On the other hand, the concept of *polylateralism* has at the same time increasingly been heralded as the best way to understand the nature and dynamics of global governance. As opposed to atomisation, analysts feel that polylateralism reflects a global architecture that, like the atomised model, was replete with different types of actors, but was more predictable and less fragmented.[23]

Rather, they foresee that agents of global civil society and subnational governments will be taking up the slack of faltering states.[24] Its proponents, in other words, do not assume that polylateralism suggests the imminent decline of the state, *per se*. However, they assume that polylateralism reflects a more 'distributed form of governance in which diverse constituencies from across the world with common interests and values (could) act effectively alongside creaking sovereignty.'[25] [26]

As one looks to the mid-21st century, an emerging reality could well be that the governance paradigm would be neither one nor the other, neither multilateral, minilateral, atomised or polylateral. Instead, the governance paradigm in a futures context might be based on 'virtual flows', where virtual interconnectedness would normally override conventional structural boundaries of any single or multiple set of fixed actors, e.g. multilateral organisations.

Contending or perceived mutual interests would determine types of interconnections and transactions, and these would reflect cohorts of interests that were increasingly identified and facilitated by AGI. It, too, could be quite possible that the highly regarded anticipatory and decision-making capacities of AGI could well intensify competing interests among such cohorts – on planet Earth and beyond.

Governance and the Dynamics of Decision-Making

In December 2021, 193 countries signed a UNESCO agreement on AI ethics, perceived to help make that technology 'fairer for everyone'.[27] Two years later, that commitment resulted in a series of high level international initiatives, including the UN, OECD, the EU and various governments including China, India, the United Kingdom and the United States.

Yet, whatever their ambitions and visions, it could be very possible that the forecast of one astute observer even before the UNESCO initiative could prove to be a crystallising example of the incongruity between traditional governance and the digital space that would determine decision-making:

> although in principle most network platforms are content-agnostic, in some situations their community standards become as influential as national laws. Content that a network platform and its AI permit or favor may rapidly gain prominence; content they diminish or sometimes even outright prohibit may be relegated to obscurity.[28]

The sheer volume of communication and data flows across borders suggests that what would be governable and who would be making decisions may no longer be dominated by conventional human planning and decision-making processes. Already by the 2020s the difficulties of controlling intrusive communications resulting in cybercrimes and cyber threats to security were obvious. Growing numbers of incidents in conflict situations, for example, demonstrated that life threatening decisions were by no means left solely to human calculations.

Box 3.2 And, Yet, Whose Decision?...

On 5 March 2016, 21 family members sat down to dinner in West Mosul, Iraq. None of them knew that at that moment, their neighbourhood was in the cross hairs of an American Unmanned Combat Ariel Vehicle (UCAV) – also known as drones. According to a *New York Times* investigation in December 2021, "The U.S. airstrike killed them all." This was early evidence that such drones had and increasingly will have had capacities to identify and destroy targets without any human intervention. No longer could one presume that drones were always controlled by 'pilots in cockpits' thousands of miles away. Artificial intelligence had made it possible for killer drones not to be dependent upon human control.[29]

This burgeoning prospect would not be new. As far back as 1951, suggested Stuart Russell, an eminent professor of Artificial Intelligence, 'When Alan Turing warned that once the machine thinking method had started, it would not take long to outstrip our feeble powers. At some stage therefore we should have to expect the machines to take control.'[30] As Russell subsequently mentioned,

> ...a few of the reasons the various "sceptics" have given for paying no attention. One I didn't mention is perhaps the worst excuse of all: some AI

> researchers – after 70 years of insisting to the naysayers that AI is possible – are now saying there's no need to worry because we won't actually achieve general-purpose AI. This is like the bus driver speeding towards the cliff edge saying, "Don't worry, we'll run out of petrol before we get there." This is no way to manage the affairs of the human race. [31]

This is not to suggest that the impacts that AGI will have on decision-making will be inherently negative. To the contrary, more and more cohorts – consisting of varying combinations of state, urban, private sector, individuals, networks, etc. – will have benefitted from *informatised* worlds.

Thanks to AGI, innovations such as tactile communications and advancements in the *metaverse* will most likely have begun to create a sense of greater virtual proximity between the individual and policy planners and decision-makers. Greater integrated data might result in more holistic analyses of decisional options and opportunities, and also play a significant role in identifying appropriate levels of decision-making. In many ways, the result could well be that organisational constructs would become flatter, freer flowing and more sensitive.

One way or another, AGI could evolve to become be an intellect that far exceeded the 'cognitive performance of humans in virtually all domains of interest'.[32] AGI might well lead to unprecedented control over decision-making and decision-makers in whatever cohort, organisation, or sector. Indeed, the sorts of decision-making assumed in the 2020s might find itself increasingly in contention with the artificial.

Of course, governments in particular had already been wary of the possible governance implications of artificial intelligence by the mid-2020s and indeed well before. They believed, though, that they could control its growing spectrum of interventions; they could guide its use and would be willing to support its development and eventually benefit from its creation.

An added complication could be that the holistic and integrated nature of AGI outputs might not necessarily encompass or incorporate those of other systems. Indeed, many systems at government levels, the private sectors and a variety of networks and so on may discover that the findings and solutions that were provided to decision-makers and planners frequently went against or contradicted the findings of other systems.

Systems of governance could well continue to reflect tensions between the human being, in this case those who had governance responsibilities, and technology. What one might eventually witness could be growing though periodic dominance of the latter over the former. And, what might have begun to emerge was 'a post-bureaucratic world' in which hierarchies would be replaced by networked systems ('netcentric') over which a whole new concept of leadership appeared, 'one that is more complex than putting people first'.[33]

This certainly might be the case on Earth and perhaps even more so in outer space, where it is clearly more likely that there would be greater dependence upon 'machines' and cyborg-equipped humans.

Yet, even in an emerging post-bureaucratic world, profound uncertainties about the respective roles of humans – who ostensibly still were the presumed planners and decision-makers – and supposedly supportive automated systems would most likely continue. The twists and turns of debates over such uncertainties that might take place in the 2050s most likely would have been recognised by similar debates 30 years before.

The prospect that artificial intelligence systems, which once had been aligned with their creators, might destabilise governance and resource allocation processes in a destructive way could clearly be one consistent theme.[34] That technology would steal a march, for example, on politics was another. And, what, for example, in 2015 was 'hardly a blip on the current political radar' might eventually become an abiding concern that artificial intelligence and biotechnology could soon overhaul societies and economies – and bodies and minds, too – fundamentally.[35]

From a governance perspective, such debates would most probably also be reflected in the practical day-to-day issues concerning ways that resources for societies as a whole would be identified and distributed. As in the past, so, too, in the future, those ways would determine the nature of humanitarian crises, their dimensions and dynamics.

The Resource Distribution Process in a 2050 Context

There were those who saw that the state construct in the 21st century was faced with 'the crisis of supplying a civilization on a dying planet'.[36] That proposition, however, depended upon the assumptions made about what would be required to sustain that civilisation, or what Chapter 2 referred to as 'human agency' on Earth and beyond. It, too, reflected possible ebbs and flows of shifting governance paradigms. From multilateral and minilateral to atomised and polylateral to cohorts based on virtual flows, ownership, control and distribution of resources would ultimately reflect a particular global architecture at a particular point in time.

Whether or not the world will have to contend with a global supply crisis, it would be more than likely that transformations in emerging governance structures will inevitably impact upon the nature of resources and supply chains and vice versa. It could well be the case that as mid-century approached, uncertainties would increase about who owned and controlled such resources and how they were distributed. And, here, the key issue for those who would have humanitarian roles and responsibilities would concern the extent to which ownership and control reduced or intensified disparities, and, hence, societal vulnerabilities.

The Nature of Resources

The concept of resources and the term, itself, have many interpretations. There are those who feel that when it comes to human vulnerability, there are *scarce* resources and *essential* resources. The former includes basic needs for human survival, including drinking water, food and shelter; the latter are indispensable for minimum existence in a given society, and traditionally has included such things as land, sources of energy and security. There, too, are resources that determine the very nature of society and those that affect societal constructs. The first includes such things as belief systems and forms of engagement, while the second reflects allocation, prioritisation and participation processes. Arguably they are all distinct, but on the other hand they are closely interrelated and intertwined.

Perhaps an emerging difference in that proposition could be that the types of resources and their sources in each category and collectively will have changed significantly between the beginning of the century and its mid-way point. Earlier some experts had forecast that with a global population that would be 28 per cent larger in 2050 than in the second decade of the century, 71 per cent more resources per capita would be used unless the global use of metals, biomass, and minerals were used more efficiently.[37]

However, reflecting on foreseeable changes in the nature of human agency, as discussed in the previous chapter, it could well be that food and food production will have changed significantly as could the sources and purification of water and types and availability of energy. Shelter may have been increasingly available due, for example, to more sea and outer space-based as well as sub-terranean housing. And, as for those resources that will inevitably be essential for societal constructs, transformative technologies will more than likely be of fundamental importance.

As for resources, themselves, all in various ways may depend upon new or previously little used materials. Perhaps from planetary and interplanetary perspectives, the changes in energy sources could have greatest impact. By 2050, a combination of nuclear fusion and space-based solar power could quite possibly provide energy across virtually all human habitats at all times. Both would require high levels of maintenance and complex resources. Nuclear fusion would rely upon helium-3, abundant in outer space, and space-based solar power arrays would require regular inspections and, when necessary, expensive repairs of the panels and the microwave transmitters that brought space-based energy to Earth or indeed to other human habitats.

The provision of essential materials such as calcium and magnesium to provide desalinated water and the use of minerals such as graphite, lithium and cobalt to meet the growing demand for clean energy technologies have been forecast to increase by nearly 500 per cent by 2050.[38] Energy transitions in turn will have had to significantly increase demands for metals such as copper, nickel, cobalt and lithium, all essential for the production of renewable power generation capacities.

Clearly, means of production are themselves 'resources' as well as outputs. For that reason, robotics and AGI will most likely be deemed to be a resource of ever-growing importance and the ways that they could affect the nature of time and human agency more generally would inevitably reflect a transformative and ever more fundamental resource when it came to determining societal constructs.

That the types of resources and access to them will have increased by mid-century would seem quite likely. In so many ways, their impacts would be intricately linked to societal transformations across the globe and beyond; and, by 2050, access to them may well be less Earth dependent. Some may be more virtual than conventionally tangible, and some such as AGI may well have escaped the control of human distributors.

Owners and Occupiers

In 2015, an obscure law was passed in the United States Congress and was signed by the then US President, Barack Obama. The law did not receive much publicity, but there were those who regarded it as one of the most revolutionary laws in the history of our planet. The law allowed private companies to mine asteroids.[39] In principle it ran contrary to the 1967 'Outer Space Treaty', which recognised that outer space was a publicly owned resource. The Obama act, however, allowed private companies to mine asteroids. 'Technically the law doesn't say a private company can own an asteroid but it can take possession of anything they extract from it.'[40]

In the world of 2050 as in that of 2015, it is more than likely that important distinctions between those who owned the sources of wealth and those who occupied such sources would continue. An owner, for example, might not have the necessary capacities 'to mine' the source, but nevertheless owned it. On the other hand, those who occupied sources of wealth due to concessions made by the owner benefited but did not own. Of course, there would be those who were both owners and occupiers as well as those who occupied but who had no or very minimal access to any resources at all.

Now in a world that veered from the polylateral to the multilateral to the atomised to virtual reality cohorts in a constantly shifting entanglement nexus, those who were owners and occupiers shifted with varying degrees of unpredictability, too. 'Overloaded states' and a state construct perceived as unable to meet global survival needs more generally might well result in a shift in importance between ownership and occupation. More and more, non-state occupiers with capacities to identify and exploit resources, accumulate and trade might be able to generate wealth which directly and indirectly would impact upon survival needs on Earth and elsewhere. To do so, they would not necessarily have to own, but their multidimensional capacities and outputs would be recognised as a justifiable rationale to occupy.

An example noted earlier were the financial and economic prospects of mining in outer space that offered rewards few could resist.[41] Who would be the owners and the occupiers in a cosmos of immense opportunities might remain a confused picture by mid-century. As noted above, the 1967 *magna carta* of outer space, i.e. the United Nations sponsored Outer Space Treaty, made it clear that outer space, including the Moon and other celestial bodies were 'not subject to national appropriation by claim of sovereignty, by means of use or occupation, or by any other means'.

Twelve years later, a so-called 'Moon Agreement' went further by forbidding any private ownership of extra-terrestrial real estate. However, by 2023, with 86 states having attempted to go into outer space and over 10,000 private sector corporations having been described as 'outer space focused',[42] it was telling that probably only 18 states – none who had space capacities – would have signed that 1979 Moon agreement.

There seems little dispute that outer space colonisation will probably have become a thriving reality by the 2050s. The two issues that seem to remain uncertain is the overall number of humans that will be temporarily or permanently based beyond Earth in the solar system, and whether the habitats that will accommodate them will be large space stations providing artificial gravity or planets such as Mars and planetary moons or both types.

As for numbers of humans, estimates range from 1 million habitants on Mars alone by 2050 to 'first hundreds, then thousands and eventually hundreds of thousands of people not just visiting space but living and working there'.[43] Yet, whatever the estimate, a key factor in determining human involvement in outer space will be the costs of launching people and payloads. Once that cost will have dropped, the flow from Earth into the cosmos will truly begin. Already, analysts anticipate that by 2040 costs of transportation into outer space will have dropped from thousands of dollars per kilogram to tens of dollars.[44]

Those inhabiting outer space would most likely reflect a fluctuating admix of state and non-state-based institutions. The latter will probably consist mainly of those from the private sector engaged in mineral mining, tourism and infrastructure maintenance as well as manufacturing enterprises and solar farms. Their sheer numbers, established presence, operational systems, related technologies and most of all economic impacts will determine who were the dominant players. Ownership was less relevant; capacities to dominate were – particularly in circumstances where the definition of ownership, *per se*, remained an intergovernmental quandary.

Box 3.3 Who's at the Asteroid Mining Table? And, Who Is Not?

By 2053 the cost of mining asteroids had dropped significantly. 30 years before the price of mining platinum from asteroid miles from planet Earth was estimated to be approximately US$1 billion per tonne. Now, it was less than U$ per $28,500 tonne.

It was evident that governments of what were then developed states were eager to support the efforts of a growing number of private sector corporations to undertake mining in outer space. NASA, for example, had been tracking over 6,000 asteroids, which helped private corporations identify potentially valuable and accessible mining opportunities.

The data base, Asterank, had already shown that mining just the ten most cost-effective asteroids – i.e. those that were closest to Earth and of greatest value – would produce a profit of around US$1.5 trillion. Bearing inflation in mind, that figure proved to be the case, though the amount transferred automatically into cybercurrencies meant that truly accurate figures were difficult to ascertain.

For many on Earth, asteroid mining had led to the creation of sufficient solar power satellites that had resulted in clean energy which was available to over 65 per cent of the planet; and, for those concerned about the exploitation of human beings – particularly children – for example, in cobalt mining in what had been the Democratic Republic of the Congo (DRC), Zimbabwe and South Africa, asteroid mining clearly reduced such abuses.

The downsides for those on planet Earth began with the erosion of those economies that had until recently been dependent upon Earth-based mining. As the results of asteroid mining began to flood the markets on Earth, not only was there a rapid devaluation of global raw materials, but also global struggles for resources and power were increasing.

Throughout all of these economic and social disruptions, it was the private sector that had been emerging as the most dominant force. Despite the initial reliance of governments to support outer space exploration, it was the capacities of a few mega-multinationals to mine, ship and trade that determined how asteroids were used. Their dominance was further reenforced by those in other sectors such as the pharmaceuticals that had become dependent upon materials provided from outer space. They, too, were determined to maximise those benefits.

The only resource regulation to which all had to adhere was that celestial bodies could not be owned by a single country. However, it was becoming all too clear by mid-century that ownership did not determine who was sitting at the decision-making table. What until relatively recently had been assumed to be the purview of governments and related intergovernmental organisations had by mid-century become dominated by the few. It was the perspectives and consequent interests of those few who intentionally or not tended to dominate a critical facet of global interests.

Back on Earth, a similar pattern may well emerge. States, for example, could find themselves faced with growing numbers of displaced peoples who occupied lands which states ostensibly owned, but over which they were unwilling or unable to assert their authority. While states nominally owned infrastructures involving essentials like roads, rivers, airwaves, national forests and so on, their ability to maintain the value of such resources may increasingly depend upon how cohorts sequestered, utilised and maintained them. Like outer space habitats, ownership could well become increasingly dependent upon those who were the occupiers.

Controllers and the Controlled

The sheer financial and economic prospects of mining in outer space could offer rewards few could resist.[45] While ownership, *per se*, may not have been possible, the lure for prospectors would most likely be irresistible. One asteroid, for example, Davida, is estimated to hold an estimated $17 trillion worth of metals. The issue will inevitably be the control of such resources. Who has access to them? Who controls and mines them and who distributes them?

Whatever the specific value, the probability might well be that occupation of such geophysical masses would leave vast amounts of resources in the hands of a growing number of commercial and other non-state actors. They may not own portions of meteors, asteroids or other moons and planets, but they will have the capacities to commercialise resources to determine how and to whom they will be distributed.[46]

Whether in outer space or on planet Earth, it could well be that the 'overloaded state' would in a generation's time be part of or dependent upon cohorts of multiple actors. The state might continue to have varying degrees of regulatory control. However, resource allocation even when it came to resources for healthcare, pensions, education and even security might be less state dependent and determined.

Control, in other words, might be shared or bypassed, but when it comes to resource distribution and recipients, control might well be determined by those who have direct access to resources and not necessarily those who ostensibly have formal authority over them. A contemporary case in point are the tensions created between the state and those who create digital currencies such as 'bit coins' and 'cryptocurrencies'.

Digital currencies were designed to work as a medium of exchange, or currency, through unregulated computer networks. They have not been reliant on any central authority such as a governments. In fact, governments often have given up efforts to control them, or in some instances have come to arrangements where bit coins and cryptocurrencies are recognised as means of exchange. For a number of states, both had become a recognised threat, and controlling them regarded as a never-ending game of cat and mouse, where the mouse frequently won.[47]

More and more can one foresee the prospect that control in a growing number of instances may increasingly bypass the state and its multilateral components. 'The corporates' and urban authorities, for example, might increasingly fill resource gaps that in no small part reflect the overstretched resource commitments of the state. More and more, non-state cohorts could find themselves working alongside states or completely divorced from them. Control, however, would neither be certain or fixed, but based upon ever fluctuating interests – perceived self-interests and mutual self-interests.

Of course, when reflecting upon the nature of control in a 2050 context, the ever-increasing intervention of artificial intelligence is certainly relevant. Whether focus is on state-based operations or those of parallel actors, the irrefutable fact will increasingly be that who controlled and who were the controlled would reflected a fluctuating balance between human capacities and AGI.

The relevance of artificial intelligence would be fundamental to plausible future prospects of human agency, as described in Chapter 2. As suggested there and certainly relevant in the context of who controls and who is the controlled, AGI, despite all its benefits, could clearly open the way towards 'increased reliance on complex autonomous analysis…(which) could marginalise the value of human review'.[48]

In so doing, one of its consequences might be an '*informatised* threat' where societies were increasingly losing control of data transmission. In turn, the prospect that AGI could result in 'the singularity' where the combined capacities of computing would frequently result in the fact that human cognition could no longer keep pace with the speed of decision-making.[49]

On a growing number of occasions, AGI – already by the 2030s – would most likely demonstrate levels of intelligence that had advanced well beyond human capacities, and in very fundamental ways assumed control and determined some of the most basic elements of the resource prioritisation process.[50] Resource priorities might well be determined for reasons that bypass human agency.[51]

Whether through AGI or cohorts of actors that may or may not involve the state, there are two certainties as one looks to the future. The first is that who will be the controllers and who will be the controlled will be far more fluid and unregulated in a generation's time. The second is that the consequences of control will most likely have unprecedented impacts upon planet Earth and beyond.

Box 3.4 Who Controls the Global Climate?

In a meeting of the UN's Fourth Committee (Special Political and Decolonisation) in October 2014, committee members had pointing to the array of benefits that they were receiving from outer space. These included various dimensions of sustainable development, monitoring of climate change, disaster preparedness, conservation and agriculture. And, yet, given all those 'fruits of the marvellous progress of science,' several states from what was then the developing world emphasised the importance of ensuring 'that outer space technology did not become an instrument of dominion and a vehicle for imposing certain cultures and values on others'.[52]

These concerns became ever more evident as the full impacts of various geoengineered innovations by richer countries were becoming increasingly apparent. One example was Solar Radiation Management (SRM), designed to reflect varying degrees of the sun's light and heat away from Earth, resulting in atmospheric cooling.

Climate geoengineering had been viewed by many scientists as a freak show in otherwise serious discussions of climate science and policy. However, the feckless response of the world community to burgeoning greenhouse gas emissions had led to increasingly serious consideration of the potential role of geoengineering as means to avoid a climate emergency. Rapid melting of the Greenland and West Antarctic ice sheets, for example, demanded stopgap measures such as SRM to buy time.

Despite the moratorium on geoengineering adopted by the 2010 United Nations Convention on Biological Diversity in 2010, states with the capacities had eventually decided to put theory into practice. Towards the end of the 2020s, it was decided that such stopgap measures should be used, particularly since the 1.5-degree climate change target was still not making much progress; and, to varying degrees of interest, policymakers in the

United States, China, Germany, India and Russia had decided to undertake the experiment.[53]

As SRM began to be introduced to varying degrees across the geopolitical boundaries of those states and a few others, e.g. Japan, it transpired that at long last positive steps towards implementing internationally recognised approaches to climate change were beginning to have positive impacts. However, due to SRM, between 1.2 and 4.1 billion people found themselves confronted with significant changes in rainfall patterns and for many negative changes affecting local crops or livestock for food or for income.[54] *At the same time, there was growing concern about the security implications. Would SRM efforts result in regional changes in weather patterns that would result in conflict? And, for those who could recall, what relevance would that 1978 UN ENMOD Convention (Convention on the Prohibition of Military or Any Other Hostile Use of Environmental Modification Techniques) really have under such circumstances two generations later?*

Ultimately who was in control of the global climate? Who were the controllers and who were the controlled?

Resource Distribution and Emerging Disparities

As has always been the case, resource distribution would continue to reflect the priorities determined by those in control. However, as one looks to the 2050s, control will most likely be far more dispersed than three decades before. In a world that veered between multilateralism, minilateralism, atomisation and polylateralism, the importance of state-based governance systems intended for resource prioritisation and distribution would most likely decline. The array of different types of actors with access to resources and powers to distribute them would make resource prioritisation and distribution far more uncertain.

An analogue is the unanticipated end of the 'Roaring Twenties' in the United States. It was the last gasp of wealth and excess for the relatively few, when on 28 October 1929 – the day of the Great Crash – the New York Stock Market collapsed. All those assumptions about the durability of the stock exchange collapsed with it. Seemingly resilient businesses, including 659 major banks, went bankrupt, unemployed workers marched in angry protest – and some of the wealthiest investors in the world found themselves on the fringes of poverty.

Returning to possible futures, there might well be governments that could afford to distribute resources to the vulnerable through such mechanisms as a 'universal basic income', a payment made without imposing any requirements on the recipients. Jobless economic growth could become a kind of new norm,[55] and yet for those who still will have jobs the disparities between their wealth and the new norm would most likely increase significantly. As so often the case in the past, such disparities could well result in vulnerabilities that frequently put the affected on the margins of survival.

Those responsible for resource distribution, whether government or non-state actors, may also have to deal with the complexities posed by competition between habitats across space and the needs of those on Earth. The former – outer space habitats – most likely will require resources to meet the demands created by interplanetary activities. These would include resources not only for survival systems but also for cross planetary trade, travel, resettlement, exploration of exoplanets and security measures.

For the latter – Earth – a disconcerting proportion of outer space assets that were anticipated to provide resources for a wide swathe of technologically unemployed people could find themselves on a downward spiral. The emerging reality could be that, while many might have to rely solely on governments for their survival, it could well be that most governments may lack the resources or were unable to keep up with the momentum of intensifying societal disparities. And, those non-state actors may find that they have neither the interest nor capacities to intervene.

Compounding that possible Earth-based prospect are those tensions between needs on Earth and those in space-based habitats. How might this sort of competition affect how and to whom resources would be allocated? Already, in the early part of the 21st century there has been growing concern that the demands of outer space would alter the very nature and protection of human rights and inevitably who gained and who was deprived of essential resources.[56]

In considering the resource distribution process and possible disparities, critical questions of rights and security will also have to be addressed. Such issues would have to take into account human engagement across the oceans of space. As on planet Earth, the question that needs to be answered is whether there will be adequate agreed frameworks and means of enforcement – provided and enforced by whom – to protect the positive and constrain the negative?

This sort of concern raises the issue of conflicts arising out of resource scarcity that would not be unlikely. For example, despite all the potential benefits noted earlier about the range of water creation and purification processes, it is estimated that 215 international rivers and more than 300 water basins that bordered multiple countries could in many instances become sources of conflict. Such conflicts might well be state-sponsored or instigated; others, mixed coalitions of interested parties; all, however, would inevitably reduce access to resources for some and increase them for others.

Box 3.5 Geoeconomic Fragmentation and Unanticipated Disparities

As far back as 2023, the International Monetary Fund (IMF) had warned that the world could soon fragment into rival economic blocs, recalling some of the worst days of the Cold War. From economic slowdowns and climate change to cost-of-living crises and high debt levels, the international system, so it was feared, would descend into prolonged chaos. This, asserted the IMF, would be a collective policy mistake that would leave everyone poorer and less secure, or, what it had called, 'geoeconomic fragmentation'.[57]

To varying degrees the warning about geoeconomic fragmentation began to ease as various arrangements were made to push the climate change agenda further along and cost of living crises were bottoming out. Over the next decade, there was relative stability, certainly when it came to some of the richest states in the world, including China, India and Indonesia.

Towards the end of the 2040s, however, despite a brief moment of seeming stability, it was becoming evident that a growing number of states in many parts of the world were beginning to fracture. Of the 193 states recognised by the United Nations in 2023, at least 73 reflected structural fragmentation and loss of consistent patterns of control. 14 out of 32 upper income countries were failing states, 11 middle income and the remaining 38 were described as lower income.

Such fragmentation was resulting in increasing atomisation where initiatives and loosely defined authority were less and less vested in conventional government systems, and non-state actors were often assuming authority and control in ways unpredictable and by no means consistent. What, too, was becoming increasingly surprising was that the nature of vulnerability and suffering was changing.

The breakdown in trade and financial systems was inevitable, but it was not only the poor who were dragged down into further poverty. Those who had assumed that, despite the increasing turmoil in the trading and banking systems, they would be able to withstand the chaos were being proved wrong.

In considering who will distribute resources, how and why, the possible consequences of AGI is once again an unavoidable theme. Predictions and warnings, resource settlements and arrangements as well as resource priorities and processes will increasingly be influenced, if not directed, by AGI. It could be that such technological benefits would reflect socio-economic status which in turn reflected technologically enhanced capacities to anticipate and adjust. In times of possible crises, types of assistance and access to them might distinguish between those who are technologically prepared and those who are not.

Such systems, some might argue, could result not only in controlling information but also in 'prioritizing certain affected populations over others, operating in particular areas over others, or otherwise manipulated in ways that could be detrimental to affected populations'.[58] That is not to suggest that the latter had been forgotten, but societally determined qualifications frequently would secure priority assistance.[59]

In other words, one could argue that those who were at the top of the resource priority process could well be those who benefited from cognitive enhancements. That, by implication, is what that Gene Equality Project experiment in May 2059 made evident. Those who did poorly, lacked the 'societal status' that would prove a platform for success.

Despite good intentions and potential universal applicability, that philanthropic effort to bring cognitive enhancements to low-income communities did not seem to work. Those in control or benefitting from transformative technologies had intentionally or unintentionally the ability to create and control socio-economic divides and related resource distribution. Many among the elite may have been concerned that the 'have-nots' would reflect a caste system that was determined by those with cyborg-type capacities generally determined and sustained by AGI.

Conclusion: The Prioritisation Process

No one is suggesting that the resource prioritisation process in the future will inevitably reflect the relatively dystopic views laid out in this chapter. Yet, there is a case to be made that the search for resources, the ways that they are prioritised, maintained and distributed can intensify vulnerabilities, which in turn can transform threats into humanitarian crises.

Such perspectives, however, are not intended to predict what governance and resource distribution will be in the future. Rather, they are there to propose types of issues that those interested in humanitarian planning and policymaking might have to support or counter in *planning from the future* for the future.

Here, again, the purpose is not about prediction, but instead about sensitising readers to the 'what might be's' – to ask them to consider how they would deal with complex change, how anticipatory and adaptive they would be when confronting uncertain futures.

And, if humanitarian crises ultimately reflect the ways that societies structure themselves, govern and allocate resources, then how might they deal with types of threats discussed in the following chapter? The reader will see that they are not predictions, but yet another way to test the anticipatory and adaptive capacities of the reader when confronted with plausible portraits of an ever more complex future?

Notes

1. This story is based on a *New York Times* feature dealing with stories of the future and is from Ted Chiang, 'Kids are still winning: DNA tweaks won't fix our problems', *New York Times*, 27 May 2019.
2. Samuel P. Huntington, *The clash of civilisations and the remaking of world order*, Simon and Schuster, 1996, p. 45.
3. Ibid., p. 49.
4. Signed in 1648, The Peace of Westphalia ended the Thirty and Eighty Years Wars and created the framework for modem international relations.
5. Selina O'Grady, *And Man created God: A history of the world in the time of Jesus*, Picador, 2012, p. 104.
6. Gavin Menzies, *1421: The year China discovered the world*, Bantam Books, 2003, p. 454.
7. Charles Rybeck, Lanny Cornwell and Phillip Sagan, 'A national security enterprise response: Digital dimension disruption', *PRISM*, 7 (2), 2017.

8 Linton Wells II, 'Cognitive-emotional conflict: Adversary will and social resilience', *PRISM*, 7 (2), December 2017.
9 PWC, *The World in 2050: The long view – how will the global economic order change by 2050* #world2050 – 2016.
10 This report only provided background material, and did not support or deny the futures perspective used here. African Union, *Delimitation and demarcation of boundaries in Africa*, 2nd Edition, Commission of the African Union, Department of Peace and Security, August 2014.
11 This report only provided background material, and did not support or deny the futures perspective used here. Kirill Krivosheev, *Crises in Central Asia belie the region's ability to democratise*, Carnegie Endowment for International Peace, 13 July 2022.
12 This report only provided background material, and did not support or deny the futures perspective used here. Mykhailo Minakov, *Eastern Europe's authoritarian belt*, Wilson Center, A blog of the Kennan Institute, 6 October 2020.
13 Tom Symons, *The nation state goes virtual*, NESTA, 2018. See also Richard Rosecrance, *The rise of the virtual state: Wealth and power in the coming century*, Basic Books, 1999.
14 Philip Rowley, 'The biggest idea you've never heard of: Virtual nations', Futures @ Omnicom Media Group, 25 May 2021.
15 Henry A. Kissinger, Eric Schmidt and Daniel Huttenlocher, *The age of AI: And our human future*, John Murray Press, Kindle edition, 2021, p. 83.
16 John Micklethwait and Adrian Woolridge, *The wakeup call: Why the pandemic has exposed the weakness of the West – and how to fix it*, Short Books, 2020, p. 64.
17 Charles Leadbeater and Jennie Winhall, *Building better systems: A green paper on systems innovation*, The Rockwell Foundation, October 2020, p. 10.
18 See, for example, 'Trying to get the hang of IT', *The Economist*, 20 March 2021, or Oliver Letwin, *Apocalypse how*, Atlantic Books, 2020.
19 Phil Rowley, 'The biggest idea you've never heard Of: Virtual nations', 25 May 2021
20 The UN 'system was constitutionally unfit to deal with transnationality and that "sovereign" states…, even acting in concert, were unable to address a host of transnational problems such as… technological disasters and systems collapse, pandemics, opioid proliferation, resistance to antibiotics,… and, of course, climate change and its cortege of threats to survival.' Antonio Donini, 'UN 2.0', *Global Governance* 26 (2020), p. 266.
21 United Nations General Secretary, *Our common agenda: Report of the Secretary-General*, United Nations, 2021.
22 Aarishi Tirkey, *Minilateralism: Weighing the prospects for cooperation and governance*, ORF Issue Brief No. 489, Observer Research Foundation, September 2021.
23 Examples used to describe polylateral trends included such initiatives as the GAVI Alliance, created in 2020, focused on providing vaccinations for children in lower income countries, combined the efforts of the Bill & Melinda Gates Foundation, the World Health Organization, UNICEF, the World Bank and various vaccines industries in developing countries. The International Science Council is another case to which analysts referred. The ISC brought together scientific bodies relevant to international policy issues, and another type of polylateral example was the World Benchmarking Alliance. Principally concerned with private sector contributions to the Sustainable Development Goals, it nevertheless reflected a global community of practice which sets standards for corporate performance on the SDGs. The Research Data Alliance was regarded as another example. It was a community-driven initiative launched in 2013 by the European Commission, the US National Science Foundation, the National

Institute of Standards and Technology and the Australian Government's Department of Innovation.

24 Nathan Gardels, 'Planetary politics when nation states falters', *Noema*, 3 September 2021.

25 Ibid.

26 Anne-Marie Slaughter, www.noemamag.com/networked-planetary-governance/ 'We don't wait for the big players – we just go do it,' stressed one proponent of polylateralism. 'I'm not saying we should work against states – just that we should not necessarily start with them. What's key is to get people away from thinking strictly in terms of "international" which connotes government-to-government interaction and state versus non-state, and instead to think in terms of the interconnected global.'

27 Gabriel Ramos, UNESCO's Assistant-Director-General of Social and Human Sciences, 'AI for all', *New Scientist*, 4 December 2021, p. 27.

28 Ibid.

29 Azmat Khan, 'Hidden Pentagon records reveal patterns of failure in deadly airstrikes', *New York Times*, 18 December 2021.

30 Alan Turing's statement was noted by Professor Stuart Russell in the December 2021 BBC Reith Lecture, Lecture 4: Beneficial AI and a future for humans, www.bbc.co.uk/radio4

31 Op. cit., #26, Stuart Russell. During the lecture he referred to one of the hazards of AI, if not well understood, in a fictional anecdote: *Suppose, for example, that COP36 asks for help in deacidifying the oceans; they know the pitfalls of specifying objectives incorrectly, so they insist that all the by-products must be non-toxic, and no fish can be harmed. The AI system comes up with a new self-multiplying catalyst that will do the trick with a very rapid chemical reaction. Great! But the reaction uses up a quarter of all the oxygen in the atmosphere and we all die slowly and painfully. From the AI system's point of view, eliminating humans is a feature, not a bug, because it ensures that the oceans stay in their now-pristine state.*

32 Nick Bostrom, *Superintelligence: Paths, dangers, strategies*, Oxford University Press, 2014, p. 22.

33 Donald Sanders in book review of Brigette Tasha Hyacinth, 'The future of leadership: Rise of automation, robotics and artificial intelligence', MBA Caribbean Organisation, *PRISM*, 3, 2017, p. 179.

34 Owen Cotton-Barratt et al., *Global catastrophic risks*, Global Challenges Foundation, 2016.

35 Yuval Noah Harari, *Homo deus: A brief history of tomorrow*, Penguin Random House, 2015, p. 437; see, also, #15 Henry Kissinger et al.

36 Umair Haque, *The collapse economy*, Eudaimonia & Co., 24 November 2021.

37 'Smarter use of natural resources can inject $2 trillion into global economy by 2050' – Erik Solheim, UNEP, 17 March 2017.

38 World Economic Forum in collaboration with the Boston Consulting Group, Mining and Minerals in a Sustainable World 2050, 2015.

39 Andrew Griffin, 'Asteroid mining made legal after Barack Obama gives US citizens the right to own parts of celestial bodies', *The Independent*, 26 November 2015.

40 For full discussion, see Keith Cowing, 'Can Congress authorize mining on asteroids?', *NASA Watch*, 24 September 2015.

41 According to the *New Scientist* (16 January 2016, p. 8), an steroid mining firm, Planetary Resources, 'has revealed the first object 3-D printed from meteorite ore, a

scale model of one of its spacecraft parts. The rock was found on Earth, but in future the company plans to mine and manufacture in space'.

42 John Koetsier, 'Space Inc: 10,000 companies, $4T value … and 52% American', Forbes, 22 May 2021. The author notes that 'most of the 10,000+ companies are clustered in just five sectors, according to a new report from SpaceTech Analytics. Navigation and mapping is the largest, with 2,820 companies, followed by Cloud Solutions at 2,406, and manufacturing at 1,048.

43 Rich Smith, 'Why this space expert thinks that "hundreds of thousands of humans could live in outer space by 2050" ', *The Motley* Fool, 2 May 2021 is a review of Robert Jacobson's *Space Is Open for Business* and why Jacobson thinks the next 30 years could be a renaissance for space companies and a big opportunity for investors who want to get in on the ground floor of the space business.

44 'What might space look like in 2050?', *RAND Review*, RAND Corporation, 5 January 2023.

45 According to the *New Scientist* (16 January 2016, p. 8), an asteroid mining firm, Planetary Resources, 'has revealed the first object 3-D printed from meteorite ore, a scale model of one of its spacecraft parts. The rock was found on Earth, but in future the company plans to mine and manufacture in space.'

46 David C. Cantillo et al., 'Constraining the Regolith Composition of Asteroid (16) Psyche via Laboratory Visible Near-infrared Spectroscopy', *American Astronomical Society. The Planetary Science Journal*, 2 (95), 12 May 2021.

47 Anshu Siripurapu and Noah Berman, 'Cryptocurrencies, digital dollars, and the future of money', Council on Foreign Relations, www.cfr.org/backgrounder/cryptocurrencies-digital-dollars-and-future-money, 28 February 2023.

48 Matthew Price, Stephen Walker and Will Wiley, 'The machine beneath: Implications of artificial intelligence in strategic decision-making', *PRISM*, 4, 2018, pp. 96 ff.

49 Elsa B. Kania, *Battlefield singularity: Artificial intelligence, military revolution, and China's future military power*, Center for a New American Security referenced in *PRISM*, 8 (3), 2019, p. 31.

50 Keith Dear and Ali Hossaini, The AI Special Issue, *RUSI Journal*, 164 (5/6), July/August 2019, see, also, Beazley, *Risk and resilience: Spotlight on technology risk*, 21 September 2021.

51 Mark Hunyadi, Professor for Moral, Social and Political Philosophy, Université Catholique de Louvain, noted in the *Geneva science and diplomacy anticipator's annual report on science trends at 5,10 and 25 years* that 'From a more ethical point of view, what I fear for the future of humanity, since it is a bit your question and it is mine too, is that by dint of constantly valuing calculation, what will count [in the end] is calculation, neglecting questions of meaning. My fear is that little by little, we will come to eliminate the human being himself, his dispositions and his aptitudes, precisely the search for meaning, imagination, spontaneous creativity.' *The GESDA 2021 Science Breakthrough Radar*, p. 24, radar.gesda.global

52 'Outer space benefits must not be allowed to widen global gap between economic, social inequality, fourth committee told, concluding debate on item', *United Nations*. United Nations, 17 October 2014. Web 27 April 2015.

53 One of the largest experiments in this area was the Lohafex which was an Indian-German experiment in 2009 which involved dumping six tonnes of iron solution into the South Atlantic to encourage plankton to bloom – trapping carbon which would then be sent to the seabed when the organisms died.

54 David Shukman, 'Geo-engineering: Climate fixes "could harm billions"', BBC News, 26 November 2014, quoting Professor Piers Foster, University of Leeds.
55 Jerome Glenn and Elizabeth Florescu, Pew Research Center see Future Work/ Technology 2050 Real-Time Delphi Study – *2015–16 State of the Future, Journal of Socialomics*, January 2016. doi: 10.4172/2167-0358.1000171
56 Those negative implications have led a growing number of international experts to press for such initiatives as the creation of legal principles that would be relevant for human rights, taking into account the demands that settlements in outer space might require. See, for example, A. Ferreira-Snyman and G. Ferreira· 'The application of international human rights instruments in outer space settlements: Today's science fiction, tomorrow's reality', *Potchefstroom Electronic Law Journal (PELJ)*, 22 (1), 2019, http://dx.doi.org/10.17159/1727-3781/2019/v22i0a5904
57 Kristalina Georgieva, *Confronting fragmentation where it matters most: Trade, debt, and climate action*, IMF Blog, 16 January 2023.
58 International Committee of the Red Cross, Statement to High-Level Panel on 'Improving humanitarian effectiveness through new technologies and innovation: Opportunities and challenges', United Nations Economic and Social Council – Humanitarian Affairs Segment, 10 June 2020.
59 'Time and time again we've seen that people who are already marginalised are the ones who experience the worst harms from large-scale artificial intelligence systems.' Kate Crawford, author of *Atlas of AI*, in interview with Timothy Revell, *New Scientist*, 21 March 2021, p. 47. See, also, relevant discussion on Takaful by Tate Ryan-Mosely, 'Algorithms intended to reduce poverty might disqualify people in need', *MIT Technology Review*, 13 June 2023.

Bibliography

African Union, *Delimitation and demarcation of boundaries in Africa*, Commission of the African Union, Department of Peace and Security, 2nd Edition, August 2014.

Arenas, Javier Garcia, 'The future of the middle classes: Technology and demographics will bring change, but they will not disappear', Caixabank, 13 September 2019.

Bostrom, Nick, *Superintelligence: Paths, dangers, strategies*, Oxford University Press, 2014.

Cantillo David C. et al., 'Constraining the regolith composition of Asteroid (16) psyche via laboratory visible near-infrared spectroscopy', *American Astronomical Society. The Planetary Science Journal*, 2 (95), 12 May 2021.

Cotton-Barratt, Owen et al., *Global catastrophic risks – 2016*, Global Challenges Foundation, 2016.

Cowing, Keith, *Can congress authorize mining on asteroids?*, NASA Watch, 24 September 2015.

Daheim, Cornelia and Wintermann, Ole, *2050: Future of work: Findings of an international Delphi Study of The Millennium Project,* Bertelsmann-stifung, March 2016. www.bertelsmann-stiftung.de, March 2016.

Ferreira-Snyman, A. and Ferreira, G., 'The application of international human rights instruments in outer space settlements: Today's science fiction, tomorrow's reality', *Potchefstroom Electronic Law Journal (PELJ), PER* 22 (1), 2019, http://dx.doi.org/10.17159/1727-3781/2019/v22i0a5904

Gardels, Nathan, 'Planetary politics when nation states falters', *Noema*, 3 September 2021.

Geneva Science and Diplomacy Anticipator's Annual Report on Science Trends at 5,10 and 25 Years – The GESDA 2021 science breakthrough radar – radar.gesda.global, 2021.

Georgieva, Kristalina, *Confronting fragmentation where it matters most: Trade, debt, and climate action*, IMF Blog, 16 January 2023.

Glenn, Jerome and Florescu, Elizabeth, 'Future work/technology 2050 real-time Delphi study of the Millennium Project – *2015–16 State of the Future*', *Journal of Socialomics*, 05 (03), January 2016. doi: 10.4172/2167-0358.1000171

Griffin, Andrew, 'Asteroid mining made legal after Barack Obama gives US citizens the right to own parts of celestial bodies', *The Independent*, 26 November 2015.

Hanson, Russell L. and Zeemering, Eric S. (Eds), *Cooperation and conflict between state and local government*, United States Institute of Peace, Legitimate state monopoly over the means of violence. www.usip.org/guiding-principles-stabilization-and-reconstruction-the-web.../le

Harari, Yuval Noah, *Homo deus: A brief history of tomorrow,* Penguin Random House, 2015.

Haque, Umair, *The collapse economy*, Eudaimonia & Co., 24 November 2021.

Huntington, Samuel P., *The clash of civilisations and the remaking of world order*, Simon and Schuster, 1996.

Hyacinth, Brigette Tasha, 'The future of leadership: Rise of automation, robotics and artificial intelligence', MBA Caribbean Organisation, *PRISM*, 3, 2017.

International Committee of the Red Cross, *Statement to high-level panel on 'Improving humanitarian effectiveness through new technologies and innovation: opportunities and challenges',* United Nations Economic and Social Council – Humanitarian Affairs Segment, 10 June 2020.

Kania, Elsa B., 'Battlefield singularity: Artificial intelligence, military revolution, and China's future military power', Center for a New American Security, *PRISM,* (8) 3, 2019.

Khan, Azmat, 'Hidden Pentagon records reveal patterns of failure in deadly airstrikes', *New York Times*, 18 December 2021.

Kissinger, Henry A., Schmidt, Eric and Huttenlocher, Daniel, *The age of AI: And our human future*, John Murray Press, Kindle edition, 2021.

Koetsier, John, 'Space Inc: 10,000 companies, $4T value … and 52% American,' *Forbes,* 22 May 2021.

Krivosheev, Kirill, *Crises in Central Asia belie the region's ability to democratise*, Carnegie Endowment for International Peace, 13 July 2022.

Leadbeater, Charles and Winhall, Jennie, *Building better systems: A green paper on systems innovation,* The Rockwell Foundation, October 2020.

Letwin, Oliver, *Apocalypse how*, Atlantic Books, 2020.

Menzies, Gavin, *1421: The year China discovered the world*, Bantam Books, 2003.

Micklethwait, John and Woolridge, Adrian, *The wakeup call: Why the Pandemic has exposed the weakness of the West – and how to fix it*, Short Books, 2020.

Minakov, Mykhailo, *Eastern Europe's authoritarian belt*, Wilson Center, A blog of the Kennan Institute, 6 October 2020.

O'Grady, Selina, *And Man created God: A history of the world in the time of Jesus,* Picador, 2012.

Oomen, Barbara and Baumgärtel, Moritz, 'Frontier cities: The rise of local authorities as an opportunity for international human rights law', *European Journal of International Law*, 29 (2), May 2018, https://doi.org/10.1093/ejil/chy021

Price, Matthew, Walker, Stephen and Wiley, Will, 'The machine beneath: Implications of artificial intelligence in strategic decision-making,' *PRISM*, 4, 2018.

PWC, *The world in 2050: The long view – how will the global economic order change by 2050,* #world2050, 2016.

Ramos, Gabriel, UNESCO's Assistant-Director-General of Social and Human Sciences, 'AI for all,' *New Scientist*, 4 December 2021.

RAND Corporation, 'What might space look like in 2050?', *RAND Review*, 5 January 2023.

Razeen, Sally, *What if cities ruled the world*? – part of the World Economic Forum's Strategic Foresight team and the Global Agenda Council on the Future of Government developed three scenarios of how the world of governance could evolve by 2050: City States, e-1984 and Gated Communities.

Rosecrance, Richard, *The rise of the virtual state: Wealth and power in the coming century*, Basic Books, 1999.

Rowley, Philip, 'The biggest idea you've never heard of: Virtual nations,' *Futures @ Omnicom Media Group*, 25 May 2021.

Ryan-Mosely, Tate, 'Algorithms intended to reduce poverty might disqualify people in need', *MIT Technology Review*, 13 June 2023.

Rybeck, Charles, Cornwell, Lanny and Sagan, Phillip, 'A national security enterprise response: Digital dimension disruption,' *PRISM*, 7 (2), 2017.

Siripurapu, Anshu and Berman, Noah, 'Cryptocurrencies, digital dollars, and the future of money', *Council on Foreign Relations*, 28 February 2023. www.cfr.org/backgrounder/cryptocurrencies-digital-dollars-and-future-money

Smith, Rich, 'Why this space expert thinks that "hundreds of thousands of humans could live in outer space by 2050" ', *The Motley Fool*, 2 May 2021.

Solheim, Erik, 'Smarter use of natural resources can inject $2 trillion into global economy by 2050', *UNEP*, 17 March 2017.

Symons, Tom, *The nation state goes virtual*, NESTA, 2018.

Tirkey, Aarishi, *Minilateralism: Weighing the prospects for cooperation and governance*, ORF Issue Brief No. 489, Observer Research Foundation, September 2021.

United Nations, *Our common agenda: Report of the Secretary-General*, 2021.

United Nations. 'Outer space benefits must not be allowed to widen global gap between economic, social inequality, fourth committee told, concluding debate on item', *United Nations*, 17 October 2014. Web. 27 April 2015.

Wells II, Linton, 'Cognitive-emotional conflict: Adversary will and social resilience,' *PRISM*, 7 (2), 2017.

World Economic Forum in collaboration with the Boston Consulting Group, *Mining and minerals in a sustainable world 2050*, 2015.

4 Towards the Brink

'Well our argument starts from the fact that I'm not at all optimistic we're going to go on for a huge length of time,' said the Nobel prize winning physicist, Roger Penrose. 'The probability that something will trigger a nuclear catastrophe is not that tiny – in fact, I think that we're lucky to be around now. But maybe other civilisations will be more sensible and settle down. In fact I think that some version of SETI (the search for extra-terrestrial intelligence) should look for different civilisations, successful ones that survived very late in the previous aeon. That may be more promising in some respects. But maybe we, maybe others, will learn to send signals into the next aeon. Probably gravitational wave signals are the best bet, but very low variations in the electromagnetic field could get through too. And we might be able to get them to do better than we have, by saying, "No, you stupid idiots, that's what we're doing!" '[1]

Portraits and Their Purpose

Portraits of the future offer examples of crises which have few precedents and are certainly not on the risk registers of those institutions that have humanitarian roles and responsibilities. These portraits may seem unusually dystopic, and they are intended to be. They may seem to be predictions, but rest assured, they are not.

Their purpose is two-fold: they should provide readers with opportunities to consider the relevance of their present crisis approaches when faced with ever more complex humanitarian threats; and, they also should provide opportunities to see what might be needed to deal with increasing complexity, now and in the future.

In a world in which the types, dimensions and dynamics of humanitarian crises are already increasing and are more than likely to continue to do so – in many instances, exponentially – it has to be acknowledged from the outset that anticipating plausible future crises is inherently difficult for many reasons. Three come immediately to mind.

The first reflects one of the premisses that underpins *Humanitarian Futures*, namely, humanitarian crises ultimately reflect the ways that societies structure themselves and allocate resources. Therefore, suggesting what sorts of humanitarian crises could occur in the future presumes an appreciation of how societies

DOI: 10.4324/9781003471004-5

might evolve, how, for example, transformative technologies may change their structures, resources and dynamics. That poses a significant conceptual challenge.

What in this context the 2020–2022 Covid-19 crisis eventually made all too apparent was that social, financial and political inequalities and disparities determine vulnerabilities that leave portions of the affected far more impacted than others.[2] While catastrophic threats such as nuclear war or a large asteroid collision would not differentiate between levels of vulnerability, the sorts of crises explored here will. They reflect humanitarian crises where there are portions of populations around the world that will find themselves at the very brink of survival when others clearly may not. The latter may suffer, but the former may not survive.

The Covid-19 crisis also suggests a second point that further complicates efforts to speculate about future crisis threats. Certainly, the pandemic as well as the 2022 Russian invasion of Ukraine and the Israel-Palestinian conflict provided compelling cases for appreciating that the dimensions and dynamics of future crisis threats will be increasingly interconnected and interrelated. At the same time, it also was and increasingly will be evident that the consequences of humanitarian crises in a Gestalt sense will be greater than the sum of individual crisis events. How might one account for that?

A third and perhaps the most self-evident concerns the difficulty of anticipating the dynamics of crisis events. They may be the consequence of what has been described as the 'butterfly effect', where the proverbial flapping of that butterfly's wings can eventually be the triggering factor responsible for a storm in some other part of the world. There, too, is the compelling though disconcerting 'black swan theory' where an event reflects a situation deemed to be totally unanticipated, though generally with severe consequences.[3] Then, there is the so-called 'elephant in the room' where all too evident crisis drivers are ignored or overlooked. And, of course, there are always those presumed 'unknown unknowns'... .[4]

Future Humanitarian Crises: Types, Dynamics and Dimensions

Throughout recorded history, there have always been those with dystopic views who have paraded their concerns in various ways about the very survival of the planet, let alone human species. Whether via religious tracks, tales and mythologies, science fiction or early scientific assumptions, there were and continue to be myriad speculations about the demise of planet Earth and its inhabitants. Now, as one looks towards the mid-21st century, there probably will have emerged an unprecedented number of social and natural scientists, policymakers and analysts who warn of potentially catastrophic, if not existential, threats to both. Their warnings are regarded as plausible but probable, though by no means certain. They perhaps reflect H. G. Well's own uncertainties when he spoke at the Royal Society in 1902:

> Humanity has come some way, and the distance we have travelled gives us some insight of the way we have to go. All the past is but the beginning of a beginning; all that the human mind has accomplished is but the dream before the awakening... . It is impossible to show why certain things should not utterly

> destroy and end the human story… and make all our efforts vain… something from space, or pestilence, or some great disease of the atmosphere, some trailing cometary poison, some great emanation of vapour from the interior of the earth, or new animals to prey on us, or some drug or wrecking madness in the mind of man.[5]

Portraits of Vulnerability

The previous chapter's focus on governance and resource distribution should already have provided some insights into the sorts of deprivation that could lead large swathes of human beings to the brink of life-threatening crises. Might such threats create or expose devastating differences between wealth and poverty, increase social inequalities and intensify vulnerabilities? Alternatively, might they expose vulnerabilities of those deemed wealthy and leave those less well-off to remain temporarily unaffected?

The portraits to be explored here will have one common characteristic. Increasingly, the impacts of the threats that they portray will spill across borders, sectors and societies more generally. Interconnectedness and interrelatedness will mean that vulnerabilities will be less and less isolated phenomena, and more and more will challenge the supposed security of wealth and status and the vulnerabilities ostensibly determined by poverty.

There is a plethora of triggers for such crises. From those that are outer space-based to those that are the result of structural fragmentation on planet Earth, crisis drivers are many. Hence, the examples proposed here are just a few of myriad possibilities. None are predictions, though by no means implausible, *portraits of the future*.

A Typology of Crisis Drivers

Any effort to paint portraits of the future cannot ignore the devastating impacts that climate change and the collapse of biodiversity are already having on the planet. Their possible effects are all too evident. Whether the elimination of urban or rural space by flooding or the stifling impact on the very air we breathe, whether intensifying droughts and heat waves, climate change and the destruction of biodiversity are and will in the foreseeable future continue to threaten even the most basic needs for human and animal survival.

Similarly, nuclear weapons are another threat that cannot be ignored when it comes to human survival and survival of the planet. There are other stark portraits of plausible crisis threats that can be added to the list, including bioengineered pandemics, cyberthreats and indeed global indebtedness. However, the purpose of the portraits of the future that follow are intended to take readers beyond the evident and the present into a world that is far less familiar. Once again, the purpose for doing so ultimately is to provide a basis for testing their capacities for anticipating and adapting to crises, unconstrained by existing standard operating procedures and established mindsets.

The portraits of the future that will be displayed here will reflect humanitarian crisis threats that could stem from *technological hazards*, *structural fragmentation*, *systems collapse* and *'natural hazards'*.

Each, of course, is interrelated and interconnected, but each, too, has its own specific characteristics and particular outcomes. And, while various aspects of these have been explored by a wide range of experts concerned with vulnerability and existential survival, few have been explored in terms of their humanitarian consequences, *per se* – the sorts of impacts that would require humanitarian intervention to save the lives and essential livelihoods of directly affected and highly vulnerable populations.

Technological Hazards

It is most likely that transformative technologies will continue to have profound impacts upon societies for the duration of human existence. As proposed in the two previous chapters, technologies over the next generation will have exponential impacts not only upon some of the most fundamental dynamics of governance and resource distribution, but also upon the very nature of human agency and space.

Transformative technologies, therefore, could also change the very nature of the drivers of vulnerability and those who are vulnerable. In a growing number of instances, such technologies might become humanitarian crisis drivers because planners and decision-makers had failed to understand the full impact of technologies' consequences, or mis-prioritised them or knowingly used them to benefit some at existential costs to others.[6]

Such capacities could well result in policies that were inherently discriminatory, where one portion of a population was provided essential resources, benefits, security and support at the expense of others. The rationale underpinning those sorts of decisions need not necessarily be malevolent, but rather the results of a logic focussed on prioritised outputs with maximum efficiency in the most appropriate time.

In this instance such rationality might also have reflected unintended competition between humans and, for example, advanced AI, or in this instance, Advanced General Intelligence (AGI), for policy planning and decision-making control. Humans ostensibly would maintain overall control, though perhaps with less certainty and consistency. Increasingly evident would be that 'machines' could analyse and provide prioritised options far more quickly and comprehensively than their human counterparts. Options and solutions proposed by the former may well be better analysed and assessed than those proposed by the latter. That does not mean that AGI outcomes would necessarily be sensitive to potential vulnerabilities that their recommendations would be creating. From a humanitarian perspective, it could well be that accepting their advice will have resulted in crisis vulnerabilities, possibly taking the affected to the very brink of survival.

Box 4.1 Ensuring Pristine Oceans
Technological Rationality and Its Human Consequences

It was 2048. An estimated 38 per cent of the 47 million people who had lived for generations along the coastlines of Indonesia, Myanmar and Vietnam were trapped in pockets of hunger and starvation with limited access to potable water. To policy planners in those nations' capitals, it was all too evident that they would soon be facing localised famines that eventually could result in country-wide upheavals.

The trigger for these looming catastrophes was an urgently implemented international agreement in 2043, referred to as the 'High Seas Treaty'. To protect the oceans that were rapidly deteriorating – with all its global consequences – it was agreed by a substantial majority of UN member states that 42 per cent of the world's oceans would become 'protected areas'. That meant that fishing, shipping and related activities would also be severely restricted along agreed coastal areas.

In retrospect what also was becoming evident was that the process which had resulted in the final treaty was deeply flawed. The treaty clearly and persuasively focused on the abiding objective – ocean protection. Yet, its strategy had failed to take into account its broader implications. In other words, it did not adequately consider the impacts not only on the coastal communities of the three countries, but also the spill overs of displaced peoples from Myanmar and Vietnam into Cambodia, Laos and Thailand.

The reason goes back to the long and arduous negotiating process that had resulted in the High Seas Treaty, itself. After almost five years of debates, stalled compromises and conflicting priorities, participants in the 2043 Intergovernmental Conference in Ocean Protection and Marine Diversity agreed at long last on one solution. That solution was to accept the neutral arrangements created and guided by a highly regarded AGI strategic development process.

Now, however, what an increasing number of signatories began to realise was that from the AGI system's point of view, human interests were not part of the calculation for achieving the ultimate objective. To the contrary, when it came to ensuring that oceans attained a pristine state, the AGI strategy regarded humans as at best a hinderance and at worst a major cause for the seas' deteriorating conditions.

As the AGI strategy with the support of agreed robotic cohorts was being implemented, the lives of more and more coastline inhabitants were rapidly coming under threat. Signs of starvation and mass displacement were increasingly evident. Those policy planners and decisionmakers, ostensibly in control of AGI processes, found that the highly focused AGI programmes had ignored the lateral dimensions so essential for human survival.

Over reliance on technological rationality is but one of the humanitarian hazards that have to be considered in a futures context. Equally as disconcerting are persistent failures to appreciate the full consequences of any single technological innovation. Too often, hazards result from the propensity to see individual technological 'breakthroughs' as single, independent innovations – an inclination rife with hazards.

Interrelationships between different technologies are missed, misperceived or consciously ignored. Such 'stove piped' analyses could mean that the negative as well as positive consequences of interrelated technologies would be lost – that the positive impacts of one could not only be bypassed but could intensify the negative effects of others, with ensuing humanitarian impacts. Swathes of people might find that a single technological innovation may be transformative, but alone may well have created *exclusions* where loss of livelihoods and essential means of survival fall prey to its implementation.

Augmented reality (AR) is a case in point. AR blurs the difference between 'physical' and 'digital' worlds and by the 2030s, despite all its positive potential may well have the capacity to undermine human psychology and be a harbinger of disinformation. From a mid-21st century perspective, AR would be

> ...so pervasive that it becomes necessary to find ways to preserve a shared experience of reality in order to avoid compromising societal cohesion. The ability to create virtual experiences that are indistinguishable from reality makes it increasingly easy to manipulate people for commercial or political purposes...[7]

With AI innovations such as 'Chatbot' and 'Bing' in the early 2020s, there clearly has been a resurgence of concern across the planet that such technological transformations would begin to dominate ways that human beings understood the world in which they lived and would actively determine decisions that needed to be made to deal with increasing societal complexities.

Such concerns could trigger a range of proffered solutions. Some might be designed to ensure national control over on-going systems and others to establish international norms. All in various ways would most likely result in efforts to constrain those corporations responsible for designing and promoting such systems. Creating and enforcing legislation that would impose limits on the use of such technologies could in various ways happen – nationally and internationally. Humans, therefore, would in principle continue to determine and dominate global and interplanetary systems and behaviour.

However, what also has to be taken into account are the possibilities that in a foreseeable future bioengineering and algorithmic innovations would already determine the thought processes of a growing number of human beings. 'Brain enhancement', as described in the previous chapter, would involve implants in the human brain which could create capacities to draw upon vast amounts of data for problem solving and prioritising solutions.

Though in principle available to all, it would not be implausible that they would be provided to those with perceived societal value and status, which in turn would reflect significant social and economic divides.

It also is not implausible that a number of metaphorical 'Cyborgs' with brain implants would intentionally create vulnerabilities that in earlier times were referred to as 'cyber threats'. Now, when far more advanced, they might well be able to establish control over the priorities and decisions of those, wherever they might be, with contending interests. The result could well be that intentionally distorted or misprioritised information flows might for cyber victims result in calamities reflected in financial collapse, unintended conflicts, under resourced infrastructures and dissipation of vital assets.

In a humanitarian context, cyber manipulation could have a seeming endless list of consequences. They could deliberately distort information that would undermine production systems, resulting in resource scarcities and eventual impoverishment. They could subvert social service systems that might well lead to large swathes of populations deprived of adequate healthcare and indeed means of survival. And, they, too, could lead to initiatives that pitted one community against another or one state against another – all too possibly resulting in humanitarian consequences arising from conflicts, including mass displacement, breakdowns in means of livelihoods and lack of access to essentials for survival.

Box 4.2 Cognitive Manipulation, Brain Control Weaponry and Humanitarian Consequences

By 2051, cracks in the Mongolian state were becoming increasingly evident. Social unrest, reflected in more and more demonstrations and violence, were becoming norms, and as upheavals intensified, the poverty that affected approximately 29 per cent of the population was intensifying, taking a growing proportion of the population to the very brink of survival.

The government in Ulaanbaatar, Mongolia's capital, had few resources to deal with a humanitarian crisis of that proportion, and hoped to be able to rely on its neighbours, China and Russia, to provide vitally needed assistance. However, for both potential donor countries, there were long-running geopolitical differences that would to a very significant extent determine their respective 'humanitarian' responses'. These differences were about the Mongolian boundaries that divided the two countries.

China, for reasons historical and geopolitical, had always intended one day to absorb 'Outer Mongolia' into its Inner Mongolian province. Despite its 1946 commitment to respect Mongolia's independence and territorial integrity, China had actively begun to pursue its objective to have Mongolia absorbed into the People's Republic. Russia, on the other hand, saw Mongolia as an essential buffer between itself and a seemingly endlessly expanding China. Their positions were irreconcilable.

In Mongolia it was increasingly evident that government attempts to provide health services or food assistance were almost non-existent, that as the winter approached there was less and less fuel and other essentials. Yet, despite that burgeoning reality, neither China nor Russia had made any commitments about the provision of assistance.

China's delay was in no small part due to its hope that the ensuing crisis would result in the Mongolian government's collapse, opening the gateway for China's longed-for absorption – the massive provision of assistance to eventually be used as a tantaliser. However, the fact that Russia, under the circumstances, had as yet made no commitment was difficult to understand, particularly given its determination to maintain Mongolia as a buffer state.

What neither Russia nor Mongolia understood was that China was employing a brain control technology that had been changing the plans and priorities of Moscow's most senior leaders. It was a technology that was able 'to undermine an adversary's will and resolve, undermine perception and command capabilities to weaken fighting spirit and manipulate decision-making'.[8]

Russia's perceived disinterest in Mongolia's 'humanitarian fate' and China's delay in providing direly needed assistance led, as Beijing had calculated, to Mongolia's collapse. Outer Mongolia and Inner Mongolia would soon be merged – ultimately at the expense of almost 900,000 people who were victims of starvation and disease.

Though China had taken the lead in cognitive manipulation, it was not alone. A plethora of states and non-state actors had been going down similar tracks, and their abilities to distort the prioritisation and decision-making processes of those who lacked such capacities were clear.

Structural Fragmentation

As discussed in the previous chapter, governance constructs may well evolve in various ways over a generation's time. Historically, such transitions build upon the fragmentation of existing orders before they evolve into new forms and systems of governance. The period between the collapse of the Roman empire and the creation of the Byzantine empire, the 17th century's Thirty Years war and the eventual creation of the post-Westphalian nation-state, the period between the violent end of China's Qing Dynasty in 1912 and the eventual creation of the Chinese communist state are but three examples of the sorts of upheaval and turmoil that generally precede the restoration of some form of order.

From a humanitarian perspective, the issue is who would get caught up in that change process? Who will have the capacities to survive or indeed even flourish in those periods of fragmentation and who might not?

As one searches for answers, a reasonable starting point is the proposition that governance, *per se*, will be less and less state determined and authority and control would increasingly fall into the hands of different types of actors. The corporate world, for example, would most likely have increasing access to and control over resources both on this planet and beyond, and would not be reluctant to join coalitions to protect them – possibly with sophisticated cyber weaponry. Control, too, could be reflected in ethnic coalitions where those who belonged benefited, but those who did not were excluded. Technologies, too, could become exclusionary whether within states or outside them – those who were technologically empowered and those who were not.

In other words, from the perspective of fragmentation, human vulnerability would intensify because of parallel or competing forms and sources of governance and authority as well as the prospect that in certain circumstances there may be neither.

There are many assumptions that continue to be made about traditional governance structures. Even in a more polylateral world order, the role of the state, though probably diminished, will continue to be an important component. Here, however, the assumption is that over the next generation, more and more states will lose their capacities to control. As also suggested in the previous chapter, many will undergo geopolitical fragmentation, where some states will decompose into independent territories, while others may continue to be geopolitically unchanged, but have lost significant power, authority and control.

Those post-Second World War multilateral institutions intended to foster and promote world political and economic order might in a generation's time have very little sway over that fragmenting world order. In fact, their increased irrelevance might well be regarded as a symbol of the era. Core functions such as the IMF's monitoring of the world monetary system and the World Bank's focus on lending funds to middle and lower-income countries would have little relevance in a world in which predictable control over traditional and more and more virtual resources were collapsing.

Predictability and certitudes would be the victims of fragmentation and their collapse would further drive the fragmentation process. It goes without saying that such economic and financial possibilities would most likely reflect dysfunctions underway in the UN's Security Council and General Assembly. As for UN agencies and programmes, lack of any certainty about financing as well as contending interpretations about principles and erratic access to fluctuating geopolitical boundaries might further mirror the impacts of fragmentation.

And, as that period of fragmentation intensified, new types of vulnerabilities and consequent humanitarian crises could well emerge. For those who normally would have felt secure in a relatively predictable, if not stable world order, resources could have dramatically declined with little access to alternatives. Perhaps many governments and the institutions that defined their purpose, e.g. security, welfare, laws and legal enforcement, might begin to erode, frequently replaced by fractious quasi-state groupings. Laws might become more fungible, currencies less and less stable and means of security equally so.

That erosion process would reflect structural fragmentation, where 'norms' would be determined increasingly by interests groups based, for example, upon ethnicity, religion, social status and functional linkages, or, indeed by AGI based cognitive compatibilities. Survival or threats to survival might depend more and more upon the capacities of such non-state groupings to assert their respective powers than upon states' efforts to amalgamate and control.

The humanitarian consequences of fragmentation could take many forms and strike social and economic classes that hitherto would have been presumed to be resilient. Closely linked to losses of livelihoods and now the very basic means of survival could well be the ways that human rights were interpreted. Those who resisted the presumed benefits of the virtual state might find themselves deprived of their assets. There might emerge a 'cybernetically underclass', those who were unable to adapt to technological change and whose value therefore was perceived as nil.

As in the past, so, too, in a hypothetical future, minority and deprived groups with inadequate means could find themselves the victims of brutal massacres or at least life threatening deprivation. The historical precedence are of course all too evident. However, if one looked for a difference between the relative stability of the present polylateral world order and a plausible future, it could be that human rights and access to resources were less protected by the state but increasingly by cohorts of contending interests.

Box 4.3 From Slumscapes to No-Man's Lands
A Violent Continuum

Unfortunately, for many of the urban poor, their plight was at best a distraction. At worst, it resulted in the informal creation of what were called 'slumscapes' or, swathes of urban space to which an estimated 9 per cent of all urban poor, or 1,280,000 people, were consigned.

Yet, for those urban authorities that created slumscapes, their intention was not to provide permanent living space, but rather slumscapes were regarded as first steps before forced displacement. Where the displaced went was of little interest. All the authorities wanted to know was that those urban poor would not continue to be a drain on resources – no matter how minimal – and would not sully the city's reputation as an example of positive modernity.

The national government which ostensibly had authority over cities within its geopolitical boundaries found itself trapped in a dilemma. Cities were becoming quasi-independent. The wealth that they generated made the government more dependent upon them than vice versa, and the growing numbers of interlinked urban networks across borders compounded the difficulty for the government to assert its authority. Not only were those in the networks rich, but they also had adopted sophisticated security measures to protect themselves.

For the government, the dilemma was increasingly evident and its potential consequences profoundly disruptive. On the one hand, those cities and their powerful trans-border urban networks would not tolerate the prospect of large numbers of the impoverished moving into their respective zones. And, yet, the movement of the displaced was creating an equally as difficult problem.

Neighbouring states were making it clear that the government had to stem the flow of displaced before they became refugees. Refugees would 'not be tolerated'. At the same time, in-country urban authorities were making it equally as clear over and over again that the displaced should not be allowed to return, not even to the squalid slumscapes.

Government options were limited. There were few places where the displaced could go. Rural areas principally comprised successful agricultural lands and various self-contained 'industrial islands'. Neither offered substantive opportunities to consign the displaced. Cross border intergovernmental collaboration was obviously out of the question, and the only alternative at the time was to herd an estimated 1,280,000 impoverished persons into what were known as 'no-mans-lands' (NMLs).

NMLs, like slumscapes, were one of the few areas where the government had no vested interests other than that they belonged to the state. Barren wastelands much of which were virtually deserts had minimal infrastructures, few sources of potable water and energy and virtually no employment opportunities. Given the increasing persistence of those informal urban networks, the only option for the government was to create impenetrable barriers that would isolate the displaced.

These barriers now defined NMLs. While the government initially provided a modicum of assistance, it was clearly inadequate. Emerging, were growing clusters of gangs roaming the barren wastelands in search of subsistence. Conflict was intensifying the plight of the displaced, and disease and starvation were taking their toll.

As rumours about conflicts in the NMLs began to make their way into the capital, one minister was overheard to say, 'Of course, the government has no control over these urban goliaths. We had no other option. Well, at least those burgeoning conflicts might resolve the displacement problem... .'

If the polylateral world order plummeted into increasingly unpredictable atomisation, then hitherto unimagined types of fluctuating partnerships and alliances could well be the result.

Now, would it be too farfetched to imagine that with greater atomisation, there might well be increasing competition between states and non-state actors over resources as well as influence? Take, for example, the prospect of intense competition between global corporations and states that actually could result in violent confrontations, or conflicts arising from a combination of competing cohorts of corporate, state, and cyber connected ethnic and religious groupings.

Assuming that a growing proportion of production and livelihoods could depend to a significant extent – e.g. 25 per cent – upon resources from beyond the planet, fragmented governance and ever more space dependent corporations might also result in trade chaos and conflicts between a plethora of contending interest groups, far more complex and unpredictable than those solely Earth-based.

Those whose livelihoods would have become dependent upon predictable flows of resources might have to face very basic uncertainties. For example, to what extent would those unpredictable ebbs and flows of trade result in the collapse of Earth-dependent production systems which would leave the lives and livelihoods of specific groups dangerously exposed?

When it came to human vulnerability, seemingly relentless uncertainties would mean that access to resources – particularly the most basic resources such as shelter, food, potable water and clothing – were unpredictable. Much would depend upon who was accepted in which cohort, but that, too, was complicated by the ebbs and flows of persistent fragmentation and realignments.

Box 4.4 Interplanetary Fragmentation and the Callisto Crisis

A total of 32 rubber-inflated domes dotted the barren landscape of Callisto, the second largest of Jupiter's 87 moons. These simple constructs belied the reality that below the surface were terraformed habitats occupied by approximately 19,700 people.

The Callistolite community included a wide range of engineering and mining experts and their families. Supported by so called 'digital humans', the principal purpose of the Callisto community was to provide helium-3 isotope to be used as fuel for fusion reactors for habitats on two planets, Mars and Earth, as well as the largest space station to date, built by the Chinese government.

Originally created by a consortium of private and public sector organisations, the community had clearly become dependent upon four multiglobal corporates for adequate resources to survive, indeed well beyond survival! and in turn the corporates dominated a market that eventually would be calculated in terms of trillions of dollars. The importance of the Callistolites meant that every aspect of their needs were assured by so called 'corporate mentors'.

Now, however, by mid-century what once had been tightknit private-public partnerships were beginning to fray. States, frustrated by their inability to control and benefit from this lucrative trade, attempted to assert their authority over 'the helium-3 oligopoly'. There was no consensus among the states, themselves, about ways 'to guide', or, control the corporates. Both on Earth and via interplanetary intervention, at least 12 out of 126 states with developed space-based interests attempted to reverse that public-private sector power relationship.

Perceived self-interests meant that, whether for reasons either good or bad, no way to resolve the disagreements had emerged. Neither side backed down. The threat of conflict between the corporate conglomerates and those states with the capacities led to a standoff. Neither side was willing to challenge the other to gain access to Callisto. Access to Callisto was blocked.

Now, five weeks since the standoff, the first signs of malnutrition were appearing. Under the circumstances, there was really no way to prevent the decline in food and essential resources. Of even growing concern was that the chemicals required to maintain adequate oxygen levels could not be provided... .

Systems Collapse

The consequences of the collapse of a system are rarely due solely to the impact of any single system, but rather to the cascading impacts that one system's failure can trigger. That said, one system's failure in and of itself can nevertheless be a plausible threat.

Take, for example, the 'systems collapse' of the international banking system in 2007–2008. It offers a poignant example of potential 'systems collapse'. It demonstrated an inherent contradiction in the very nature of banking, per se, in a rapidly changing investment environment; it revealed the inconsistencies in governmental and intergovernmental approaches to respond to the crisis in coherent and consistent ways. Ultimately, it, too, brought to light the ways that such failures could trigger vulnerabilities that might have life impacting effects not merely upon the poor, but also those who otherwise assumed degrees of economic security.

As relevant are the implications of satellite communication failures. The collapse of a satellite communication system may be the result of cyberattacks, space debris, satellite collisions with other satellites or meteors or equipment deterioration. There are myriad reasons. In any event, their overall consequences are perhaps one of the most disconcerting examples of systems collapse and ultimately their humanitarian impacts.

Satellite collapse would disrupt virtually all aspects of global communications such as internet access, broadcasting, data transmission, phones and television. It, too, would clearly impact on navigation systems such as the Global Positioning System, means of transportation – including air and sea transport – scientific research, data identification and collection, weather forecasting, climate monitoring and the list goes on and on.

With such plausible threats stemming from the collapse of a satellite system, it would be surprising if it already did not rank high on most risk registers. One would also hope that their consequences would be assessed in terms of their more immediate as well as longer-term humanitarian implications. Disaster monitoring, including disasters triggered by natural events, as well as refugee flows, logistics operations, crisis anticipation and operational planning are all examples of the consequences of a systems collapse, in this case the vital links between a satellite communications system and humanitarian challenges.

The more complex the system, the greater is the ensuing disruption from its collapse.

Box 4.5 Trans-stellar Competition and Systems Collapse

The Democratic Republic of the Congo was no longer a single federal state. Since 2042, the highly centralised DRC had become a loose-knit amalgam of 12 semi-independent republics under the banner of the Congo Confederation. The people of those republics no longer had to suffer seemingly endless battles waged by federal leaders determined to maintain their authority from Kinshasa.

At long last the relentless conflicts and suffering had been replaced by a grouping of republics that were achieving societal wealth and growth which in turn had left myriad analyses of regional poverty well into the annals of a bypassed history.

One of the key drivers for this profound transformation was the impact of the mineral, tetrataenite. That recently discovered mineral in the Congo Confederation's state of Kasai had become of critical importance for creating magnets essential for a wide range of products, from drones and cyber systems to neural implants and satellites.

In the past, the majority of the provinces that had once comprised the DRC had had little benefit from the former republic's vast amounts of minerals. They were exported beyond the DRC to manufacturers more often than not in China, India, Europe and the United States.

Now, stability and relative harmony had been emerging because a considerable portion of the economic benefits of manufacturing was being undertaken by those former DRC provinces – those semi-autonomous states – fuelled by Kasai's abundance of tetrataenite. With the interchange between minerals and manufacturing, not only were economic benefits ever more evident, but so, too, social stability within and across the Confederation's components were developing in ways unimaginable in the times of the DRC.

Yet, as one began to approach the end of the 2040s, competition was emerging that few had anticipated. A potato-shaped asteroid referred to as Psyche-18 was found to contain US$ 7 quintillion worth of gold. However, even more valuable was the amount of tetrataenite that would almost double that amount. And, at the same time, the cost of robotic space mining and Earth-outer space transport systems radically dropped in price. Outer space mining began to compete with Earth-based markets and in more and more instances to dominate the market.

What was becoming increasingly evident was that the interface between minerals and manufacturing in the Confederation was being threatened. The competition for tetrataenite from Psyche sent the Kasai's income plummeting, but equally as threatening was that magnet manufacturing was more and more undertaken by manufacturing industries located on various outer space locations, principally Mars.

Still, by 2051, most of states in the Confederation and their related industries and social structures were able to keep their heads above water. Soon after, however, competition between the Confederation's components and Psche-18 and its related extra planetary manufacturing began to gnaw at the former. First Kasai and then the others began to collapse. Eroding financial security was beginning to be reflected in food deprivation and collapse of essential infrastructures needed for health, transport and energy systems.

Though not necessarily intended, the mining of asteroid Psyche-18 had brought down a confederated system that had transformed the horrors of the DRC into a stable, economically sound alternative. Now, conflict-related displacement and the very means of survival foretold instability and systems collapse.

One type of system can be replaced by another often without adequate attention paid to the consequences of the transition, itself. In a related vein, the challenges of moving from one system to another may be purposely bypassed, and the potential 'transition risks' consciously ignored. Alternatively, the transition from one system to another might be regarded as too risky, resulting in maintaining an earlier system that has less and less relevance. Or, clearly, knowledge about systems under focus may still be being developed, and systems collapse may precede in the interim.

As to the first, there has been a persistent concern that geo-engineered systems such as solar radiation management (SRM) might be introduced without adequately taking into account its consequences. This sort of transition risk, as noted in the previous chapter, was recognised by the UN's Fourth Committee (Special Political and Decolonisation) in 2014, and the concern was that SRM, which could serve the interests of wealthier states, would do so at the expense of those states that had alternative, less expensive systems in place.

The prospect that moving from one system to another is deemed too risky may result in the collapse of the perceived safe option and the failure to prepare the way for another. Often the decline or collapse of systems can result from unfinished research or analysis of systems threats and opportunities.

All such prospects in one way or another have serious humanitarian implications. Failure to anticipate infrastructure weaknesses such as dams, roads, water and sewage systems can be life threatening, and, despite an upsurge in the attention given to the societal consequences of AI systems, too few have focused on their humanitarian implications. Introducing and maintaining systems without adequate preparation or analyses of their implications can drive large portions of societies to that brink – too often not appreciating their consequences until it is too late.

Box 4.6 Plutonium Leakages and the Systems Transition Risk

It was uncertain why there was such an unprecedented upsurge in lung disease and cancer in the towns and rural areas along the banks of the Columbia River. The fact, however, was that in a portion of the United States renowned for its commitment to ecological and human well-being, an estimated 50,000 people had been diagnosed with one or both diseases over the course of two months. That meant an increase in cases of 42 per cent beyond the norm. It was a shocking statistic for a region of 2.5 million in total, and more than disconcerting for policy planners responsible for them.

What few had foreseen was that the Columbia River in the US state of Washington was riddled with plutonium. And, it was that plutonium by 2042 that was taking its toll on the local populations.

Just under a century before, in 1950, plutonium that had initially been created for the production of nuclear weapons had been buried in 42 miles of unlined pits in what became the Hanford complex. That complex followed the bend of the Columbia River and contained an estimated 120 million gallons of high-level waste and another 444 billion gallons of contaminated liquid.[9]

To everyone's horror, in 2017, one of the tunnels created to bury low-level waste collapsed. Clearly over 3/4s of a century, the system had weakened. The leakage had to be stopped urgently and further collapse prevented as quickly as possible. According to the US government's Department of Energy, the most effective way to stop the leakage was to dump tens of thousands of tonnes of dirt where the collapsed tunnel had been.

What had not been taken into account was that the dirt once placed in the weakened unlined pits would also become low level radioactive waste. Now, towards the end of 2037, the threat intensified as increasing amounts of plutonium flowed into the Colorado River. The numbers of victims surpassed those who had been affected twenty years before.

A major system had collapsed, which eventually was acknowledged. However, what became all too evident was that inadequate attention continued to be given to trying to understand not only the cause of the crisis but also the possibility that there might be alternative ways of dealing with it.

Natural Hazards

Natural hazards might be triggers, but they are not disasters, per se. It is the man-made context which explains why natural hazards transform into humanitarian threats and crises.

Climate change is clearly an example of fundamental changes in physical environments that have been altered by the ways that human beings have used and increasingly exploited natural resources, including air, water, soil, woodlands and on and on. The consequences of this sort of 'natural hazard' is clearly recognised and similarly its humanitarian impacts. As the head of the International Federation the Red Cross/Red Crescent Societies already noted in 2019, 'By 2050, 200 million people every year could need international humanitarian aid as a result of a cruel combination of climate related disaster and the socioeconomic impact of the climate change.'[10] This would be nearly twice the estimated 108 million people who needed help in 2019.

Yet, beyond this generally accepted truth, there are others that also need to be recognised for their potential humanitarian consequence. Certainly, one is the collapse of biodiversity. Though closely linked to climate change, biodiversity loss is in and of itself a natural hazard because without it the very substance of much that is essential for human existence.

The World Health Organization, for example, had estimated that traditional medicines based upon local plants were successfully used by 60 per cent of the world's population. Although synthetic medicines have been increasingly available for many purposes, the global needs and demands for natural products persist. Medicinal products and biomedical research would continue to rely on plants, animals and microbes to understand human physiology and to understand and treat human diseases.[11]

Covid-19 was deemed to be a clear case in point:

> a reminder of the intimate and delicate relationship between people and planet. Biodiversity loss, ecosystem degradation and other human-driven disturbances are increasingly linked to the occurrence, risk and spread of zoonotic and vector-borne diseases. In many instances, climate change acts as a threat multiplier.[12]

From the perspective of plausible humanitarian crises, human disregard for loss will inevitably lead to a growing number of pools of vulnerability. Uncontrolled urban sprawl as well as rural areas could well find themselves facing severe malnutrition and infectious diseases. The latter would most likely become sources of pandemics, pathogens carried across borders that could eventually be spread around the world, for example, by avion flocks.

Of course, geological time-bombs, such as the prospect of a major landslide in the Canary Islands is another example of a so-called natural hazard. Once unleashed, these sorts of phenomena could create gigantic tidal waves far bigger than any normal tsunami. Crossing at speeds of up to 500 miles per hour and in many places at heights equivalent to at least two Empire State buildings, scientists have predicted that over a period of 8 hours these mega-tsunamis could devastate cities in the United States such as New York as well as on the West African coastline and the coastal regions of Western Europe.

The ripple effects of a mounting number of natural hazards will inevitably lead to humanitarian crises because humans ignored or misunderstood their potential consequences. Many future disasters, in other words, will form part of a challenging terrain of seemingly improbable events, which may not have grabbed the attention of those concerned with humanitarian threats.

Box 4.7 The Nature of Sand and Societal Polarisation

'Still, no one has really done anything about it,' commented the former head of UNEP's Global Resource Information Database. 'Here we are 30 years after we signed a global agreement on reconfiguring the use of sand, and few governments, private sector or community organisations have done anything to reduce its use.' He then went on to say that 'our entire society is built on sand. It is the world's most consumed raw material after water and an essential ingredient to our everyday lives. If we don't protect it, we on this planet will all be losers.'

Even in 2050, despite mounting warnings, sand continued to be the primary substance used in infrastructures and virtually all technologies across the world, and it now really was beginning to run out. Whether exponential increases in urban infrastructures, lunar space elevators, windows, computer screens, brain implants or even land regeneration projects, the global rate of sand usage had increased fourfold since 2019. That far exceeded the natural rate at which sand was being replenished by the weathering of rocks by wind and water. And, at the same time, while many essential minerals were being transported from various sources in outer space, the importation of sand in adequate amounts was just not financially feasible.

What choices did the global community have? Many impoverished peoples along river embankments or coastlines relied on 'sand mining' for basic incomes. The options between preserving the environment or ensuring production of even the most basic technologies, of supporting local and global corporations or protecting natural resources remained at best wavering. There were, of course, numerous meetings with what was officially designated as the 'Global Survival Alliance' as far back as 2026.

Yet, as one senior official observed, 'After years of consultation, no big plans, no standards on how sand should be extracted, no land planning on where you should extract and where you should not extract, no monitoring of where it is coming from in most of the places and no enforcement of laws because relevant authorities continue to ponder ways to reconcile such basic resource contradictions – between development needs and the protection of the environment, between economic growth and planetary security.'

And, all the while, availability of vital sand was being depleted. The poverty of those dependent upon sand mining brought them increasingly towards the precipice of survival. Less anticipated was the result that many globally priced goods, dependent upon sand-related products, were becoming out of reach to middle-class people in some of the wealthiest countries. These changes to the global incomes ladder generated intensifying polarisation between a new 'middle class poor' and governments that had failed to come to decisions about ways to preserve that essential source of societal building blocks – sand.

Another plausible natural hazard could be the result of 'space debris' penetrating the Earth's atmosphere. While the term is generally interpreted as the 'junk' which results from human interventions such as satellite collisions, space debris also includes natural phenomena such as pieces of cometary and asteroidal material called meteoroids.

As opposed to asteroids and comets which ostensibly can be diverted from the planet,[13] it is increasingly assumed that such space debris could result in expanded holes in the ozone layer and increased radiation, both leading to significant destruction of agriculture and exponentially expanding health threats such as cancer.

Perhaps even more likely is that the demographic swing from rural to urban will have made the impacts of space debris far more destructive than in the past. When urban conurbations were smaller and less populated and rural areas more extensive, space debris might have gone unnoticed. (Even a single meteor might have gone relatively unnoticed.[14]) However, as debris that ranges from the size of a car to that of a snowflake roar through the Earth's atmosphere at up to 28,000 km/hour, they can become projectiles.[15] City centres could become inadvertent targets, and the calamity arising from the 2001 destruction of New York's World Trade Center is a small reminder of a much larger humanitarian consequence that could be.

Box 4.8 Space-Based Pathogens

The United Nations had warned that one of the most pressing problems facing modern medicine was the mutation of bacteria becoming resistant to antibiotics. The UN had estimated that by 2050, such resistance could claim up to 10 million lives a year – more than double the current toll. It so happened that the United Nations had been right. Even by 2050, however, ways to deal with the rapid change of bacterial pathogens remained uncertain.

The one thing though that had become very evident was that the bacteria which could cause diseases in humans could also be infected by viruses – bacteriophages. This meant that when the virus's descendants went on to infect other bacteria, they would transfer bacterial genetic material, too – at a rate several thousands times faster than any other known process.[16]

Though there had been varying degrees of success to address this potentially existential issue, the underlying assumption of scientists seeking to deal with those rapidly transforming pathogens was that they were essentially Earth-based. Their rapid development, the virologists believed, stemmed solely from dynamic transitions among bacteriophages on the planet.

Only recently had that assumption begun to be challenged. A group of astronomers and cosmologists put forth the proposition that bacteriophages might also be generated in man-made materials now clustering as space debris in Lower Earth Orbit. As such debris came crashing on to planet earth, they brought with them other forms of rapidly transforming viruses.

Now, there was growing concern that the United Nations' original prediction might have been too low.

Dimensions and Dynamics of Crisis Threats

From the local to the global, all societal phenomena, including humanitarian crisis drivers and crisis threats, reflect and will continue to reflect highly complex 'messes', namely, multiple complex systems that are in a constant state of flux. The words of two well-known risk analysts ring all too true:

> People are not confronted with problems that are independent of each other, but with dynamic situations that consist of complex systems of changing problems that interact with each other… *messes*. Problems are abstractions extracted from messes by analysis. Therefore, when a mess, which is a system of problems, is taken apart, (i.e., analysed), it loses its essential properties and so does each of its parts. The behaviour of a mess depends more on how the treatment of its parts interact than how they act independently of each other.[17]

To that extent all crisis drivers and crises, themselves, share this common attribute. In a related vein, the proposition that crises are not bound by time or space but are in constant flux also reemphasises the point that very few, if any, crises are isolated phenomena. Here, again, this was evident in the aftermath of the 1755 Lisbon earthquake.[18] Three centuries after, where virtually all phenomena directly and indirectly spilled over into others in an ever more globalised world, the proposition should become increasingly difficult to ignore.

When considering the dimensions and dynamics of plausible crisis drivers in the future, it is important to recognise that the impact of such drivers have not only significant catastrophic consequences in and of themselves, but their impacts are compounded by the ways that they trigger or mesh with other crisis drivers. The interacting nature of crisis drivers is an inherent feature, and is captured in terms such as *cascading risks*, *synchronous failures* and *simultaneous crises.*

If there is any difference between the use of such terms in a generation's time and now, it will be because the very locations in which they might be felt and the sheer complexities arising from hitherto unaccounted for or unknown types of triggers will have been at play. The dynamics may in many instances be recognisable, but their exponentially increasing consequences far less so.

Interacting Nature of Crisis Drivers

By 2050 it is probable that the number of crisis drivers will significantly increase. Hundreds of millions and in some circumstances billions of lives might have to contend not only with ever more complex crisis drivers but also with the consequences of the ways more and more crisis drivers interact from longitudinal (viz, timeframes) as well as latitudinal (viz, crisis interactions) perspectives.

Of course, the interacting nature of crisis drivers is more than evident when it comes to climate change and the collapse of biodiversity. Flooding, air pollution, weather variability, declines in agricultural and water availability are just a few of the severely interconnected consequences of both. Yet, when it comes to dealing with various types of crises more generally, all too often their possible interconnections are ignored or at least not adequately explored. What policy planners and decision-makers also too often fail to recognise is that the impacts of interacting crisis drivers inevitably create greater havoc and disruption in their totality than their individual impacts otherwise would.

Box 4.9 The Waters of the Third Pole and Interacting Crises

The Hindu Kush-Himalayan (HKH) region extends some 3,500 km from Afghanistan in the west to Myanmar and China in the east, and runs through Pakistan, Nepal, India, Bangladesh and Bhutan.

It continues to be the world's greatest source of natural hazards. They range from earthquakes, floods, mass land movements, deltic flooding, natural contamination, fires and atmospheric brown clouds. When linked to human intervention and related impacts upon agriculture, health, water quality, population growth, demographic shifts, the HKH region had already by 2045 witnessed an estimated 500 million people directly affected by unprecedented food insecurity, new forms of disease, mass displacement, major habitat and infrastructure collapse, demise of livelihoods and intensification of conflict.

The reason for such humanitarian crises is due to vast amounts of meltwater. HKH is one of the most geographically active zones on Earth and the mountains are still growing as India continues to push northwards into Eurasia. Such is the size, elevation and climate of this region that it hosts the largest areas of glaciers, snow and permafrost outside of high latitudes, which is why it has become known as the Third Pole.

The Third Pole holds huge reservoirs of frozen fresh water that are the sources of ten of the world's greatest rivers. This so-called 'water tower of Asia' represents one of the most extreme natural and cultural environments of the world. The drainage basins of these rivers cover an area of 8.6 million square kilometres, which is equivalent to the size of Brazil, and provide water for an estimated 4.3 billion people or around 43 per cent of the world's population. That population directly and indirectly benefit from the water, food and energy provided by the river basins that originate in the HKH region.

All the main rivers originating in the HKH region are fed to some degree by glacial meltwater, with 40–45 per cent of the river flows in the Indus and Tarim coming from melting.

The proportion of glacial melt in river flows has been increasing well beyond initial scientific assessments as the majority of glaciers in the HKH region continue to recede due in no small part to climate change. Increased melting has been increasing the volume of water in rivers and that has now led to wider spread flooding. At the same time, as glaciers have been receding and, in some instances, disappearing, the amount of meltwater has been significantly decreasing.

> *With decreasing groundwater, recharge rates have also been declining substantially. This, in combination with reduced surface flows and variations in summer monsoon precipitation, has been leading to highly significant water stress in many parts of the HKH region and associated river basins.*

Cascading Risks from a Futures Perspective

Cascading risks, here, will be described as the result of a chain of events compounding the impacts on a whole system, including people, infrastructure, the economy, societal systems and ecosystems.[19] 'They are the new reality,' noted two well recognised experts. 'Fault and event trees can be compiled in order to investigate the vulnerability paths by which cascading impacts are propagated.'[20]

From a futures perspective, plausible cascading risks would include drivers, the dimensions and dynamics of which trigger multiple 'lines of dominoes' that are widely disbursed, difficult to anticipate, where connections are highly complex and where interactions and their consequences are inconsistent and unpredictable.

The list of plausible crisis drivers that, like dominoes, will cascade into each other appears endless. Such cascading risks could be triggered by threats to the biodiversity of Earth's ecosphere, global economic depressions and the imposition of stifling cultural or religious eras such as the dark ages. They, too, include what might be called the smaller messes, those that also stem from myriad possibilities, from resource-related conflict to the interplay between natural hazards and industrial phenomena, from nuclear accidents and extensive radiation poisoning to urban infrastructure collapse.

And, yet, they all share common characteristics. Cascading risks may initially be geographically defined but ultimately have no boundaries. Their consequences spill across geo-political and socio-economic systems in ways complex, uncertain and unpredictable. One kind of crisis driver inevitably triggers others, and their ripple effects eventually but not instantly become global. They are transformative; they may take their toll in terms of millions of lives affected and livelihoods lost. They would include the ripple effects that stem from a natural event, e.g. a tsunami, that would in turn trigger a major industrial accident, e.g. destruction of a nuclear energy plant, which would result in mass displacement, unemployment and deep poverty.

Another example would be the plausible consequences of a nuclear exchange between Pakistan and India. It has been suggested that it might well lead in some still undetermined but plausible future to the deaths of 20 million people in both countries. In its aftermath, five million tonnes of soot could lift high into the atmosphere and shroud the sunlight. Surface temperatures drop to minus 1.3 centigrade. Corn production in the US falls significantly as does rice production in China. And the result, according to ICAN's Ira Helford, in her presentation at the Norwegian Government's conference on nuclear threats, is one billion dead.[21]

Box 4.10 Cascading Impacts of Magma Blobs

Most recent figures were that around 280,000 people had been killed over the past two days, with an estimated 180,000 awaiting medical attention and at least 78,000 unaccounted for. That grim news permeated across South America and beyond, but more particularly in the states of Colombia and Paraguay where cascading crises were ramping up death tolls at a pace few could imagine.

A cascade of crises affecting both countries was initially triggered by a volcanic explosion near the town of Mesa de Herveo, about 129 km from Colombia's capital Bogotá. According to the geologists and engineers who had been on site, the explosion was no ordinary volcanic event but rather the result of an energy company's deep drilling into magma layers in order to capture the energy from so-called magma blobs. That energy would provide heat that would generate virtually 1/3 of the country's energy for what was described as 'permanent' and 'at no cost'.

Puncturing one of those blobs, however, had led to lava and poisonous gas flows that were far greater than those from normal eruptions, and spread for hundreds of miles in matters of minutes. Such dangers had been recognised by geologists and engineers as well as by the government for many years, but the opportunity to produce so much energy at such consistent levels and so cheaply made the 'unlikely risks' of magma mining acceptable.

Tragically, the experts proved right. At least 100,000 in the town that bordered the volcano had become victims of that miscalculation. However, the tragedy was compounded by the fact that the poisonous gases resulting from the magma explosion, were stalling aircraft in flight. In fact, two aircrafts on their way to Paraguay's capital, Asunción, were 'frozen'.

Both crashed, with the loss of 532 passengers and crew, and one plummeted down into the huge hydroelectric dam, the Itapúa, on the Parana River between Brazil and Paraguay.

Water from the collapsed dam roared across at least 1,460 square kms of agricultural lands and villages. How many people had lost their lives remained uncertain, but it was assumed that the figure would be at least 2,000. Whatever the actual number, the loss resulted in violent protests against local and central authorities – for once again, local populations felt justified in condemning the dam's construction as had previous generations.

No one initially assumed that their tragedy had begun with deep drilling into a volcano more than 3,442 miles away.

Synchronous Failures in 2050. *Synchronous failures*, or, intersystemic crisis drivers are 'where multiple stresses interact within a single social-ecological system to cause a shift in that system's behaviour'.[22] Such stresses can in turn lead to crises that can propagate across multiple system boundaries even on to a global scale. According to Homer-Dixon, the term's creator, synchronous failures reflect 'the convergence of stresses that's especially treacherous and make synchronous failure a possibility as never before. In coming years our societies won't face one or two major challenges at once, as usually happened in the past. Instead, they'll face an alarming variety of problems – likely, including oil shortages, climate change, economic instability, and mega-terrorism – all at the same time.'[23]

One of the key characteristics of a synchronous failure is the number of 'blind spots', or unanticipated issues that are inherent in systems' collapse. The unintended consequences – an inevitable part of all crises – become even more apparent when it comes to synchronous failure. A small though very relevant example are the consequences stemming from the Eyjafjallajökull volcano erupted in Iceland in April 2010. While it was a relatively small eruption, it caused enormous damage to air travel across western and northern Europe over an initial period of six days. Few had anticipated such consequences, neither aircraft manufacturers nor airline companies had considered let alone prepared at all for such a small example of a synchronous failure also is a reflection on the nature of blind spots.

That such 'blind spots' can lead to broad systems collapse was evidenced in Mumbai in 2005 when the city and surrounding areas suffered a multi-sector systems failure. When it came to the city's essential services, all went down at once – due in no small part to planners' earlier decision to remove a mangrove ecosystem that served as a buffer between land and sea. In a torrential rainstorm the lack of that buffer exacerbated the rainstorm's impact, leading to simultaneous collapse of essential services, including the mobile phone and electricity systems. Two years before, in Ottawa, a 'software bug' in the US state of Ohio's First Energy Company collapsed, affecting transmission lines, which in turn brought all the city's essential services to a standstill.

The cause of the system's failure was due to overgrown foliage along the transmission line, and within a very short span of time affected 10 million people in Ontario and another 45 million in 8 US states. In both cases, broad system's collapse occurring synchronistically is inevitably compounded by blind spots.

Nuclear weapons, *per se*, could certainly fit into the category of a synchronous-type threat. It clearly provides a good example of a 'convergence of stresses', where anticipated as well as unanticipated factors, can generate crises on a global scale. When considering the wide range of options in the world of nuclear, biological and chemical threats, it is the nuclear in its various guises that would appear to generate the most obvious ultra-mess. This in no sense is to suggest that biological and chemical threats could not have devastating and often enduring effects upon billions. Rather the nuclear issue, perhaps more clearly, demonstrates unanticipated as well as anticipated issues that are inherent in systems' collapse.

The consequences of a nuclear event would seem difficult to limit. The immediate deaths of hundreds of millions, if not billions, of lives, the destruction of governance structures, economies, most forms of social services, food production and water systems would be simultaneous, and the inevitable 'nuclear winter' would result in soot lofted into the stratosphere causing a multi-year cooling and drying of the world.

The threats discussed under the heading of synchronous failures underscore two points. The first is that threats have to be seen far more globally, interconnected and interrelated than in the past; secondly, no matter how seemingly improbable the threat may be, their effects can be existential for a significant portion of human beings in large portions of the planet, if not for the planet as a whole.

Box 4.11 Synchronicity and the Overshoot

Seventy per cent of the members of the recently formed Global Science Council now believed that the sixth mass extinction was underway. The 2048 Millennium Ecosystem Report (MER) said it all. All the warnings that had been made for the past half century about the interaction between key ecological hazards were coming to the fore – interacting in ways that was potentially existential on a global scale. However, what this third edition of the MER had failed to take into account were the unprecedented numbers of human beings that were already being driven to and over the brink of survival.

Human populations by mid-century were larger than initially forecast, 10.6 billion people were taking basic means of human survival well past safe and sustainable levels. Forests had rapidly disappeared despite endless warnings of the eventual consequences when it came to carbon absorption. Deserts were expanding well beyond what even some of the most pessimistic forecasters had imagined, agricultural lands had been increasingly degraded, in no small part due to the persistent use of biochemical fertilisers, water scarcity across the globe was becoming a new norm, and ocean acidification was a recognised but unresolved threat. That 1.5 degree climate target had never really been achieved.

All reflected multiple crisis drivers which were interacting across the world's essential and all-pervading socio-ecological system. Their synchronicity now presented the Earth's population with a threat to the very survival of the human species. There seemed little possibility that the full consequences of those crisis drivers could be sufficiently reduced in time.

Of course, there continued to be initiatives intended to reduce the consequences of such synchronicity. These, however, were at best 'tactical' but with no commitment to an overarching strategy. Efforts to dredge plastics from the oceans, to establish space-based solar panels, to attempt to have governments restrict the destruction of forests were all examples of tactical adjustments.

What the world now faced goes back to warnings by scientists in the early part of the century. Already then, there were warnings that the Earth was approaching 'overshoot'. In other words, if the number of human beings continued to grow exponentially, continued to consume all available resources and expand in all 'suitable habitats', humanity will have exceeded the very carrying capacity of the Earth. The only way to draw back from the edge of that ultimate existential threat was to radically reduce consumption, waste and ultimately promote radical population reduction.

Of course, none was adequately achievable. Few decision-makers and policy planners dared venture into such politically uncertain territory. Overshoot was inevitable.

Now, across the globe – north and south, east and west – over 180,000 people were dying each day for reasons directly attributable to ecological crisis drivers. This figure was about day-to-day deaths, and did not include those who were losing their livelihoods nor who had to contend with disease, water impurity and malnutrition as well as suffocating heat waves.

For decision-makers, the challenge was to deal with both the immediate and the longer term, and the will to do so was not apparent.

Simultaneous Crises

Clearly related to synchronous failure are the consequences of simultaneous crises. During the first two decades of the 21st century, the number and types of crises faced by the international community increased significantly, if not exponentially. All too often crisis drivers might have been ignored or relegated to categories such as 'of marginal significance' or 'let's wait and see', but as the statistics made evident, a widening array of crisis threats and crises had been emerging, and in an increasingly inter-related world, often those crises, though occurring independently and simultaneously, impacted others.[24]

Geographical proximity may have little consequence when it comes to simultaneous crises. A case in point is the parallel occurrence of financial volatility in developed and some middle-income countries and severe droughts in lower-income countries. The former, the 'financially liberated' are generally speaking willing to accept the risk of fluctuating assets, everything from bonds and market shares to house prices and lifestyles. Hence, market collapse as was evident in 2008 can directly and indirectly threaten the very well-being of 'the liberated'.

The latter, drought-affected, have generally had resources, e.g. extractive resources, that formed the basis of varying degrees of trade between developed countries and themselves. Now, it could be foreseen that with a major decline in agriculture, those resources would be needed even more by some middle and lower-income countries to offset the disruptions caused by radically declining agriculture. However, the downward spiralling markets of many developed economies could well have made it more difficult for farmers to access the funds they would need to maintain normal production levels.

While both drought and financial crises may be occurring within approximate timeframes, not only could they be taking place in different geographical locations, but as types of crises they are distinctly different. And, yet, both, though simultaneous and separate, will compound the impact of the other.

It, too, is evident that the plethora of crises makes determining how to prioritise responses extremely difficult. If one looks at the increasing number of famines that had been occurring in many countries in the Middle East and southern Africa between 2019 and 2022, when it came to response, which were prioritised and why? In a related vein, potential threats may not be recognised as such, but when they are, often the prospect of spillovers overs are ignored and instead siloed perspectives tend to dominate. Furthermore, the impacts of simultaneous crises may become apparent at different times.

Though earlier the Hindu Kush Himalaya (HKH) portrait was used as an example of cascading risks, it, too, can be used as a good example of simultaneous crises. At least six types of natural phenomena: floods, earthquakes, mass movements, hazards in deltas and coastal zones, arsenic contamination, and fires and atmospheric brown clouds occurred at different times, but rarely addressed as interlocking phenomena.

When combined with the effects of human activities, these phenomena could plausibly lead to severe humanitarian crises in the HKH region. These six hazards could trigger crises resulting from food insecurity, mass migration, destruction of human habitats and infrastructure, damage to industry and livelihoods, and exponential increases in disease and conflict.[25] And, yet, their cumulative impacts and interrelatedness might too often be ignored, miscalculated or misunderstood.

Borrowing from the concept of synchronous failures, simultaneous crises can eventually result in multiple stresses that could readily impact a 'single social-ecological system', and in so doing go well beyond the effects of simultaneous crises. Might simultaneous crises eventually lead to crises that can propagate across multiple systems, even on a global scale? For now, however, the category of simultaneous crises serves to ask what such draining events might look like if they occurred in parallel?

For those with humanitarian roles and responsibilities, the sheer magnitude of such simultaneous events demonstrates the importance of ensuring effective local, national and regional capacities. However, in pointing to this self-evident truth, there will be a critical factor to bear in mind in anticipating and communicating risk. 'Local', per se, in the longer term will have less to do with geo-physical space, and far more to do with interactions driven by web-based systems, including teleportation, tactile communications and atomised networks. How this will work into preparedness and response planning will be a core element in preparing for crises in general, and certainly for crises that strike simultaneously.

Box 4.12 Simultaneous Crises

An unparalleled global financial crisis, a bioengineered 'superbug' and a meteor's destruction of a space-based communications network – none implausible, all possibly happening simultaneously.

Debt was being used not surprisingly to drive economic growth, allowing immediate consumption and investment against the promise of paying back the borrowing in the future. Global credit had grown from $109 trillion to $312 trillion. Hence, spending that would have taken place normally over a period of years was accelerated based on the availability of debt.

Now, within one year, the debt-credit dynamics made the financial markets more complex, opaque and system-wide leverage exploded. As a result, an emerging financial crisis was becoming more threatening, and what ensued was unprecedented, so severe that it pushed the global economy to the brink of a depression far worse than that of 1929.

Fear of financial and economic collapse required government rescue efforts that should have been far greater than those of 2007–2008. However, the leadership and cooperation needed as well as the sacrifices that would result from seemingly draconian measures were unacceptable to many key high and middle-income countries.

It was inevitable that unprecedented levels of unemployment would ensue along with the collapse of industries. The majority of governments, whatever their levels of development, could not generate adequate resources required for any significant forms of recovery. Lack of agricultural investment, infrastructural decline, reduction in medical services and consequent social unrest all presaged a major global crisis.

In the midst of the financial crisis emerged a 'designer bug'. In the words of experts, 'As ill-equipped as we may be to fight newly emergent natural pathogens, we are even less prepared to cope with engineered pathogens. In the coming decades, it may become possible to create pathogens that fall well outside the range of infectious agents modern medicine has learned to detect, treat, and contain.'

Efforts to stem the impact of the laboratory-created pathogens and to restore global financial stability were inevitably dependent upon effective communications across myriad institutions and experts. However, added to this scenario was the collapse of communications networks based in outer space.

Due to a collision with a passing meteor several of the essential communication systems would be disabled for a period lasting days, if not weeks. The possibility of such a collision happening was increasingly accepted. That it had happened at the same time as the financial crash and the bio-engineered super virus was by no means implausible.

It was part of a situation of simultaneous crises, which left those with humanitarian roles and responsibilities facing an unprecedented pandemic at a time when the collapse of the international financial system had led maybe billions without means of survival – and when communications were unstable at best.

No one had anticipated the impact of these simultaneous crises. How could one have assessed whom might be affected? What sorts of systems were in place to deal with such multiple threats? Was it even possible to say at the time who could provide assistance?

Drawing Back from the Brink

Possible – perhaps. Probable – who knows? Yet, having taken the reader to the brink of various futures-focussed humanitarian catastrophes, it is now time to see what lessons might be learned in order to draw back from the edge of those dystopic cliffs.

For example, how does the reader now think about the future? What is the reader's speculative framework? How should strategists concerned with human vulnerability define future, and for what purposes? What are the underlying assumptions that underpin that definition? What are realistic timeframes for policy planners and decision-makers to begin to prepare for a future in which it is more than likely that the types, dimensions and dynamics of humanitarian crises will increase exponentially?

To what extent do they focus on the prospect of the very nature of vulnerability significantly expanding? Might the lack of attention to sand depletion serve as yet another example of policy planners' and decision-makers' failure to focus adequately on the types of crisis threats that increasingly will demand the attention of those concerned with threats to life and livelihoods?

On a strategic level, when it came to efforts to promote pristine oceans, the governments of Indonesia, Malaysia and Vietnam were so singularly fixated that they had accepted the highly focused programmes and processes of their AGI systems. AGI had ignored the lateral dimensions so essential for human survival, and the three governments were willing to bypass tortuous and complex negotiations, and chose instead AGI's technological rationality. Are such scenarios plausible?

Both suggest a common theme that might be recognised in principle but not always in practice, namely, that policy planning and decision-making are not only overly focused on the immediate but all too often on a single or single set of factors. All too often the interconnections between these and a much wider range of potential crisis drivers ignored, excused away or forgotten.

Siloed perspectives are by no means a new theme. Yet, given the growing complexities that will mark future vulnerabilities, conceptual silos pose ever more serious hazards. How can such hazards be overcome in order to identify, mitigate and prepare for increasingly integrated and interrelated humanitarian threats?

Siloed solutions can also be exclusionary, even those, or perhaps, particularly those that are technologically defined and implemented. That certainly was the case when and where rational motives led to solutions that excluded those that were most likely to be in greater need and included those that would be less vulnerable – all for seemingly rational reasons.

Assumptions about the changing nature of human agency and space also need to be explored by those seeking to anticipate and mitigate potential humanitarian threats. With that in mind, the reader should consider the implications and consequences of new types of materials and resources on potentially vulnerable communities. Clearly, that issue was ignored when asteroid mining had crippled a good portion of mining-dependent communities in what had once been the Democratic Republic of the Congo.

And, can the reader assume that conventional state structures and international institutions ultimately will be relatively consistent providers or even 'providers of last resort', or, will those with humanitarian roles and responsibilities have to face the prospect that preparedness and response will require constructs that are far more atomised or at least more polylateral? That certainly was suggested when witnessing the rationale for violent displacement in no-man's lands, or the abandonment of vulnerable communities on Jupiter's moon, Calisto.

Reflecting on the response to the existential crisis that had been underway on Calisto, an increasingly inescapable issue arises – who and what is 'the humanitarian actor'? Self-interests and a growing awareness of mutual self-interests may well be the ultimate determinant as the dimension and dynamics of crisis threats rapidly expand. Crisis impacts will be less and less isolated events. They will spill over in various ways, intensifying existing vulnerabilities and creating new ones – irrespective of geographical locations and economic strength.

When a synchronous failure was triggered by policy planners reluctance to understand the consequences of overshoot, and when the depletion of water in China's Shiyang River generated displacement and conflict in South Asia as well as the Far East, and when simultaneous crises wreaked havoc in cities and farmlands bordering the Columbia River in North America, the case for more global and longer-term approaches for anticipating and dealing with exponentially increasing types, dimensions and dynamics of humanitarian crises would seem to be all too apparent.

The last four chapters, which discuss the theme *Destination – Planning from the Future*, provide practical strategies for policy planners and decision-makers to move well away from the brink towards more effective ways to identify, monitor and mitigate humanitarian threats, now and in the future.

As will be seen, one step in that direction is an appreciation of an increasing *entanglement nexus* which will mean that humanitarian action will increasingly be driven by mutual self-interests. A second step is to appreciate how a changing and more polylateral global architecture can be used to enhance humanitarian anticipation and response.

That said, so much effective humanitarian threat identification and mitigation will depend upon the capacities of *the organisation*. What that means in practice will be a third step that will lead into that final step, that Helenus alternative to make *planning from the future* actionable.

Notes

1 Interview with Nobel Laureate, Roger Penrose, in Michael Brooks, 'The context', *New Scientist*, 19 November 2022, p. 46.
2 See, for example, Delan Devakumar, Geordan Shannon, Sunil Bhopal, Ibrahim Abubakar 'Racism and discrimination in Covid-19 responses', *The Lancet*, 1 April 2020, https://doi.org/10.1016/S0140-6736(20)30792-3; Jun He et al., 'Discrimination and social exclusion in the outbreak of COVID-19', *International Journal of Environmental Res. Public Health* 2020, 17 (8), 2933, https://doi.org/10.3390/ijerph17082933
3 Nassim Nicholas Taleb, *The black swan: The impact of the highly improbable*, Penguin Books, 2008
4 'Reports that say that something hasn't happened are always interesting to me, because as we know, there are known knowns; there are things we know we know. We also know there are known unknowns; that is to say we know there are some things we do not know. But there are also unknown unknowns—the ones we don't know we don't know. And if one looks throughout the history of our country and other free countries, it is the latter category that tends to be the difficult ones.' Donald Rumsfeld, the US Secretary of Defence, in a 12 February 2002 press conference regarding the Iraq invasion.
5 From H. G. Well's lecture at the Royal Institution, London in 1902. See reference to that speech by Martin Rees, *In the future: Prospects for humanity*, Princeton University Press, 2018, p. 14.
6 The UN Secretary General, Antonio Guterres, noted in 2023 that 'globalization and technological change are modifying the risk landscape. Data on disasters show that the biggest dangers in the past were related to droughts or earthquakes, wars or pandemics. The numbers of disasters and their severity are likely to increase significantly because the exponential increase in the speed and scope of technological development is very recent, while technology itself continues to receive quaint attention as a source of risks from accident and misuse. Taking a close look at the history of technological progress makes recent accelerations more salient.' Simon Institute for Long-term Governance & UNDRR – 2023, *Existential Risk and Rapid Technological Change.*
7 'Human factors of AR, trends – quantum reality & advanced AI – augmented reality', The *GESDA 2023 science breakthrough radar*, Geneva Science and Diplomacy Anticipator's Annual Report on Science Trends at 5, 10 and 25 years, p. 53.
8 Wang Zhaowen and Fu Mighua, *Analysis of cognitive domain warfare in informatised warfare*, www.81.cn/jmywyl/2015-07/28/content_6602887.htm, as referenced in Elsa B. Kania, 'Minds at war: China's pursuit of military advantage through cognitive science and biotechnology', *PRISM*, 8 (3), 2019, p. 87.
9 The technical elements of this portrait is based upon Michael Lewis, *The fifth risk*, Allen Lane, 2018, pp. 72–75.
10 John Engedal Nissen, *Danish Red Cross the humanitarian price of climate change and how it can be avoided: Hurricane Dorian, Abaco, Northern Bahamas*, September 2019, www.ifrc.org

11 World Health Organization, *Biodiversity and health*, 3 June 2015
12 World Health Organization, *Nature is our greatest source of health and well-being*, 5 June 2020
13 As of late 2022, the most likely and most effective method for asteroid deflection involves, according to NASA, a kinetic impactor designed to redirect, for example, asteroids as reflected in its 2022 DART Mission. Astronomers think 1 million or more space rocks are relatively near planet Earth, and just 9,700 had been identified by 2014. NASA had reported then to have a handle on the biggest, most dangerous asteroids – the ones at least 0.6 miles (1 km) wide, which might end human civilisation if they hit the Earth. Researchers have now identified roughly 95 per cent of the 980 behemoths thought to cruise through Earth's neighbourhood. None of them appear to pose an impact risk for the foreseeable future.' 'NASA is developing an Asteroid Redirect Mission (ARM) – a first-ever mission to identify, capture and redirect an asteroid to a safe orbit of Earth's moon for future exploration by astronauts in the 2020s.' 'Responding to potential asteroid redirect mission targets', *NASA News*, 14 February 2014.
14 A relatively recent example of an asteroid approaching an urban area was asteroid 2012 DA14 which landed near the Russian town of Chelyabinsk, with 1.156 million inhabitants. The asteroid was 17 metres in diameter, weighed 10,000 metric tonnes and was equivalent to approximately 470 kilotonnes. While only 1,100 people were injured.
15 Peter Schultz, Brown University, Meeting of the American Geophysical Union, San Francisco, 14 December 2015.
16 The reference to the dynamics of bacteriophages comes from Gilead Amit, 'Tiny hitchhikers on viruses could promote resistance to antibiotics', Science & Technology, *The Economist*, 9 August 2023.
17 Russell Ackoff as quoted by Can M. Alpaslan and Ian I. Mitroff, *Swans, swindlers: Coping with the growing threat of mega-crises and mega-messes*, Stanford Business School Press, 2011, xiii.
18 While spillover from the event was slower than it would be in more modern times, it is nevertheless interesting to note that the Portuguese earthquake had direct impacts upon the politics of the time, including the decline of popularity of King Joseph I and his advisors, rising discontent in the Portuguese colonies and the emergence of the study of seismology as well as significant impact on the Age of Enlightenment.
19 Daniel Quiggin, Kris De Meyer, Lucy Hubble-Rose and Antony Froggatt, *Climate change assessment – 2021*, Research Paper, Environment and Society Programme, Chatham House, September 2021, p. 35.
20 D. Alexander and G. Pescarole, 'What are cascading disasters?' *UCL Open: Environment* (1), 03, 2019.
21 Ira Helford, 'Wider impact: Long-term effects on health, environment and development', *Oslo Conference*, 4 March 2013.
22 Brian Walker, Reinette Biggs, Anne-Sophie Crépin, Carl Folke, Eric F. Lambin, Garry D. Peterson, Johan Rockström, Marten Scheffer, Will Steffen and Max Troell, 'Synchronous failure: The emerging causal architecture of global crisis', *Ecology and Society*, 20 (3), 2015, p. 6.
23 Thomas Homer-Dixon, *The upside of down: Catastrophe, creativity and the renewal of civilization*, Souvenir Press, 2006, p. 16.
24 Thomas Homer-Dixon and Johan Rockstrom, 'What happens when a cascade of crises collide?', *New York Times*, 13 November 2022.

25 Humanitarian Futures Programme, *Humanitarian crisis drivers of the future – waters of the Third Pole: Sources of threats, sources of survival*, www.humanitarianfutures.org – Library Section.

Bibliography

Alexander, David and Pescarole, Gianluca, 'What are cascading disasters?' *UCL Open: Environment*, 1, 03, 2019.

Alpaslan, Can M. and Mitroff, Ian I., *Swans, swindlers: Coping with the growing threat of mega-crises and mega-messes*, Stanford Business School Press, 2011.

Amit, Gilead, Tiny hitchhikers on viruses could promote resistance to antibiotics, Science & Technology, *The Economist*, 9 August 2023.

Brooks, Michael, 'The context', *New Scientist*, 19 November 2022, p. 46.

Devakumar, Delan, Shannon, Geordan, Bhopal, Sunil and Abubakar, Ibrahim, 'Racism and discrimination in Covid-19 responses', *The Lancet*, 1 April 2020. https://doi.org/10.1016/S0140-6736(20)30792-3

GESDA, 'Human factors of AR, trends – quantum reality & advanced AI – augmented reality', The *GESDA 2023 Science Breakthrough Radar*, Geneva Science and Diplomacy Anticipator's Annual Report on Science Trends at 5, 10, and 25 years.

He, Jun, He, Leshui, Zhao, Wen, Tie, Xuanhua, and He, Ming, 'Discrimination and social exclusion in the outbreak of COVID-19', *International Journal of Environmental Res. Public Health*, 17 (8), 2933, 2020. https://doi.org/10.3390/ijerph17082933

Helford, Ira, Wider impact: Long-term effects on health, environment and development, *Oslo Conference*, 4 March 2013.

Homer-Dixon, Thomas, *The upside of down: Catastrophe, creativity and the renewal of civilization*, Souvenir Press, 2006.

Homer-Dixon, Thomas and Rockstrom, Johan, 'What happens when a cascade of crises collide?', *New York Times*, 13 November 2022.

Humanitarian Futures Programme, *Humanitarian crisis drivers of the future – waters of the Third Pole: Sources of threats; sources of survival,* www.humanitarianfutures.org – Library Section.

Kania, Elsa B., 'Minds at war: China's pursuit of military advantage through cognitive science and biotechnology', *PRISM*, 3 (8), 2019.

Lewis, Michael, *The fifth risk*, Allen Lane, 2018.

NASA, 'Responding to potential asteroid redirect mission targets', *NASA News*, 14 February 2014.

Quiggin, Daniel, De Meyer, Kris, Hubble-Rose, Lucy and Froggatt, Antony, *Climate change assessment – 2021*, Research Paper, Environment and Society Programme, Chatham House, September 2021.

Rees, Martin J., *In the future: Prospects for humanity*, Princeton University Press, 2018.

Schultz, Peter, *Brown University, meeting of the American Geophysical Union*, San Francisco, 14 December 2015.

Taleb, Nassim Nicholas, *The black swan: The impact of the highly improbable*, Penguin Books, 2008.

Walker, Brian, Biggs, Reinette, Crépin, Anne-Sophie, Folke, Carl, Lambin, Eric F., Peterson, Garry D., Rockström, Johan, Scheffer, Marten, Steffen, Will and Troell, Max, 'Synchronous failure: The emerging causal architecture of global crisis', *Ecology and Society*, 20 (3), 6, 2015.

World Health Organization, *Biodiversity and health*, 3 June 2015.
World Health Organization, *Nature is our greatest source of health and well-being*, 5 June 2020.
Zhaowen, Wang and Mighua, Fu, *Analysis of cognitive domain warfare in informatised warfare*. www.81.cn/jmywyl/2015-07/28/content_6602887.htm

5 The Entanglement Nexus

Despite distrust and contending interests, the United States and what was then the Soviet Union agreed in 1984 to collaborate in developing and maintaining what was to become the International Space Station. Over the ensuing four decades, Russia, the United States, and most members of the European Space Agency and Japan, collaborated in programmes that included space medicine, astronomy and meteorology.[1] *These shared initiatives did not include all the activities that continue to be undertaken on the ISS. Clearly there were state undertakings that were and are not shared. Nevertheless, as one observer noted, the Russian cosmonauts and the American astronauts, along with those from other nations, always dine together.*

This perceived model of international collaboration was sullied in relatively subtle ways. When it comes to national security and fears of technology transfers, it has not been able to shed political baggage. The ISS is in that sense two different space stations: one Russian, the other American. For many who monitor the activities aboard the ISS, the reality is that 'the ISS feel more like a truce than a partnership. Astronauts and cosmonauts may ride the same rockets to the station (for now) and eat dinner together at the same table, but as far as the countries themselves are concerned, this friendship has well-defined limits. Indeed, the very existence of the ISS depends on making these limits to collaboration explicit to all the countries involved. And despite this soft divide, neither space station could exist without the other. The reality is that the system we have has become mutually interdependent.'[2]

That interdependence does not guarantee permanence nor does it mean that it will automatically lure other states into it. China is developing its own equivalent, and there are a variety of US companies that are preparing hardware for private space stations. 'But the ISS will always serve as a reminder that international collaboration in space for the betterment of the entire species is *possible, no matter how unlikely it may sometimes seem from the ground.'*[3]

Introduction

We're all humanitarians now – well not quite. Nevertheless, there clearly has been a growing awareness and acceptance of the interdependencies and interrelatedness that can explain resilience, vulnerabilities and ways to mitigate the latter.

DOI: 10.4324/9781003471004-6

When readers were asked to consider 'the what might be's' in a futures context, the prospect of ever more complex interdependencies and interrelatedness were key themes. Not to take such propositions into account would bring them, as future planners and decision-makers, closer and closer to the brink. They would have failed to appreciate the growing entanglements which increasingly frame human and societal behaviour. For reasons better or worse, intentional or unintentional, intensifying entanglement needs to be a core consideration for those who recognise the importance of *planning from the future* to anticipate and mitigate ever more complex humanitarian threats.

The Entanglement Nexus

Issues such as climate change, the erosion of biodiversity, pandemics and vulnerable cyber systems have fostered an increased awareness of varying degrees of interconnected and interrelated relationships. By no means is this to suggest that there has been a paradigmatic shift in the nature of humanness. Human behaviour for the most part continues to reflect varying degrees of self-interest on an individual as well as societal scale – somewhere between Maslow's hierarchy of needs, Mitrany's approach to functionalism and Burton's human needs that drive conflict.[4]

It does suggest, however, that evolving patterns of institutional and sectoral interests, growing numbers and types of actors involved in cross geographical and cross sectoral transactions and an emerging rebalancing of the political and the functional are leading to a growing acceptance that 'my interests are increasingly dependent upon yours' and are reflected in an *entanglement nexus*.

The entanglement nexus is about connectivity. It assumes that over the next generation there will be an exponential increase in the number of formal and informal means and structures of human engagement. *Ad hoc* and permanent systems and networks, coalitions, associations and functional groupings, interactions reflecting virtual states – the list goes on and on. The essential point is that the connections, enduring or temporary, will intensify, and their intentions reflecting an increasing range of collaborative and competitive motives.

For the purposes of this book, entanglement may not only explain the motivations underpinning humanitarianism in the future, but also the nature of humanitarian action and who actually is a humanitarian. Eventually, might emerging global patterns of interests and behaviour alter what are deemed to be humanitarian principles? Could such changing perceptions result in regulated obligations that would define preparedness and response, and also who would be responsible for their implementation and when?

The answers might in the first instance lie in an appreciation of the evolving patterns of entanglements that reflect the perceived importance of interdependencies, why they will increasingly matter and how should they be fostered.

Evolving Patterns of Entanglements

What do a referendum in Crimea, an economic downturn in China, a drought in New Zealand, a policy change in Brussels, and cow herders in West Africa

> have to do with farmer protests in France? [The answer:] Understanding how seemingly unconnected events and policies led French farmers to protest on the streets illustrates just how tightly globalization links all kinds of people and industries, whether they realize it or not.[5]

Both the question and answer go to an increasingly evident fact that more and more the local is global and *vice versa*, global is local, and local impacts other locals. In other words, global dynamics increasingly affect the local (e.g. communities, cities, regions) not necessarily constrained by traditional geopolitical boundaries; and, the dynamics of such local groupings can have impacts upon the wider global system as well as local in one area impacting locals in others and eventually spilling over into global. This emerging reality is but one step towards recognising increasing entanglement that marks in myriad ways ever tightening global interrelationships.

By no means are such patterns utopian. Though it will be argued here that entanglement probably could have more positive benefits in dealing with global threats and crises in the future, it clearly has dystopic dimensions as well. A single cyber-attack, for example, can disrupt systems in any part of the world. Trade restrictions on one country can cripple its economy with ripple effects across the globe, a bioengineered virus in one part of the world can become a global pandemic or the persistent use of fossil fuels by energy producers can add to temperature rise more globally. Proximity is less and less geographical. Whether the impact be one or a combination of societal, economic or security factors, an 'entangled particle' can wreak havoc on others on planet Earth and elsewhere.

All these self-evident downsides are neither new nor should be a surprise to the reader. It is more than likely, however, that the fine balance between the positive and the negative could tilt in favour of the former. While this perspective might be surprising for those who witnessed the turmoil and agonies suffered by so many throughout the early 2020s, the assumption underpinning that tilt is still valid.

The basic reason goes to the heart of intensifying interdependencies and increasing types and numbers of non-state actors. In multilateral constructs, as modern history clearly demonstrates, the state ultimately had been the principal determinant of interests and geopolitical action.

Now, however, if one looks at patterns of interacting networks, increasing cross-sectoral engagement, growth in global communications, trade and financial interdependencies, changes in the nature of governance and the related nature of *polylateralism* (as discussed in *Chapter #3: Governance and Resource Prioritisation from a Futures Perspective*) there is a trend towards greater interaction, if not always collaboration – not necessarily for reasons of good will, but certainly for reasons of necessity.

The terms 'interconnected', 'interrelated' and 'interdependent' all reflect so much of what is the present global architecture. Yet, even these terms do not adequately define the intensity of the interrelationships which more and more bind human beings together, for better or for worse, intentionally or not, with negative and positive consequences. The fact of the matter is that human beings have become entangled in a nexus of relationships that are increasingly entwined and inescapable. As evidenced in the energy sector, 'Increased self-sufficiency may give countries an increased sense of resilience but could also make them vulnerable; an interconnected global market can ease disruptions caused by extreme weather or political instability.'[6] This reality pervades and will continue to do so. Its logic seems irrefutable.

Interacting Networks. In a study undertaken in 2020–2021 concerning an international architecture for managing global threats, researchers noted that international and global non-state and multisectoral institutions and networks, including though not necessarily dominated by states, had risen by 46 per cent between 1992 and 2021, 44 per cent of those involved environmental issues.[7] That trend reflected increasing perceptions that global security and survival depended upon recognised common interests, and that the pursuit of both depended upon a wide range of representative organisations well beyond traditional multilateral structures.

Here, however, the issue is not about the nature of systems and organisations, which will be discussed in the next two chapters, but rather about perceptions, sense of inclusion and exclusion, awareness and evidence that affect the probability and consequences of entanglement.

The exponential increase in the number of multinational enterprises (MNEs) – deemed to be the 'global Goliaths' – is a clear example of intensifying entanglement.[8] In 2000, there were an estimated 38,000 MNEs across the globe with approximately 350,000 affiliates. Two decades later, that figure increased to around 60,000 with more than 500,000 foreign affiliates. In total, they then were responsible for at least 33 per cent of global output in addition to a further 12 per cent of gross output by foreign affiliates. More than half the world's exports and 49 per cent of its imports could be attributed to MNEs – contributing to approximately 28 per cent of global GDP.[9]

While their operations have generated considerable criticism and the difficulties of controlling them certainly so, their influence has impacted the global economy and societies more generally in so many ways. Even when it comes to cross-national standards affecting such things as accountancy, administration and organisational design and operations, these non-state goliaths determine and are determined by essential interconnectedness.

> Moreover, since multinational corporations are often large, they pose unusual challenges to national and regional governments who seek to maintain political autonomy and yet are often anxious to seek the investment, technology, and managerial skills of foreign firms.[10]

Global insurance, for example, requires insurers across the world to cooperate efficiently in order to issue and service insurance policies in local markets. Arranging multinational insurance needs common frameworks across global networks in order to devise insurance policies and manage claims internationally. This presents multiple challenges through different laws, languages, processes and systems of the different parties involved. Nevertheless, the importance attested to such networks once again points to a level of entanglement that has intensified significantly over the past two decades.

In a related context, an increasing number of insurers have played positive climate change roles by lowering insurance costs for those insured willing to undertake effective climate change management. This continues to be tested in several countries in Africa where 'there appears to be clear scope for a dynamic interaction between insurers and governments where symbiotic use and generation of climate risk information can advance mutual goals'.[11]

Growing interdependencies in the corporate sector now and increasingly will make the traditional multinational corporations no longer unique as global players. Generally speaking, there are few foreseeable products that will not require materials, manufacturing or markets that go beyond the competencies or resources of any single company and increasingly any single country.

There have been arguments that contest this assertion, one being the proposition that technologies can make products and production more 'local', not requiring transnational dependencies. For example, it has been suggested that the increased use of 3D printing will enable manufacturing to be done 'locally' and would not require resources or components needed to go transnational. Rather, the increasing use of 3D printing, according to some, would shorten supply chains, hence, reducing global trade.[12]

This perspective has been refuted by others such as the OECD and the World Bank. They have used the example of 3D printing to counter what appears to them as conventional wisdom. 'Such new technologies will inevitably lead to an increase in world trade as it allows to reduce production costs.'[13] In other words, technologies generally will continue to increase interdependencies and interactions, and that will increasingly become a perceived norm across the globe, including what continues to be referred to as 'the global South'.[14]

The scientific community is another case in point. Certainly since the 16th century, that emerging community recognised research interdependencies – and, now, with few exceptions, has been increasingly dependent upon the exchange of data and research methodologies and findings at a global level.[15] Between 2014 and 2018, the number of scientists across the globe grew to 8.8 million, a growth of 13.7 per cent during that four-year period. Using co-authored research as an indicator, one study found that openness among advanced science systems is strongly correlated with impact – 'the more internationally engaged a nation is in terms of co-authorships and researcher mobility, the higher the impact of scientific work'.[16]

When discussing alternative patterns of governance in a hypothetical future in Chapter 3, reference was made to the 'dispersed' and 'virtual state'. Drawing on that example, it is worth recalling that the political interests of 'citizens' of one country residing in a foreign state would be able to have their own representatives support their interests in their country of origin. Here is an additional factor reflecting another aspect of entanglement.

And, perhaps on a more dystopic note, the interconnected nature of terrorist groups and drug cartels, too, have intensified – yet, another example of cross sectoral, cross cultural, cross-dependent entanglements at a global level.[17] Greater reliance on a digital and globalised media and communications system could create new opportunities for attacks with widespread impacts. Interlinked supply chains and greater worldwide awareness could allow even conventional terrorist attacks to have global implications for economies and emergency management capabilities.

All these examples in so many ways reflect perhaps one of the greatest drivers of the entanglement process, namely, the ubiquitous internet.

If one looks at the number of users of the internet in 2021, the case for growing global entanglement is very evident. In the year 2000, an estimated 5.8 per cent of the global population, or, 361 million people were 'connected'. By 2021, that figure rose to 64.2 per cent or over 5 billion in a global population of 7.7 billion.[18] Counting the family and village uses of mobile phones, and taking into consideration the limited use of these devices among children under five years of age, humankind is now almost entirely connected, albeit in the early 2020s with considerable levels of inequality in the bandwidth as well as in the efficiency and prices of the service.[19]

Nevertheless, the burgeoning use of the internet across a wide array of socio-economic lines is obvious. The transfer of US$ 706 billion worth of remittances sent by migrant workers to family members is certainly a case in point. Nearly 1/3rd were digitally dispensed – including through cryptocurrencies and mobile money – and such internet modalities continue to be on the rise.[20]

Another aspect of the internet is social networking. No one can doubt its downsides – everything from bullying to social media addiction and fake news to cyber-attacks, nor its upsides – such as enhanced exchange of information, engaging with a more global culture and on-line learning and discovery. However, whatever its societal strengths and weaknesses, it would be difficult to argue that it has not fundamentally changed some basic aspects of societal interconnectedness.

Messages no longer flow solely from the few to the many, with little interactivity. Now, messages also flow from the many to the many, multimodally and interactively. By disintermediating government and corporate control of communication, horizontal communication networks have created a new landscape of social and political change. Online and particularly wireless communication have helped social movements pose more of a challenge to state power.

Even in those instances where governments do attempt – often, successfully – to close down networks, alternatives emerge. In China, for example, despite what has been termed its 'digital authoritarianism', new social media emerge as others are officially closed down.[21] Attempts at control might well have triggered a 'splinternet' – a 'Balkanised internet' – where many national or regional networks do not speak to one another and may even operate using incompatible technologies.[22] However, the likelihood of a fractured internet world is in some instances countered by economic realities, and, as one specialist has noted:

> I think China could cut itself off from the global internet and likely would if there were a big enough domestic crisis… [but] I do believe that China will continue to rely on the global internet. The Chinese diaspora is everywhere in

the world. Nobody wants connections to home cut off. Businesses will still rely on selling their products overseas.[23]

Efforts were clearly underway by the 2020s and even before to constrain and guide social networks more generally. However, whatever the battles that persisted between states, technology companies and internet users, the fact was that, from a global perspective, social media underpinned by an increasingly sophisticated Internet was a clear example of intensifying entanglement at a global level and beyond.

The internet, social networking and the *metaverse*, global supply chains in the service as well as manufacturing sectors, flows of scientific research, increases in virtual and physical transnational travel, satellite dependencies, expanding cultural linkages and even crime are just some of the factors that not only reflect global entanglement, but also are responsible for its exponential growth. All in their varying interdependent, ways have been significantly changing the perceptions of relationships and their interrelated consequences across the globe and one day into outer space.[24]

This sort of interconnectedness was clearly evident in the aftermath of the 2011 Fukushima Tsunami. The tsunami's impact on Japanese production disrupted global supply chains affecting the auto industry, telecommunications and consumer electronics, particularly in the United States and Europe. On the other hand, lower Japanese growth resulted, albeit temporarily, in lower world energy demand and prices.[25] Floods in China in 2020 affected 54 million people, 14 millions of whom were displaced and destroyed somewhere in the region of 1 million hectares of agricultural land. The crisis resulted in the highest importation of maize and soybeans in over a decade. Australia, Canada and the United States were the initial providers, soon to be replaced by Kazakhstan and Russia.[26]

An all too evident case in point were the unprecedented levels of global interconnected and interrelated interests so apparent in the wake of Russian attacks on the independent state of Ukraine in 2022. In its aftermath, there were those who foresaw a return to a 20th century 'Cold War' in which functional global links were limited comparatively speaking to a few major commodities, e.g. petroleum, and where state authority was dominated by traditional geopolitical interests.[27]

And, though the invasion was horrifying in so many ways, it reflected three aspects of interacting systems which had few Cold War precedents: direct and immediate global impacts; the complexity of severing functional linkages; and, the increasingly fluctuating balance between the political and the functional.

Prior to the war, Ukraine had been the world's largest producer of sunflower oil and, combined with Russia, over 36 per cent of wheat exports, making it the world's largest exporter of wheat. In a matter of three weeks, a combination of sanctions imposed on Russia and the decline of production in war-affected Ukraine had led to increases in the price of bread and other basic foods, particularly in Middle Eastern and North African countries, all highly dependent on grain from

Ukraine.[28] More generally, the United Nations said that the war's overall impact on the global food market alone could cause an additional 7.6 million to 13.1 million people to go hungry.[29]

The war also made evident that, despite the fury which it generated and the consequent stream of sanctions from a plethora of institutions, including churches, the private sector, intergovernmental institutions such as the European Union as well as governments, it had proven difficult for them to be implemented. Sanctions on commodities such as oil and gas, palladium for catalytic converters and titanium, crucial for the aerospace industry, were too disruptive for many countries to impose them quickly or in their entirety. Ways to circumvent some of the most critical would continue until alternatives were found in other parts of the world.

In no sense is this to suggest that such sanctions were not well intended and that many were not enforced. Rather, it is to say that myriad networks upon which the global community depended meant that some of the most critical interdependencies could not be easily severed, that alternative interacting networks needed to be found to ensure economic and societal stability as well as political interests. Basic means of survival – be it food, healthcare or adequate shelter – were becoming a concern in higher income as well as in middle and lower income countries.

The fact that 143 governments had condemned Russian violations of international law more generally and certainly International Humanitarian Law clearly reflected varying degrees of moral as well as political outrage. At the same time, the global reactions and responses also underscored another emerging reality, namely, that political interests were ever more dependent upon and driven by functional interests. The latter more often than not reflected interconnectedness and interdependencies that went beyond geopolitical boundaries.

Rebalancing the Political and the Functional. 'We have no eternal allies, and we have no perpetual enemies,' said Lord Palmerston in a speech before Britain's House of Commons in 1848. 'Our interests are eternal and perpetual, and those interests it is our duty to follow.'

A century later, functional entanglements were beginning to intensify across virtually all continents. Despite the West's mid-20th century anti-Communist containment policy that restricted relations with the Soviet Union, much of Eastern Europe, China, Korea and Vietnam for at least two decades, functional institutions on both sides of the containment boundaries were pursuing interests that can be deemed as functional, supported by political interests or by-passing them:

> The members of the Western alliance set up an export control organisation CoCom to limit the flow of strategic materials and technology to communist countries. [However] scholars have given relatively little attention to the efforts of companies and other business organisations to promote their commercial interests in this divided world. Neither have they been particularly keen on looking at the impact of government policies on micro level business operations. The companies were naturally eager to defend their interests, because trade with

> the socialist countries was often profitable. Furthermore, companies usually tend to oppose policies that restrict their freedom of action.[30]

The balance between those systems that are intended primarily to pursue political objectives and those designed to deal with functional issues such as commerce, the sciences, education, technology, health, sports and so on is central to understanding the dynamics of entanglements. And, while that balance fluctuates, it is evident that in an increasingly 'polylateral world order', functional interests will more overtly define the objectives of the political. Less and less does the political dominate and define the boundaries and objectives of the functional.

That said, functional interests have always in modern history and well before been enmeshed in the objectives of the state and *vice versa*. Functional interdependencies and interests defined politics and were defined by politics in so many ways. Functionalism has always been intertwined with politics. In fact, many such as Karl Marx defined the very construct and processes of political institutions as functionally driven, and by no means was he alone.[31]

In reflecting on the interaction between governments and those with functional interests during the 2020–2021 Covid crisis, one well known economist pointed out that the World Bank and the IMF wanted to support flagging economies and

> used the full powers of the state to do so; central bankers justified their interventions by the need to maintain the integrity of financial markets… and the state can still use its power to do huge things but it can only use them in the service of the powerful and the wealthy. As soon as their crisis is over, those powers will be put back in their box.[32]

Whether that 'box' is the inevitable destination for the state in the aftermath of a crisis is perhaps an exaggeration. Nevertheless, it suggests once again that the assertion of influence through functional interconnections in the political process is a reality that cannot be ignored. Whatever aspects of the multilateral construct, juggling and rebalancing between the functional and the political are increasingly evident.

Even ostensibly functional organisations such as the Universal Postal Union, the World Maritime Organization and the World Health Organization reflect that tension between both. The International Atomic Energy Agency (IAEA) in the midst of the Cold War is yet another example. Despite nuclear weapons being recognised as a central feature in US–Soviet rivalry, the IAEA successfully 'created a transnational community of experts to build the foundations of nuclear technology exchange, safety measures, and safeguards'.[33]

In highly politicised efforts by major political powers to reshape the multilateral construct, 'the fact that globalization's interconnections have placed private sector and civil society at the front lines of geostrategic competition, rather than solely governments', suggests that rebalancing.[34] 'The hope that "functional agencies" in international organisations could help de-politicise controversial issues by treating these as neutral, technical challenges was not entirely unfounded; but nor could it eliminate the frictions of international high politics.'[35]

The OECD's extensive analysis of the impact of scientific advice on government policymaking is another case in point about tensions between the functional and the political.

In this instance, many scientists who had been focussing on research findings for dealing with Covid-19 felt that they had to modify the ways that those findings were presented in order to have maximum impact upon government decision-makers. According to the analysis, it became evident that scientists increasingly felt that they had to adjust the ways that they conveyed their 'functional' findings if they were to have impact. They would have to make them more 'politically accessible' if their interests and concerns would be acceptable to those with political responsibilities. This is not to imply that they abandoned their integrity, but rather that they recognised that the functional had to be sensitive to the political – *had to be intertwined* – if the former were to achieve their objectives.[36]

That fluid rebalancing also has considerable significance when it comes to the entanglement nexus. More and more actors reflecting an increasing range of non-state interests are recognising their interconnectedness at global levels, not necessarily dependent upon the state, but aligned with it. A former Governor of the Bank of England suggested that sort of entanglement when in 2020 he spoke about the forthcoming COP-26:

> Private finance is now increasingly focused on the opportunities and risks in the transition. Every major systemic bank, the world's largest insurers, its biggest pension funds and top asset managers are calling for the disclosure of climate-related financial risk through their support of the Taskforce for Climate-related Finance Disclosures (TCFD). Investors controlling over $40 trillion in assets (across Climate Action 100+, UN PRI, and the Net Zero Asset Owner Alliance) want to see transition plans to a low carbon world from their portfolio companies. This is backed by the critical roles that Multilateral Development Banks, Development Finance Institutions and National Development Banks are playing to accelerate their support to low carbon growth.[37]

Of course, states' involvement in issues of potentially global consequence is profound and will continue to be so in the foreseeable future. Whether virtual, dispersed or traditional, the state will remain a key factor when it comes to political processes and alignments. Yet, what will determine both will increasingly be functional issues reflecting interdependencies of increasing numbers of non-state actors whose interests are inherently functional. It will be characterised by a *polylateral* global architecture.

The consequences of cyber system's collapse, pandemics, climate change, the use of outer space are for the most part functional issues affecting human life and framing political agendas. They, too, are indicative of a growing awareness that more and more functional issues – threats and opportunities – will reflect interdependencies that will in turn determine relationships between multiple actors, relationships that at times will transcend states, at times including states and at times determined by them.

The Entanglement Paradox

Entanglement is by no means a guarantee that interconnections and interdependencies result in consistent and predictable outcomes. Indeed, the paradox is that entanglements can intensify unpredictability and discrimination. Here are a few cases to consider.

In a 2018 analysis about the consequences of disasters due to flooding, researchers found that

> when a supplier is impacted by a disaster hampering its production, international trade increases the chance that other suppliers can jump in and temporarily replace it. Interestingly, the global increase of climate-induced river floods could even cause net gains for some economies such as India, South East Asia, or Australia.[38]

Another case reflecting uncertainties in the entanglement paradox stems from an analysis by the United Nations Conference on Trade and Development (UNCTAD) on Foreign Direct Investment (FDI) from emerging markets.

There is an understandable assumption that for all intents and purposes, developing countries are dependent upon direct investments made by those in developed countries, but not *vice versa.* It is interesting to note that the outward Foreign Direct Investment by the BRICS (Brazil, China, Russia, India and South Africa), for example, rose from $1.1 trillion in 2011 to $3.7 trillion in 2021, an increase of 235 per cent directly and indirectly affecting markets and employment in G7 countries.

While there can be little doubt that interconnectedness and interdependencies are recognised phenomena, it, too, has also become clear that the consequences of interdependencies needs to be further understood. How are they identified and by whom and who indeed are 'included' and 'excluded'?

For example, it was not until the aftermath of the 2008 financial crisis that the Group of 20 began to focus more systematically on an understanding of the dimensions and dynamics of economic entanglements. Its Mutual Assessment Process (MAP) is a case in point. Created in the aftermath of the 2008 financial crisis, the MAP illustrated how integrated the world economy was and how economic interdependencies had become more complex than previously understood or recognised.

That crisis made clear that MAP was needed to identify those interdependencies and associated spillover effects, giving greater attention to the

> design of domestic policy with international implications in mind. Indeed, one of the pressing global governance issues was the need to further develop a consensus on the nature of global interdependencies.

> ...We now realize that we live in an exceptionally tightly correlated world economy with the potential for highly correlated fluctuations in economic activity . To better understand the nature and channels of these international linkages and more generally to assess the need for economic policy cooperation and coordination, we need to further invest in the development of economic models [that reflect such fluctuating dependencies].[39]

At the same time, what, too, was becoming increasingly evident had been miscalculations and *exclusions* in many analyses that relate to the entanglement nexus. As researchers began to realise, despite the upsurge in global entanglements, initiatives such as the MAP, were *exclusionary* and *discriminatory*. They worked at low levels of disaggregation. Using the IMF's Global Integrated Money and Financial Model (GIMIF), as another case in point, they noted that only five stylised regions – the United States, the Eurozone (split between Germany and the rest), Japan, developing Asia *and the rest of world* were used.

Exclusionary tendencies were even evident in the ostensibly neutral findings of the sciences. It seemed that there were and may well be growing numbers of people whose views and vulnerabilities may not be included in analyses intended, for example, to identify threats and possible solutions for Covid-19. It is difficult 'to make sense of a world that is already making sense of the world', reflected one scientist sarcastically. Hence, 'What gets counted, counts!'[40]

Whether referring to sources and access at developing or developed state levels, there are significant elements and aspects of society that are ignored. They reflect examples of persistent 'data poverty', the antithesis of those who have 'privileged data'.[41] They also in all too many instances reflect data discrimination. Socio-economic backgrounds, racism, differing degrees of support for scientific investigation and unpredictable flows of migration all too often leading to misunderstandings about the nature of entanglements.

Contending perceptions about the consequences of entanglement also generate misperceptions about the nature and dynamics of entanglement. Again, in the world of the sciences, the *Science-Policy Platform on Biodiversity and Ecosystem Services (IPBES*) offers important perspectives on how misinterpretations about entangled components are perceived and assessed.

The IPBES was created to identify and prioritise key scientific information, undertake regular assessments of knowledge on biodiversity and relevant ecosystems and build capacities needed to strengthen the science-policy interface. These were apparently clear and accepted by a membership which by 2015 included 137 governments, 124 IGOs and several thousand other stakeholders ranging from scientific experts to representatives of academic and research institutions, local communities and the private sector.

However, the value of the network was compromised, according to various stakeholders, because outputs and proposals did not reflect situationally specific concerns nor accommodate the views of many of its component parts. The lead social and natural scientists were often perceived as disdainful, and these sorts of perceptions and misperceptions were particularly evident when it came to relations between the scientists and participants from lower-income countries, including governments.[42]

'Language', too, can also be exclusionary and distort entanglement. The relationships between the military, the private sector and humanitarian actors in peacekeeping operations have often failed to arrive at understandings about ways each seeks to achieve its objectives and their respective criteria for success. The reason frequently given is that too little effort is made to understand the other and too little appreciation of the benefits that each might have to offer is too frequently the result. The very terms used and the perceptions and perspectives that underpin those terms tend to diminish or exclude the objectives and modalities of each.[43]

What such weaknesses suggest is that entanglements and their broad societal implications are too often not recognised or ignored. Nevertheless, recognised, ignored or not, the rebalancing of the functional and the political, the upsurge in the types of interconnected and interdependent actors across the globe as well as their fluidity are and will continue to shape an increasingly polylateral world order.

That world order will reflect a widening array of actors, with myriad interests – some based on self-interests and others on *mutual self-interests* (MSI). The former all too often will focus on gains without an adequate appreciation of the negative and positive consequences of those gains for others as well as their potential feedback loops. The latter is based upon awareness of aligned or overlapping interests that can best be achieved through degrees of cooperation and collaboration which may result in better outcomes for all parties involved.

The relationship between the entanglement nexus and mutual self-interest, however, not only sheds light on the evolving world order, but also suggests the drivers of humanitarian action and who will be emerging as humanitarian actors.

Entanglement and Mutual Self-Interest

Increasingly, 'we will have to deal with "contending" and not "universal principles"', suggested the well-known anthropologist, Arjun Appadurai. In a world in which different power structures will emerge, with their concomitant local and regional perspectives and values, the presumption of common principles will be less and less relevant. More and more, perceptions of self-interest and possible mutual self-interest will be an approach to problem solving.[44]

Mutual self-interest (MSI) spans those activities where the self-interests of one party are dependent upon those of others and *vice versa and* are recognised as such. As Appadurai suggests, principles, of course, cannot be ignored, but in a world where values and cultural norms are varied, even fractured, recognised interconnections are predominantly functional. So implied the Nigerian Vice President, Yemi Osinbajo, when he noted how Nigeria's trade with China was not encumbered with imposed Western value systems. Cultural norms and values, he suggested, should not be criteria that determined functional, mutually beneficial interests. Political alliances, manufacturing, commerce, scientific investigation and even religious alignments may to varying degrees reflect moral assumptions, but ultimately their functional benefits tend to dominate.[45]

Over time functional benefits may eventually result in a kind of *transactionalism* where increasing interaction at social levels builds up feelings of trust and good will.[46] They, too, might reflect ethical assumptions underpinning enlightened self-interest, or, in other words, 'doing well by doing good'.[47] Here, however, the use of the term, MSI, is not to suggest or propose that inevitably it will lead to peaceful relations or mutually beneficial interaction. Rather, it is used to demonstrate the dynamics of intensifying global entanglement, where functional activities and outcomes increasingly rely on different actors exchanging goods, services and materials to achieve outcomes that are acknowledged to be mutually beneficial.

On one level, this proposition is more than evident and acknowledged. From scientific findings, the insurance and manufacturing industries to agricultural production and the tools of the internet, few are institutionally, organisationally and geopolitically self-contained. The interwoven links for each of these sectors have expanded exponentially over the past three decades. And, from that perspective, MSI is generally viewed from a 'horizontal' perspective where a product is regarded as dependent upon functional interdependencies.

Yet, what also has to be calibrated are MSI's more complex dimensions, those entangled vertically as well as horizontally. In other words, interdependencies at one level may feed into or generate interdependencies at others, consistently, erratically but always possibly.

Economic globalisation, it has been argued, may well have enhanced corporate gains, but at the same time it also has lured a large number of private sector organisations into high risk exposure.

As was evidenced by the impact upon high tech industries in the aftermath of Thailand's 2011 floods, horizontally, there clearly were interdependencies between local infrastructures, employment, resources and potential instability and the corporation. Yet, as more and more evidence also made clear, the effects of that disaster did not 'end at the factory gate', but directly and indirectly spilled over into wider social contexts. The wealth that can be generated and the subsequent social benefits, if not cohesion, that can emerge from private sector-led economic growth can as easily be dissipated and destroyed.[48]

Earlier, the consequences of the Russian invasion of the Ukraine in 2022 were used as an example of entanglement. Here, that same example demonstrates the horizontal and vertical dynamics of mutual self-interest.

From a horizontal perspective, functional interrelationships between Russia and those dependent upon its gas and oil were many. Despite the fact that Russia had its own domestic oil industry and manufacturing capabilities, it had throughout the Ukraine crisis still relied on specialised equipment and technologies from outside its borders. These included drilling rigs, pumps, wellhead equipment, pipelines and enhanced oil recovery methods (EOR). While Russia tried to develop domestic alternatives, the recognised mutuality of self-interests – despite political sanctions – saw the flow of goods continue between approximately 1600 Western corporations and Russia.[49]

Not only were commodities such as gas and oil central to significant portions of industries, for example, throughout the EU, but so, too, did they provide essential services within varying timeframes for significant portions of the populations in Western Europe. For Russia, in light of the income it generated, that trade provided services to a significant portion of the economy, including the military. There were indeed mutualities of interests that far transcended any single sector, and the verticality of those entanglements suggests how difficult – despite enormous political tensions – it proved to be to sever those ties. That said, interests may be mutual but are by no means permanent or enduring. They fluctuate according to patterns of interest – vertically and horizontally.

Related to both is the presumption that mutual self-interests generally result in relatively equitable exchange. That, too, is a perspective that needs to be explored, for the reality is that interdependencies by no means ensure equal benefits. Mutuality can result, for example, in income inequalities, in the growth of some markets at the expense of others, in inhibiting initiatives whether they be political, social or military.

Such downsides may be acknowledged, ignored or go unrecognised. Nevertheless, whether negative or positive, the dimensions and dynamics of MSI and their often fluid and unanticipated outcomes reflect levels of entanglement that will increasingly be unprecedented at local and global levels.

Entanglement, Mutual Self-Interest and Humanitarian Motives

It was March 2014, and the Ebola crisis in Liberia was raging. By the end of the month, more than 6,525 people had been infected and approximately 2697 had died. Conventional government, INGO and NGO responses were having relatively little effect, and it was not until the rubber production company, Firestone, a subsidiary of Bridgestone America, became involved that truly resourceful, innovative and effective responses were triggered.[50] The company's quick and comprehensive action was focused principally upon its 8,500 plantation workers and their families on the company's plantation, and became a humanitarian initiative that eventually would set an example for those in the wider health community in Liberia and across much of West Africa.

The rationale for the corporation's response, according to Bridgestone's spokesman, was of course to save lives. At the same time, 'Had Firestone not taken swift action and enacted the appropriate protocols, our operation could have been severely impacted.'[51]

The importance of Bridgestone's operations in Liberia from a commercial perspective goes without saying. At the time, it was the largest private sector employer in Liberia and operated the largest contiguous rubber farm in the world. A disabled workforce could have resulted in potentially calamitous losses. On the other hand, there were empathetic concerns as well. The company's demonstration of empathy took many forms well beyond immediate health needs – including survivor welcome celebrations, opportunities for survivors to share their experiences and solidarity packages which included essential household items such as mattresses, bedding material and mosquito nets.[52]

Stepping back, it was interesting to consider what was the balance between mutual interests and compassion during the course of that rampaging Ebola pandemic? Were the two mutually exclusive? Alternatively, were they also reflections of a kind of entanglement that has relevance when it comes to understanding the rationale for humanitarian action? As noted by the World Bank,

> One of the most important policy messages… is that the world is so interconnected that natural disasters are not local events anymore: everybody can be affected by a disaster occurring far away. It means that risk management is more than each country's responsibility: it has become a global public good.[53]

Mutual Self-Interest versus Compassion

Four years later, on a different continent, a series of workshops took place at King's College, London, under the heading of ***Mutual Self-Interest versus Compassion***. Their purpose was to explore whether compassion and self-interest might result in mutual self-interest. Assembled were leaders from the Christian, Islamic and Jewish faiths, medical experts and specialists in neurology, moral philosophy and experienced representatives of the humanitarian sector.[54]

The diversity of views indeed reflected the diversity of participants. However, if there was a single theme that had emerged it was the difficulty of separating compassion from an overt or subliminal sense of self-interest, and that self-interest was more often than not fulfilled by consciously or unconsciously linking one's own interests with the ways that one perceived the interests of others.

The neuroscientist suggested that compassion and an awareness of mutual self-interest were possibly 'hardwired into the brain'. A consistent view from those of different faiths was that compassion could be seen as means for alleviating one's own suffering by addressing the suffering of others – a kind of 'self-compassion'. The moral philosopher and the social psychologist came to agreement on the likelihood that the interrelationship between compassion and mutual self-interest reflected one's world view, 'our *weltanschauung*'. The two were innate, and both were circumscribed by cultural and social contexts.

Participants from humanitarian organisations generally agreed with the characteristics of compassion and mutual self-interests that had been discussed. In turn, their contributions from a humanitarian perspective focussed on two interrelated issues. The first was that compassion was a term frequently conflated with others such as mercy, pity, empathy and 'helplessness'; the second was that, while mutual self-interest – 'the bargaining chip' – was more relevant to the developed world, more often than not the principal relevance of compassion from a humanitarian perspective was focused on 'the vulnerable South'.

Those humanitarian perspectives might have been understandable. Looking at the persistent poverty that differentiated high income countries from middle and lower-oncome countries in 2018, there would seem to be good reason for those with humanitarian roles and responsibilities to focus on a 'north–south divide'.[55]

Yet, that presumed divide too often ignored critical entanglements which would increasingly make both co-dependent. The interacting impacts of climate change as well as sources of pandemics were but two.[56] Others would include the bottom-line fact that increasing investments in the developing world came from multinational corporations and, as noted earlier, a growing number of countries, including the BRICS, were directly and indirectly impacting upon those in the so-called 'resilient North'.

There were many more examples of such interconnectedness and interrelationships that were proposed during those ***Mutual versus Self-Interest*** roundtables at King's College, London. By no means were they always positive. Arguably, the balance between their positive and negative consequences frequently wavered, and the former certainly did not exceed the latter.

However, there was little doubt that horizontal and vertical dimensions of entanglements did reflect global interconnectedness that was historically unprecedented. In a growing number of ways that interconnectedness led to links reflecting an expanding range of institutions, consortia, networks and alliances that crisscrossed planet Earth and beyond. Their durability certainly could not be presumed. However, more and more their actions would seem to acknowledge that to achieve their own objectives they had to be sensitive to the impact that theirs might have on others.

We're all Humanitarians Now

Over several cups of coffee, a couple of former colleagues who had served as aid workers in the 1984 Ethiopian famine found themselves discussing the types of global crises that were increasingly plausible – now three decades after they had been helping to provide humanitarian assistance in northern Ethiopia's Wollo province. Cyber systems failures, climate impacts, mass displacement, nuclear disasters, bio-engineered pandemics, rapid decline of water access – the list seemed endless. Then, considering the implications of the list, the colleague from the ICRC mused, 'Well I guess we're all humanitarians now.'

What he meant was that the sorts of crisis threats that flowed from that discussion went beyond the abilities, training and experience of most institutions and individuals in the humanitarian sector. They required capacities that ranged from industrially specific technical expertise to transdisciplinary collaboration, from different understandings about the drivers of crisis threats and their consequent effects and ways to deal with them. The range of those who might be responders would increasingly go well beyond those conventionally deemed to be humanitarians.

And, in an increasingly entangled global construct, responses to such potential threats could only be effectively identified, monitored and mitigated if there were the capacities and resources to do so – and both would depend upon a full appreciation of recognised *mutual self-interests*.

Of course, that proposition should by no means suggest that aspects of well-motivated empathy and compassion would be irrelevant – even despite the definitional complexities evident in those King's College, London workshops. However, what was becoming increasingly obvious and hopefully fully understood and appreciated was that identifying, monitoring and mitigating disasters threats in an ever more entangled world must become everyone's commitment. It must be seen as a global public good, for

> global catastrophic risk reduction is a global public good, as even a large country would only capture a small portion of the total benefit of risk mitigation. Moreover, it is an inter-generational public good, as many of the beneficiaries are future people who have no voice in the political process.[57]

It is with that hope and perspective in mind that a full appreciation of the positive aspects of the entanglement nexus should lead to more coherent and consistent approaches for dealing with increasingly complex and uncertain humanitarian threats – even those '*what might be's*' referred to in the previous chapter.

With that in mind, it is important now to focus on the sorts of multidimensional and multisectoral approaches needed to deal with such threats. The chapter that follows will propose ways that existing systems, including alliances, coalitions, networks and social movements, can be mobilised to meet the humanitarian challenges ahead. Though diverse and possibly in contention, many of these systems would nevertheless accept the importance of coalescing to deal with future crisis threats, in no small part for reasons of mutual self-interest.

Will the entanglement nexus and growing awareness of mutual self-interest in identifying and mitigating humanitarian threats mean that 'we are all humanitarians now'?

Notes

1 As of 2022, long-term crew members of the ISS by nationality are Belgium, Canada, France, Germany, Italy, Japan, the Netherlands, Russia, the United Kingdom and the United States,

2 Daniel Oberhaus, 'How Cold War politics shaped the International Space Station: A brief history detailing how the United States and Russia led the effort to create the technical marvel', *Smithsonian Magazine*, 9 September 2020.

3 Ibid. In this context, it is worth noting that on 27 April 2023, NASA stated that Russia had confirmed that it would support the station through 2028. Yuri Borisov, head of the Russian space agency, Roscosmos, said that agency, had sent letters to the leaders of the other space agencies involved in ISS, informing them that 'the ISS program is the largest and most successful international project in the field of space, and I am glad that such a unique laboratory will continue its work and will contribute to the realization of the most daring ideas of mankind in space exploration.' His translated remarks were published by Roscosmos on social media. See: Jeff Foust, 'Russia Commits to ISS extension to 2028', *SpaceNews*, 27 April 2023.

4 'Abraham Maslow's hierarchy of needs is a motivational theory in psychology comprising a five-tier model of human needs, often depicted as hierarchical levels within

a pyramid… . Needs lower down in the hierarchy must be satisfied before individuals can attend to needs higher up. From the bottom of the hierarchy upwards, the needs are physiological, safety, love and belonging, esteem and self- actualization.' Saul McLeod, 'Maslow's hierarchy of needs', 21 May 2018, www.simplypsychology.org/maslow.html. David Mitrany's 'functionalist theory' stated that economic and social needs could set the basis for a functional system of international relations guided by practical 'needs' instead of political ideology and propaganda. Mihal Alexandresus, 'David Mitrany: From federalism to functionalism', *Transylvania Review*, XVI (1), 2007.

J.W. Burton suggests that of the primary causes of protracted or intractable conflict is people's unyielding drive to meet their unmet needs on the individual, group and societal levels. For example, the Palestinian conflict involves the unmet needs of identity and security. 'Resolving Baluchistan conflict: A human needs approach', *Scientific Figure on ResearchGate*. www.researchgate.net/figure/Human-Needs-as-presented-by-Maslow-Burton_tbl1_341113614

5 World101, *Global era issues from the Council on Foreign Relations*, Council on Foreign Relations, https://world101.cfr.org › global-era-issues

6 Jason Bordoff and Meghan L. O'Sullivan, 'The age of energy security: How the fight for resources is upending geopolitics', *Foreign Affairs* May/June 2023.

7 Randolph C. Kent et al., *Towards an international architecture for managing global threats*: *Systems compendium annex*, Royal United Services Institute, 2021.

8 C. Fritz Foley, James R. Hines, Jr and David Wessel, *Global goliaths: Multinational corporations in the 21st century economy*, Brookings, April 2021.

9 OECD, Policy Notes Series, *Multinational enterprises in the global economy: Heavily debated but hardly measured*, May 2018.

10 B. Kogut, 'Multinational Corporations', www0.gsb.columbia.edu/faculty/bkogut/files/Chapter_in_smelser-Baltes_2001.pdf. The author also notes that 'there are, thus, economic and sociological definitions of the multinational corporation that differ, and yet complement, each other. In the economic definition, the multinational corporation is the control of foreign activities through the auspices of the firm. In the sociological definition, the multinational corporation is the mechanism by which organizational practices are transferred and replicated from one country to another.'

11 Swenja Surminski, Jonathan Barnes, Katharine Vincent, 'Can insurance catalyse government planning on climate? Emergent evidence from Sub-Saharan Africa', *World Development*, 153, May 2022.

'The analysis offers a new perspective on the catalyst role of insurance by focusing on the ways in which political economy factors, particularly incentives and relationships, influence this process. However, that ambition faces many challenges that go beyond availability and suitability of data. Limited trust, unclear risk ownership and/or lack of incentives are key barriers, even if there is risk awareness and overall motivation to manage climate risks.'

12 Caroline Freund, Alen Mulabdic, Michelle Rita, *Is 3D printing a threat to global trade: The trade affects that you didn't hear about*, World Development Report – Policy Research Working Paper 9024, World Bank Group September 2019; Andrea Andrenelli and Javier Lopez Gonzalez, *3D Printing: The final frontier for international trade in goods?* OECD, 9 November 2021.

13 This assumption is explained in Caroline Freund, Alen Mulabdic and Michele Ruta, 'Is 3D printing a threat to global trade? The trade affects you didn't hear about', *Journal of International Economics*, 138, September 2022, 103646.

14 Manuel Castells, 'The impact of the internet on society: A global perspective', *Change: 19 Key Essays on How the Internet is Changing our Lives*, BBVA: Open Mind, 2014.
15 A relevant discussion can be found in Suzie Sheehy, *The matter of everything: Twelve experiments that changed the world*, Bloomsbury Publishing, 2022.
16 Caroline S. Wagner, Travis Whetsell, Jeroen Baas and Koen Jonkers, 'Openness and impact of leading scientific countries', *Front. Res. Metr. Anal.*, 28 March 2018, https://doi.org/10.3389/frma.2018.00010
17 See, for example, Brenda J. Lutz and James M. Lutz, 'Globalisation and terrorism in the Middle East', *Perspectives on Terrorism*, 9 (5), October 2015, pp. 27 ff. 'While it is abundantly clear that there is no single cause that explains terrorism, it has been suggested that increasing globalisation has contributed to outbreaks of terrorist violence. If globalisation has in fact played such a role, then higher levels of terrorism would be associated with be associated with greater levels of globalisation.' Also see: Robert Saviano's *Zero, Zero, Zero*, Penguin, 2016, regarding the internationalisation of drug trafficking.
18 Internet world stats: Usage and population statistics, *World internet users and 2021 population stats.* More detailed statistics include that users in 1995 were 16 million or 0.4 per cent of global population; 2000 – 361 million or 5.8 per cent; 2005 – 1.018 billion or 15.7 per cent; 2010 – 1.971 billion or 28.8 per cent; 2015 – 3.366 billion or 46.4 per cent; 2021 – 5.053 billion, or 64.2 per cent.
19 Op. cit., #14, Manuel Castells.
20 Visa Economic Empowerment Institute, *The rise of digital remittances: How innovation is improving global money movement*, 2021, www.visaeconomicempowermentinstitute.org
21 For a discussion on the battles between the state and 'the rights of internet users', see, for example, Adrian Shahbaz and Allie Funk, *The global drive to control big tech*, Freedom House, Freedom on the Net, 2021.
22 James Ball, 'Russia is risking the creation of a "splinternet" – and it could be irreversible', *MIT Technology Review*, 17 March 2022.
23 Charlotte Jee, 'Russia wants to cut itself off from the global internet: Here's what is means', *MIT Technology Review*, 21 March 2019.
24 According to the BBC – 'Ukraine: Arnold Schwarzenegger's anti-war video trends on social media', 18 March 2022, in one day had been viewed nearly 25 million times and had been retweeted 325,000 times.
25 Vasco M. Carvalho, Makoto Nirei, Yukiko U. Saito, Alireza Tahbaz-Saleh, 'Supply chain disruptions: Evidence from the Great East Japan Earthquake', *The Quarterly Journal of Economics*, 136 (2), May 2021, https://doi.org/10.1093/qje/qjaa044
26 Kanat Makhanov, 'National disasters in China and shift in the global grain market', Eurasian Research Institute, Akhmet Yassawi University, 2020
27 Berit Lindeman and Ivar Dale, 'Sanctions on Russia may not be working, we now know why', 'European businesses and third countries are actively circumventing sanctions, providing Russia with sanctioned goods and thus helping its war effort.' Al Jazeera, 5 June 2023; Maria Snegovaya, Tina Dolbaia, Nick Fenton and Max Bergmann, 'Russia sanctions at one year', Centre for Strategic and International Studies, 23 February 2023.
28 Lotanna Emediegwu, 'Russia's invasion of the Ukraine exacerbates hunger in the Middle East and North Africa', Aid and International Development, Economics Observatory, 30 March 2022.

29 United Nations Security Council 9008th meeting, 'Conflict, humanitarian crisis in Ukraine threatening future global food security as prices rise, production capacity shrinks, speakers warn Security Council', SC/14846, 29 March 2022.
30 Niklas-Jensen-Eriksen (leader), Maiju Wuokko, Aaro Sahari, *Business, governments and international trade in Cold War Europe (2012–2014)*, Capitalism, State & Society research group, University of Helsinki, Finland. The United Kingdom was a leading economic power, whose government was the most influential European member of CoCom. Many British manufacturing companies were eager to sell more goods to communist countries or to buy cheap Soviet energy, while giant oil companies like the British Petroleum and the Royal Dutch Shell tried, in the late 1950s and 1960s, to contain the expansion of Soviet oil exports.
31 Op. cit., #4.
32 This quote comes from a review by Oliver Bullough in *The Guardian*, 10 September 2021, of Adam Tooze's *Shutdown: How Covid shook the world economy*, Allen Lane, 2021.
33 Elisabeth Roehrlich, 'International organizations during the Cold War', 3 February 2017. www.wilsoncenter.org
34 Will Moreland, 'The purpose of multilateralism: A framework for democracies in a geopolitically competitive world', *Foreign Policy at Brookings*, September 2019, p. 17.
35 Stewart Patrick, *Best laid plans: The origins of American multilateralism and the dawn of the Cold War*, Rowman and Littlefield, 2009, p. 54.
36 OECD, *Covid 19 and policy for science*, OECD Science, Technology and Policy Papers, No. 152, 3 July 2023. https://doi.org/10.1787/8f86e60b-en
37 Mark Carney, *The road to Glasgow*, speech presented at the Guildhall, London, 27 February 2020.
38 Anders Levermann et al., *Climate-related flooding may quickly disrupt global trade chains: US–China exchange especially vulnerable*, Earth Institute, 28 May 2018 news. climat.columbia.edu
39 Badye Essid and Paul Jenkins, *Understanding global interdependencies: The contribution of economic models*, Think Tank 20: Macroeconomic Policy Interdependence and the G-20, www.brookings.edu, April 2020.
40 Dr Katja Mayer, Department of Science and Technology Studies at the University of Vienna, presentation at an OECD workshop on Social Sciences and Interdisciplinary Research in April 2021.
41 Stefania Milan, Associate Professor of New Media and Digital Culture at the University of Amsterdam. Principal Investigator (PI) of the DATACTIVE project noted in an OECD workshop on Social Sciences and Interdisciplinary Research in April 2021 that 'a case in point – a year ago, according to the WHO, only two countries in Africa had access to Covid information'.
42 Anne-Sophie Stevance, Peter Bridgewater, Selim Louafi, Nicholas King, et al., 'The 2019 review of IPBES and future priorities: Reaching beyond assessment to enhance policy impact', AGRIS, FAO [2020]. Information provided by Centre de Cooperation Internationale en recherche agronomique pour le development, Ministre des Affaires Étrangers.
43 HFP, *The virtuous triangle and the fourth dimension: The humanitarian, private and military sectors in a fragile world*, humanitarianfuturesprogramme.org see: Key Findings, 2014.

44 Arjun Appadurai, 'Tactical humanism', in Jerome Binde (Ed.), *The future of values* UNESCO Publication/Berghahn Books, 2004, p. 17.

45 This was one of the main themes of Vice President Yemi Osinbajo's speech on 27 March 2023 before an audience at King's College, London.

46 Eilstrup-Sangiovanni, *Debates on European integration*, Palgrave Macmillan, 2006, p. 29.

47 Geoffrey Garrett, 'Doing well by doing good', *Wharton Magazine*, Spring/Summer 2017 gives one example of enlightened self-interest when he suggests that 'the two biggest challenges facing the Western world today are increasing economic growth and making that growth more inclusive. For emerging markets, building better infrastructure—particularly in already clogged cities—is essential to realizing their full demographic and developmental potential.'

48 Aon Benfield, *2011 Thailand floods event recap report: Impact forecasting*, March 2012.

49 Douglas Busvine, 'Sanctions aren't working: How the West enables Russia's war on Ukraine', *Politico*, 11 December 2023: ...When the European Council – the intergovernmental branch of the EU – does sanction Russian business leaders suspected of aiding and abetting the Putin regime, it has often relied on slipshod evidence that makes the decisions easy to challenge in court, POLITICO has also found. Nearly 1,600 Western multinationals continue, meanwhile, to do business in Russia. Many that announced they would pull out have struggled to do so. The Council of Europe in *EU sanctions against Russia explained* said that in certain instances 'a temporary exception is foreseen for imports of crude oil by pipeline into those EU member states that, due to their geographical situation, suffer from a specific dependence on Russian supplies and have no viable alternative options.' The Kiev School of Economics Institute noted on 16 January 2024 in *Stop Doing Business with Russia* that 1,600 multinational corporations were using a variety of means to bypass the sanctions.

50 Comment made by Dr Brendan Flannery, the head of the US Center for Disease Control and Prevention's team in Liberia, quoted by Jason Beaubien, *All things considered*, NPR, 6 October 2014.

51 Miles Moore, 'Firestone continues fight against spread of Ebola', *Rubber News*, 10 November 2014.

52 While the company's empathy was acknowledged in this instance, it had many critics over time about its general relations with indigenous peoples.

53 'China floods to hit US economy: Climate effects through trade chains', Potsdam Institute for Climate Impact Research (PIK), 28 May 2018.

54 For summary, see: Humanitarian Futures Programme, *Humanitarian motives: Mutual self-interest versus compassion*. www.humanitarianfutures.org at Key Findings. Also, HFP-King's College, London, Feinstein Institute, Tufts University and Overseas Development Institute, *Planning from the future, perspectives on organisational change*, www.humanitarianfutures.org at Key Findings, 2016, p. 18 ff.

55 In 2018, the gaps between countries – Yemen, Syria, Somalia and Afghanistan – accounted for 82 per cent of all recorded battle casualties. Of the world's 10 hungriest countries, 8 were in sub-Saharan Africa, plus Yemen and Timor-Leste. When it came to internal displacement, Iraq, Syria, Sudan, Nigeria, the Philippines and Pakistan took the lead. Of the 25 poorest countries in the world, 22 were in Sub-Saharan Africa.

56 Nicholas Stern noted in a talk on 4 February 2022 to a group of NGOs at 'The Long Humanitarian Century' forum that this fact needed to be linked to ways that global issues of climate change should be addressed.
57 Global Challenges Foundation, *Global catastrophic risks – 2016*, p. 24.

Bibliography

Alexandresus, Mihal, 'David Mitrany: From federalism to functionalism', *Transylvania Review*, XVI (1), 2007.

Andrenell, Andrea and Gonzalez, Javier Lopez, *3D printing: The final frontier for international trade in goods?* OECD, 9 November 2021.

Aon Benfield, *2011 Thailand floods event recap report: Impact forecasting*, March 2012.

Appadurai, Arjun, 'Tactical humanism', in Jerome Binde (Ed.), *The future of values* UNESCO Publication/Berghahn Books, 2004.

Ball, James, 'Russia is risking the creation of a "splinternet" – and it could be irreversible', *MIT Technology Review*, 17 March 2022.

Bordoff, Jason and O'Sullivan, Meghan L., 'The age of energy security: How the fight for resources is upending geopolitics', *Foreign Affairs,* May/June 2023.

Bukhari, Syed Shahid Hussain, Roofi, Yasmin and Bukhari, Syed Adnan, 'Resolving Balochistan conflict: A human needs approach', *Pakistan Journal of Social Sciences*, 35 (1), 30 June 2015.

Bullough, Oliver, 'Review of Adam Tooze's Shutdown: How Covid Shook the World Economy', Allen Lane, 2021.' *The Guardian*, 10 September 2021,

Carvalho, Vasco M., Nirei, Makoto, Saito, Yukiko U. and Tahbaz-Saleh, Alireza, 'Supply chain disruptions: Evidence from the Great East Japan Earthquake', *The Quarterly Journal of Economics*, 136 (2), May 2021. https://doi.org/10.1093/qje/qjaa044

Castells, Manuel, 'The impact of the internet on society: A global perspective', *Change: 19 key essays on how the internet is changing our lives*, BBVA: Open Mind, 2014.

Eilstrup-Sangiovanni, *Debates on European integration*, Palgrave Macmillan, 2006.

Emediegwu, Lotanna, Russia's invasion of the Ukraine exacerbates hunger in the Middle East and North Africa', Aid and International Development, *Economics Observatory,* 30 March 2022.

Essid, Badye and Jenkins, Paul, *Understanding global interdependencies: The contribution of economic models*, Think Tank 20: Macroeconomic Policy Interdependence and the G-20, www.brookings.edu, April 2020.

Foley, C. Fritz, Hines, James R. and Wessel, David, *Global goliaths: Multinational corporations in the 21st century economy*, Brookings, April 2021.

Foust, Jeff, 'Russia commits to ISS extension to 2028', *SpaceNews*, 27 April 2023.

Freund, Caroline, Mulabdic, Alen and Rita, Michelle, *Is 3D printing a threat to global trade: The trade affects that you didn't hear about, World Development Report – Policy Research Working Paper 9024*, World Bank Group September 2019; 9 November 2021.

Garrett, Geoffrey, 'Doing well by doing good,' *Wharton Magazine*, Spring/Summer 2017.

Global Challenges Foundation, *Global catastrophic risks, 2016.*

Humanitarian Futures Programme, *The virtuous triangle and the fourth dimension: The humanitarian, private and military sectors in a fragile world,* humanitarianfuturesprogramme.org see: Key Findings, 2014.

International Monetary Fund, *World economic outlook: War sets back the global recovery*, April 2022.

Internet World Stats: Usage and Population Statistic*s, World internet users and 2021 population stats.* /www.worldinternetstates.com

Jee, Charlotte, 'Russia wants to cut itself off from the global internet: Here's what is means,' *MIT Technology Review*, 21 March 2019.

Jensen-Eriksen, Niklas (leader), Wuokko, Maiju and Sahari, Aaro, *Business, governments and international trade in Cold War Europe (2012–2014)*, Capitalism, State & Society research group, University of Helsinki, Finland, 2015.

Kent, Randolph et al., *Towards an International Architecture for Managing Global Threats – Systems Compendium Annex*, Royal United Services Institute, 2021.

Kogut, B., *Multinational corporations*, www0.gsb.columbia.edu/faculty/bkogut/files/Chapter_in_smelser-Baltes_2001.pdf.

Levermann, Anders, et al., *Climate-related flooding may quickly disrupt global trade chains: US–China exchange especially vulnerable,* Earth Institute, 28 May 2018. news.climat.columbia.edu

Lutz, Brenda J. and Lutz, James M., 'Globalisation and terrorism in the Middle East,' *Perspectives on Terrorism*, 9 (5), October 2015.

McLeod, Saul, 'Maslow's hierarchy of needs', 21 May 2018, www.simplypsychology.org/maslow.html

Makhanov, Kanat, 'National disasters in China and shift in the global grain market', Eurasian Research Institute, Akhmet Yassawi University, 2020.

Moore, Miles 'Firestone continues fight against spread of Ebola', *Rubber News,* 10 November 2014.

Moreland, Will, 'The purpose of multilateralism: A framework for democracies in a geopolitically competitive world', *Foreign Policy at Brookings*, September 2019.

Oberhaus, Daniel, 'How Cold War politics shaped the International Space Station: A brief history detailing how the United States and Russia led the effort to create the technical marvel', *Smithsonian Magazine*, 9 September 2020.

OECD, Policy Notes Series, *Multinational enterprises in the global economy: Heavily debated but hardly measured*, May 2018.

OECD, *Covid 19 and policy for science*, OECD Science, Technology and Policy Papers, No. 152, 3 July 2023. https://doi.org/10.1787/8f86e60b-en

Patrick, Stewart, *Best laid plans: The origins of American multilateralism and the dawn of the Cold War*, Rowman and Littlefield, 2009.

Roehrlich, Elisabeth, 'International organizations during the Cold War', 3 February 2017. www.wilsoncenter.org

Saviano, Robert, *Zero, zero, zero*, Penguin Books, 2016.

Snegovaya, Maria, Dolbaia, Tina, Fenton, Nick and Bergmann, Max, 'Russia sanctions at one year', *Centre for Strategic and International Studies*, 23 February 2023.

Stevance, Anne-Sophie, Bridgewater, Peter, Louafi, Selim, King, Nicholas, et al., 'The 2019 review of IPBES and future priorities: Reaching beyond assessment to enhance policy impact', AGRIS, FAO, 2020. Information provided by Centre de Cooperation Internationale en recherche agronomique pour le development, Ministre des Affaires Étrangers.

Surminski, Swenja, Barnes Jonathan and Vincent, Katharine, 'Can insurance catalyse government planning on climate? Emergent evidence from Sub-Saharan Africa', *World Development*, 153, May 2022.

Tooze, Adam, *Shutdown: How Covid shook the world economy*, Allen Lane, 2021.

United Nations Security Council 9008th meeting, 'Conflict, humanitarian crisis in Ukraine threatening future global food security as prices rise, production capacity shrinks, speakers warn Security Council,' SC/14846, 29 March 2022.

Visa Economic Empowerment Institute, *The rise of digital remittances: How innovation is improving global money movement*, 2021. www.visaeconomicempowermentinstitute.org

Wagner, Caroline S., Whetsell, Travis, Baas, Jeroen and Jonkers, Koen, 'Openness and impact of leading scientific countries', *Front. Res. Metr. Anal.*, 28 March 2018. https://doi.org/10.3389/frma.2018.00010

World101, *Global era issues from the Council on Foreign Relations*, Council on Foreign Relations. www.educatingforamericandemocracy.org

6 Managing Humanitarian Threats in a Polylateral World

Humanity faces a stark and urgent choice: breakdown or breakthrough. The choices we make – or fail to make – today could result in further breakdown and a future of perpetual crises or a breakthrough to a more sustainable, peaceful future. So suggested the United Nations Secretary-General in 2021.[1]

> *If we are to deliver on our promises to future generations – to secure a world where everyone can thrive in peace, dignity and equality on a healthy planet – then 2021 must be the year we change gear.* ***We must think big.*** *We need to reshape the foundations and reaffirm the core values that underpin collective action.*
>
> ***Time is of essence and the choices before us are stark.*** *Our welfare, and indeed the permanence of human life, now depend on us working effectively together across borders and sectors to manage many shared risks and achieve a vital set of common goals, including but not limited to, those set out in the UN75 Declaration.*[2]

Introduction

The 2021 ***Our Common Agenda*** suggested that the United Nations had to be aware of its diminishing strengths. An essential lesson-learned from a UN perspective was that conventional multilateral systems would have to be more inclusive than originally designed. Nevertheless, that essential lesson assumed that multilateral systems would still be globally dominant, but that to be more effective, they would have 'to reflect a more inclusive and more networked multilateralism'.[3] They would have to ensure that the sciences, the private sector and communities came together at the state-based policymaking table.

The UN's position reflected a reasonable step towards a 'coalition of the willing', and so it was agreed that a 'Summit for the Future' would take place in 2024 with the formal participation of key civil society organisations. Its objective would be to attain a new global consensus on a future planning agenda in which 'countries worked together to solve global problems – that the international system works

DOI: 10.4324/9781003471004-7

fast to protect everyone in emergencies; and the UN is universally recognized as a trusted platform for collaboration'.[4]

That said, there is little to suggest that the multilateral construct, and in this case the United Nations, broadly speaking will be able to generate the creativity, consistency and coherence required to deal with ever more complex crisis threats. Rather, instead of automatically assuming that multilateralism, *per se*, will be central for dealing with the sorts of threats portrayed in Chapter 4, there are other constructs in a more *polylateral* world order, as described in Chapter 3, that are emerging and that will play major roles in addressing humanitarian vulnerabilities.

The entanglement nexus, as discussed in Chapter 5, will be a driver of polylateralism, and in turn, polylateralism will increasingly determine and be determined by how the increasing numbers and types of systems, networks, alliances, coalitions and social media across the globe may be configured and interact. Such adjustments will influence governance and society generally and will have significant consequences when it comes to anticipating who will be significant humanitarian actors. Therefore, an appreciation of their respective weaknesses and strengths would seem a sensible starting point. The former might well persist, and such limitations need to be recognised and offset wherever possible; and, as for the latter, strengths, they should be recognised and enhanced, again whenever possible, by cross institutional linkages.

And, for what purpose? Here, it is to suggest three. How diverse actors could come together in *clusters*, a metaphor to suggest ways that a wide range of institutional capacities and comparative advantages can be identified for their potential humanitarian value. Second, how such *clusters* should lead to *webs*, reflecting components' strategic and operational linkages, and finally, using the metaphor, *swarms*, to describe ways that humanitarian action could be made more systematic, targeted and coherent.

Exploring Systems, Alliances, Coalitions, Networks and Social Movements

> There is a fundamental change underway regarding how global problems can be solved, and perhaps how we govern ourselves on this shrinking planet. Emerging non-state networks of civil society, private sector, government and individual stakeholders are achieving new forms of cooperation, social change and even the production of global public value. They address every conceivable issue facing humanity from poverty, human rights, health and the environment, to economic policy, war and even the governance of the Internet itself.[5]

Whether systems, networks, alliances, coalitions, or social movements, all in their own ways reflect complex interconnections – *ecosystems* – that explain relationships that emerge in pursuit of their respective goals.[6] Like the entanglement nexus, these do not automatically foster or reflect consistency or coherence, but do suggest an acceptance of interconnectedness, interrelationships and varying degrees of interdependencies.

As one begins to explore ways that humanitarian threats are and increasingly will be identified and mitigated in an ever more complex environment, it is important to bear in mind that the sheer speed of technological transformations, the changing nature of human agency, emerging interests on and beyond planet Earth, increasing numbers of shared or contending interests and concerns, growing global entanglement – and the list goes on – will all result in a rapidly growing number of systems, networks, alliances, coalitions and social movements.

Yet, despite their increasing numbers and the prospect of changing dynamics, there are present strengths and weaknesses that will most likely persist in the foreseeable future.

Persistent Weaknesses

For the purposes of assessing their potential for effectively dealing with humanitarian crisis threats, each institutional category – systems, networks, alliances, coalitions and social movements – has particular strengths and weaknesses and together in varying degrees they also share them.

Systems and alliances and to a lesser extent coalitions all too often get bogged down in seeming inconsistencies, contradictions and complexity. The global community now faces an increasing number of 'wicked problems' – problems that are difficult 'to resolve fully due to incomplete and at times contradictory information and frequent changes in requirements and output functions in a turbulent context'.[7]

This explains in no small part why the very capacities of the multilateral sector to deal with a confluence of crises are under strain, perhaps unprecedented except in times of world wars. In the early 2020s, global economic impacts of a persistent pandemic, the Russian invasion of Ukraine and ensuing inflation along with energy insecurities, climate change and its increasingly apparent consequences across the globe, wars in Gaza and the West Bank that tested the most basic principles of international human rights law and persistent conflicts in at least 12 countries leading to mass starvation, all reflect the overburdened nature of the multilateral construct as presently defined.

Hence, one apparent and persistent weakness for many systems, alliances and coalitions stems from ***policy quagmires*** where those involved in defining and agreeing on processes and objectives are confronted with complex problems that appear simply too hard to solve. The quagmires that all too often hamper creative solutions can result in arrangements that are stuck in incremental and narrowly focused outputs. These quagmires often result in minimal policy adjustments when confronting complex pressures in an ever more polylateral world.[8]

This in turn has led to the emergence of parallel systems of action, where issues are being dealt with through networks and social movements that are much more flexible though all too often lacking adequate authority and sustainable structures. In that sense, networks such as the Internet Protocol (IP) Network and social movements, like Extinction Rebellion, can have significant influence and more flexibility in presenting their common objectives. However, because there is little formal obligation to implement or operationalise specific policies, their impacts upon policy development and implementation can by no means be assumed.

Those bodies that are not part of state-based institutions, coalitions and alliances such as the private sector may act independently, frequently adding even more complexity to already complex problems.

Closely related to policy quagmires is a second weakness, namely, that *objectives and missions* are frequently ambiguous and ill-defined. Wittingly or unwittingly, compromise to sustain some sort of coherence often results in undertakings that may suit, for example, particular sub-components of a governmental system rather than that system as a whole. Siloed government departments, over accommodating intergovernmental organisations, alliances and coalitions that tolerate 'below the surface contentiousness' can compound ambiguity when attempting to define objectives and missions.

Such weaknesses are further compounded by the likelihood that in many instances systems, coalitions, alliances, networks and social movements are deaf to potential commonalities between and among them. Ambiguous objectives and misunderstandings about their respective objectives and missions are intentionally or unintentionally barriers for identifying opportunities for mutual support. In fact, they could be sources of conflict at any level.

Planning and Prioritisation Processes such as those underpinning the UN's Sustainable Development Goals (SDGs) initiative generally have received considerable praise.[9] The coalition of what are referred to as 'partners' is extensive, consisting of a wide range of governments and intergovernmental, private sector and civil society organisations. However, like similar international initiatives such as the Global Compact in 2000, the SDGs are well intentioned, but their implementation frequently fails to confront the complexities and paradoxes that underpin their objectives.

In the case of the SDGs, criticisms range from insensitivities to microcultures and local languages, ways that implementation feeds corruption and their use as public relations 'rainbow washing'. More relevant, here, however is the fact that many potential actors, specifically governmental, intergovernmental organisations and the private sector, base their plans on outmoded methodologies and a general lack of means to measure SDG indicators. This point was noted in a report by Paris21 which found that even highly developed countries were still not able to report more than 40–50 per cent of the SDG indicators.[10] In other words, planning and prioritisation processes often have been developed without the competencies to produce relevant statistics and data.

Beyond this sort of 'technical failing' is another fundamental issue, namely, many governments regard the SDGs as a 'misuse of country ownership', 'an imposition of intergovernmental institutions'. Planning and prioritisation processes all too often reflect specific country problems and not connectivity with others. They, too, are defined by assumptions that may have declining relevance but ignored because of institutional reluctance to be diverted by the uncertainties of the future.[11] [12]

Contending objectives. Another weakness that pervades many systems, alliances, coalitions, networks and social movements are potentially *contending objectives*. The divisive consequences of contending objectives frequently result in systems' objectives being sacrificed to ensure a sense of harmony. Take a look, for example, at emerging responses to climate change. Governmental responses to this potentially existential threat have been inconsistent, often more rhetorical than actionable. In turn IGOs also frequently find themselves mimicking the same expressions of concern but not translated into actionable plans, and simultaneously generating levels of frustration and disillusion with the present multilateral construct.

What emerges is that processes that sustain harmony become an equally if not more important objective of many globally bodies. Recent efforts for dealing with climate change by the International Maritime Organization are not untypical.

The organisation consists of 175 member states, 66 IGOs with observer status and 85 INGOs with consultative status. However, despite the ostensible interest of most members to limit greenhouse gas (GHG) emissions, a few shipping lobbies such as the World Shipping Council and the International Maritime Council were able to completely stall the GHG initiative in order to keep the industry free of environmental regulations that had been agreed at the 2015 Paris climate talks. Nevertheless, while it was all too evident that the IMO's initial objective had been lost in bureaucracy, it was the negotiating process – rather than any implementable actions – which was acclaimed as a success.[13]

Funding dependencies and funded concessions. This weakness opens the way to a further one, namely, *funding dependencies and funded concessions*. Both too often determine organisational action within systems. The European Organization for Nuclear Research, CERN, is an interesting case in point. The idea that '[they] are so busy getting private sector money because governments do not have enough, that [they] are ceding to the private sector partner, and the ownership of that intellectual property' reflects a more general challenge for the subcomponents of systems, in this case, 'the organisation'.[14]

Tensions between the broad objectives of alliances, networks, coalitions, etc., and their components' interests are not unusual. And, while not always the case, it is the interests of the components which tend to dominate. The humanitarian sector – including systems at headquarters level as well as those in vulnerable countries – is a case in point.[15] This weakness also relates to the inherent *risk aversion* that certainly is reflected in many systems, alliances and coalitions and to lesser extents networks and certainly far less so, in social movements.

For example, it is not surprising that a 2022 G20 Report on Multilateral Development Banks concluded that the MDBs had to revamp their approaches to risk tolerance, because their use of overly conservative measures of risk was preventing them from unleashing hundreds of billions of dollars in new lending to help lower-income nations at a time of overlapping global crises.[16]

Both a reflection of weakness as well as strength are the growing impacts of *social media* on established institutions across the globe.

> …in less than a generation, the most successful network platforms have brought together user bases larger than the populations of most nations and even some

> continents. However, large user populations gathered on popular network platforms have more diffuse borders than those of political geography, and network platforms are operated by parties with interests that may differ from those of a nation. Operators of network platforms do not necessarily think in terms of government priorities or national strategy, particularly if those priorities and strategies might conflict with serving their customers. Such network platforms may host or facilitate economic and social interactions that surpass (in number and scale) those of most countries, despite the platforms having formed no economic or social policy as a government would have.[17]

Yet, it is evident that social networking can undermine key objectives of virtually all types of global actors. When it came to the 2019–2022 Covid-19 pandemic, one of the greatest challenges that had to be faced was disinformation about the causes of and appropriate responses to the disease. As noted in a series of studies by the OECD, while the exchange of information between the sciences and a range of actors – be they governments and intergovernmental bodies or coalitions such as the Global Evaluation Coalition – was vital, but all too frequently, confusing and uncertain.[18] However, as was also very clear, social media dramatically compounded that confusion and uncertainty. For example, 'anti-vacciners' railed against vaccination programmes, and its impact was felt across the globe.

The impacts of social media have increasingly influenced decision-making processes, distorted political positions during and in the aftermath of elections, undermined the credibility of established institutions; and even generated social movements against them and led to doubts about the nature of global threats such as climate change.[19]

However, like social media, many systems, networks, alliances and coalitions have important strengths that have to be recognised, and in this context for appreciating their value for dealing with global threats.

Fluctuating Strengths

While systems weaknesses are the playing fields of many analysts, there are positive developments which also need to be taken into consideration. Perhaps one of the most positive 'strengths', or, developments, stems from the fact that transformative technologies have created a sense of positive interconnectedness across a wide sweep of geopolitical, economic, social and geographical boundaries – the upside of the entanglement nexus.

In various ways social media and transglobal communications have opened up new ways to engage with people and communities, even those traditionally not accessible.[20] Interrelated, are various degrees of economic and commercial interdependencies and social, intellectual, cultural and scientific areas of common interests.

How might these positive considerations relate to managing global threats from a polylateral perspective?

In answer to that question, it is evident that there is a greater awareness of threats and their global implications, and that has been reflected in *increasingly global awareness* of potential spill overs and complexities. In a clearly related sense, *new forms of collaboration* and concomitantly *the triggers* that led to them reflect that awareness. And, as discussed when considering the entanglement nexus, *functional interrelationships* also determine more and more the direction of a *growing number of global actors* and their perspectives. In no small part are these stimulated and sustained by *new technologies*.

The growth of *global actors and perspectives* is evident. Over the past three decades, for example, the number of international bodies concerned with risk management has increased from 147 to 289.[21] CERN, again, offers a useful example. It may have its downsides, but at the same time it demonstrates systems thinking that goes beyond physics into the realm of a more global public good. The implication of its scientific work is understood, but that its resources are increasingly used across the globe to promote projects such as assistance to vulnerable children far less so. Cross-sectoral systems and perspectives, which will later be referred to as 'global solutions networks', are increasingly evident.

New forms of collaboration are emerging that counter the criticism that many bodies that deal with hazards lack adequately inclusive approaches for identifying and mitigating them. The Non-Communicable Disease Alliance (NCDA) is but one of a growing number of global efforts that suggest new forms of collaboration. Its focus is at the community level, where approximately 2,000 organisations (including governmental, intergovernmental and non-governmental), the private sector and research institutions from more than 170 countries seek solutions for diseases such as diabetes, heart disease and cancer.[22]

The Global Resilient Cities Network (GRCN) is an example of global collaboration not state dependent. Its objectives include highlighting ways that cities can share information, collaborate on developing innovative practices and seek project funding – all in a network that is urban and not dependent on state-based structures.

As opposed to the GRCN, the Sustainable Energy for All Alliance, or the SEforAll, is a global coalition that includes a wide and diverse range of actors that does include governments as well as the private sector, civil society and international organisations working. In partnership with the United Nations, they have garnered their capacities to focus on delivering universal access to electricity. At the same time, their intention is to double the amount of renewable energy in the global energy mix from its current share of 18 per cent to 36 per cent.

The challenges which SEforAll has to face in its efforts to achieve its objectives has led to global sub-components, resulting in a Leadership Council (LC) to create new and intersectoral partnerships, generate vital data, generate much needed finance – all complemented by high level advocacy. It is worth noting here that the SEforAll's LC triggered many hundreds of different types of organisations at local, national and global levels to deal with its complex ambitions as a collective force. It is assumed that these hundreds will eventually trigger many thousands more.

Similarly, for all the eventual achievements and parallel frustrations that stemmed from the UN Framework Convention on Climate Change (UNFCCC) and subsequently the Kyoto Protocol and eventually the IPCC agreements and the COPs, it serves as another example about the ways global collaborative initiatives can trigger an unanticipated number of diverse 'sub-systems'.[23]

For example, out of the UNFCCC emerged the Indigenous Peoples Organisation for Climate Change, the constituency of Youth and Non-Governmental Organisations (YOUNGO) and the Women and Gender Constituency. In other words, global initiatives should also be measured in terms of the systems, coalitions, alliances, networks and social movements that they trigger.

In a related vein, *new technologies* also trigger new global-oriented actors reflecting *functional interrelationships*. One example is the Global Partnership on Artificial Intelligence, an ecosystem of AI practitioners, entrepreneurs, academia, NGOs, and AI industry players and organisations focused upon common interests in controlling technology's perceived upsides and downsides.

Created in June 2020, its value was re-enforced the following year in UNESCO's Recommendation on the Ethics for Artificial Intelligence. Both underscored the importance of having a wide range of actors sharing their analysis of the evolving impacts of AI.[24] Similarly, the benefits and hazards of outer space exploration have been bringing together the private sector, non-governmental organisations and governments to address a host of contemporary or prospective developments, including asteroid mining, increasing numbers of satellite owners, the emergence of 'mini-satellites', cyberwarfare and the potential deployment of 'defensive' space weaponry to protect satellites.[25]

The Geneva Science and Diplomacy Anticipator (GESDA) is yet another example of the growing number of global cohorts that are triggered by new technologies, recognised functional interrelationships and that result in new forms of collaboration among global, regional and national actors. Its purpose is to bring together scientists from around the world to provide an overview of scientific trends from 5, 10 and 25 years perspectives, in part to contribute to global initiatives such as the Sustainable Development Goals.

And, similarly, the United Nations Development Programme's Accelerator Labs are designed to bring together an extensive range of academic and research institutions along with bodies such as the Grassroots Innovation Augmentation Network and a number of governments and private sector organisations 'to anticipate emerging signals of change and testing ways to address complex and interrelated challenges to be scaled either through UNDP programmes and operations, Governments, and/or private sector'.[26]

These sorts of initiatives have increased exponentially over the past decade.[27] All in various ways underscore a trend so important to those concerned with vulnerabilities and their humanitarian consequences, namely, an increasing awareness of potential spillovers and complexities.

New Perspectives

Yet, despite all the potential benefits that are evident from recent global cohorts, it is more than disconcerting to see that, from a more holistic perspective, the global community lacks the coherence, long-term commitment, structures and capacities to effectively manage humanitarian threats in an ever more polylateral world. All those policy quagmires, ambiguous and ill-defined objectives, inadequate planning and prioritisation processes, contending objectives, funding dependencies and funded concessions remain as drags for preparing to deal with the present, let alone the future – and this certainly includes humanitarian action.

However, there are steps that policy planners and decision-makers can begin to take now that can enhance resilience and response capacities. By no means are they 'the solution', but they do offer ways to utilise the positive elements of the entanglement nexus to prepare now for the future.

Three Metaphors: Clusters, Webs, Swarms in a Polylateral Context

When discussing the evolving nature of development, the World Bank noted that the 'development context is not stable anymore… . [It is] constantly in crisis because this is what is happening… . We are basically driven to adapt to the extreme challenges.'[28] In a more general sense, Geoff Mulgan implied the same thing when he noted that

> although we live surrounded by systems, we struggle to understand them let alone to guide and control them. I believe we need a novel approach that focuses on how to enrich and open up the shared intelligence around us.[29]

This does not mean that conventional intergovernmental systems, for example, will not continue to have value. Rather, it is to say that a growing number of systems, alliances, coalitions, networks and social movements will be less the monopoly of state-based systems, and more and more fluctuating amalgams of different types of actors in a less predictable 'polylateral' world order.

From a humanitarian perspective that means that the process of identifying potential threats as well as ways to mitigate them will increasingly be in the hands of complex and often erratic and unpredictable arrays of actors. Their respective motives, institutional interests, obligations and capacities as well as prioritisation processes may result in confused or contending outputs. Ways to avoid such downsides of the entanglement nexus are needed now, perhaps more than ever. How best to capture the positive opportunities of that nexus can be described with three metaphors: *clusters*, *webs* and *swarms*. Each is far more concerned with dynamics and linkages rather than constructs, *per se*.

Driven by plausible humanitarian threats, *clusters* of varied expertise will be increasingly likely to come together to deal with such threats, driven in no small part by a growing awareness of mutual self-interest. Principally focussed on problem resolving processes, clusters can trigger *webs* of understanding about problem-solving that could lead in turn to relatively assured and timely *swarms* of appropriate responses.

These processes, however, do not necessarily foretell of permanent constructs or enduring paradigmatic shifts over time. Rather, they suggest that in a period of growing polylateralism, there will be dynamics and linkages that will be increasingly relevant in the foreseeable future. Their consequences will certainly be of humanitarian relevance.

Clusters: Concept and Creation

The Concept

The metaphor, *cluster*, is neither to suggest a system, network, alliance, coalition or social movement, *per se*. Instead, it serves as a way to describe each or perhaps even all, but whatever its composition, clusters are principally about process – the dynamics and linkages that create them. It makes no assumptions about the characteristics of actors at the outset. Instead, it reflects the process by which attitudes about interests are identified and evolve as much as the interests, themselves.

As long as there are recognised common interests, or *mutual self-interests*, those who perceive them will be inclined to seek some sort of relationship to achieve them. Borrowing from a 2019 study on *Systems Leadership for Sustainable Development*, the process that triggers clusters begins 'in response to a complex problem that stakeholders realize they cannot solve alone'.[30]

Of course, the term, cluster, is used in various ways, not necessarily the way that it is intended here. The United Nations uses it to define actions that specific types of actors might need to use when it comes to complex humanitarian crises.[31] Related is the OECD's definition of the term, with particular emphasis on 'an agglomeration of firms in a related business, which are brought together in developed and developing economies'.[32]

The difference between those definitions and the one that is suggested here is that the constituency of any cluster reflects issues at hand, not necessarily based on any specific sector or type of organisation. Initially, its intention is not permanence and is likely to be fluid and transient at the outset. A cluster may coalesce because individual components have identified a problem, a common issue of concern and an opportunity, and those components, too, may withdraw should such objectives no longer seem advantageous or relevant to their particular interests.

As opposed to more standard alignments, clusters at the outset are not necessarily structurally entangled, nor are they necessarily bound by treaties or legal agreements. They come together to exert influence and agree on functional measures to achieve agreed objectives. It reflects as much a process as it does a tangible grouping. Fluidity and informal decision-chains are normal traits during the cluster formulation process.

Clusters of actors are not inherently static. There are dynamics that occur that affect their rhythm and sense of purpose, which in turn can result in more defined objectives and common processes. Disputes over the substance of what hitherto had been an agreed objective may lead those within a cluster to redefine the substance and purpose of the objective that had initially brought them together; a growing awareness that the sum of a cluster's interests can be 'greater than its individual parts' may transform the ways that cluster members now view their individual objectives.

Such dynamics suggest that clusters frequently go through an identification phase when efforts to clarify objectives leads to increasing rationale and commitments to coalesce.

Take, for example, how one foresight expert described his Action Foresight 'Global Swarm'. What for the purposes of this discussion will be called a 'cluster', Action Foresight consists of groupings of

> geographically, culturally and professionally distributed teams of researchers, innovators and practitioners who come together to collaborate, scale and mutualize resources for big challenges, high impact foresight projects and our shared commons.
>
> [Its] plurality of perspectives facilitate our collective creativity, enabling us to better formulate methodologies, capture discoveries, and perform analysis that best addresses the complexity of our contemporary challenges. Our collective creativity is facilitated by our plurality of perspectives and our shared vision of enabling plural futures. Our track record represents our value and ability to surface and empower subaltern and outlier perspectives and engender preferred futures.[33]

It is that 'polarity of perspectives', 'distributed teams' and emphasis on foresight which underpin the concept of clusters here. Issue focused, institutionally unconstrained, multiplicities of expertise and willingness to empower others through evidence and insights will be of increasing importance in maximising effective anticipatory humanitarian action in a polylateral world order.

Already a pattern is emerging in which some of the most functional roles of multilateral institutions, e.g. IGOs, are being assumed or at least sustained by others. When it comes to acknowledging the importance of diversity and distributed teams, the United Nations recognises that a wide mixture of non-state actors are and increasingly will be essential for agreeing on as well as implementing the objectives of core issues such as climate reduction.[34]

In a less positive though relevant example of increasing diversity and distributed teams is the response by the governments of Mexico and the United States to 'pandemic refugees' during the Covid-19 crisis. Federal and state institutions on both sides of the border appeared ill prepared, reluctant or unwilling to deal with the emerging pandemic and asylum-seeking populations. Rather than the support of traditionally recognised states, IGOs or INGO-based humanitarian actors, the crisis affected were increasingly dependent upon a growing number of *ad hoc* humanitarians, including those from religious, local community and academic institutions.[35]

The clusters of actors that have been increasingly evident in humanitarian action also reflect the transnational nature of many organisations, particularly in the private sector. In this regard, there may be no formal systems, *per se*, but that sector, for example, in Southeast Asia, has become

> …more involved in disaster risk management, especially through their business continuity plans and long-term strategic business objectives particularly in direct assistance to communities; disaster preparedness for businesses; developing new and innovative products for disasters; participation in joint projects with NGOs and international organisations; and as an avenue for corporate social responsibility like the establishment of private foundations and trusts.[36]

Of importance, too, when considering clustering is the willingness of a growing number of diverse actors to work together in a kind of *bricolage* where multiple actors 'just make do'. Making do, however, is neither random nor unskilled. Rather, it is the authority to use what is immediately available or perhaps incidentally at hand to make sense of a situation or resolve a problem.[37] Bricolage provides a perspective on triggers for dealing with everything from displacement on borders to global threats such as cyber collapse in ways that IGOs, for example, would be reluctant to adopt alone.

Humanitarian action will depend more and more upon a proliferation of different actors – *clusters* – that are not necessarily bound by alliances, coalitions or formal networks. Instead, more and more, increasing awareness of interrelatedness, interdependencies and mutual self-interests will be a significant coalescing factor that will expand the numbers and types of those who assume humanitarian roles and responsibilities. It is an identification phase in which a range of interests and actors will come together and could well catalyse into webs of action.[38]

Cluster Creation

Ever greater complexity exposing and intensifying global vulnerabilities demands consistent and indeed persistent efforts to enhance awareness across multiple sectors about ways to identify and address such vulnerabilities. Some of these efforts may stem from different bodies such as the International Science Council seeking ways to ensure that all in the scientific community have access to on-going research and findings. Others may be platforms, soon to be described on page 187, that will identify and facilitate activities relevant to humanitarian threat identification and appropriate response.

> ***Mapping.*** Myriad institutions and professional bodies have enormous amounts of knowledge and experience which too often are not recognised or understood for their humanitarian relevance. At the same time, there, too, is a considerable number of such institutions and professional bodies that are not fully aware of the activities of others even in their own areas of expertise and interest. Mapping, or, in other words, identifying existing or potential organisational

> linkages, processes, 'products', outputs and essential inputs within and across sectors would open pathways not previously known or considered.

Mapping, therefore, can provide sectoral and intersectoral benefits to participants, but its importance from a humanitarian perspective is that it could also identify clusters of diverse actors that could bring additional capacities and innovations for dealing with humanitarian threats to the fore. From astrophysicists' research institutions to product marketing in the automotive industry, there are sectoral and cross sectoral connections that can provide more nuanced understanding of crisis drivers and ways to deal with them.

The natural and social sciences, for example, clearly have contributed enormously to an understanding of the drivers of humanitarian crises – ways to avoid them as well as mitigate their impacts. Yet, it is by no means certain that their expertise is fully appreciated or adequately used or integrated across disciplines. Nor, can it be assumed that scientists, themselves, are always aware of other scientific institutions that could have direct impact on their own work. This has been evident when it comes to relationships between the social and natural sciences.[39]

The challenge for the sciences and for organisations and coalitions of organisations more generally is to have clear and systematically consolidated views of existing sectoral and institutional linkages. Mapping would therefore expand an awareness of the scope and dimensions of formal and informal connections and common interests in and across sectors. In so doing, it should result in a greater propensity to appreciate the importance of multisectoral analyses of future threats, and therefore intersectoral ways to monitor and deal with them.

Such awareness will result in an essential inflection point for clustering diverse and multidimensional sectors together to foster conceptual and operational webs of humanitarian action.[40] However, to do so will depend upon how effectively analysts will be to contend with inevitable information challenges.

Resolving the Information Challenge. Inconsistent, often contradictory data about plausible threats, their drivers and potential consequences frequently undermine effective decision-making.[41] Furthermore, decision-makers and policy planners are all too often provided with data that reflects merely one component of highly complex and interacting threats as well as means for mitigating them. Unless data is 'accessible', it is more than likely that complex threats will be handled in very linear ways.[42]

Significant efforts have been and continue to be made to ensure more coherent and 'usable' data for dealing with global catastrophic risks. In 2018, it was assumed that

> no known methodology for compiling a comprehensive, interdisciplinary view of severe global catastrophic risks. While a fully complete list of such risks may remain beyond reach, what is accessible is a "classification framework" designed specifically to draw on as broad a knowledge base as possible, to highlight commonalities between risk scenarios and identify gaps in our collective knowledge regarding global catastrophic risks.[43]

Less than five years later that was less the case. The methodology had emerged to make data compilation and information gathering highly effective. There remain other challenges that now needed to be faced: clarity of objectives, coordination, interdisciplinary methodologies and data integrity.

In the first place, the objectives for which the data can be used all too often remain unclear. For example, is there general understanding about what is meant by humanitarian threats and their plausible causes? Given the range of factors that trigger and affect humanitarian threats (particularly if one accepts that they are often reflections of normal life), what are the parameters of necessary data – the types and levels of depth required? How accessible and retrievable will such data be? And, who will determine its relevance and veracity and how?

The issue of coordination between policymakers and researchers remains fundamental as does the importance of the relationships between researchers across disciplinary, organisational and geo-political boundaries. Data which reflects multiple perspectives is crucial, and 'greater machine intelligence' will most likely play an important role in this regard.[44] Therefore, closely linked to mapping are initiatives to identify data flows from different disciplines, which in turn will identify connections, patterns and relationships that may not be apparent when studying each discipline in isolation.

When it comes to interdisciplinary methodologies, climate change has proven to be an increasingly good example of how disciplines such as meteorology, oceanography, ecology and the social sciences can come together to model and predict climate change impacts. Similarly, bioinformatics reflects mapping data flows across biology, computer science and statistics, which enables researchers, in this instance, to provide individualised approaches to medical care.[45]

Another example of cross data mapping can be found in 'smart cities' where urban planning, transportation and information technology are linked to provide integrated and holistic approaches that far exceed standard, linear approaches to city development.[46]

Yet, with all these positive trends, an issue of abiding importance is that of data integrity. How will the data be used? What and who will determine confidentiality? Who will monitor its use?

The answer more often than not is situation and context specific. Nevertheless, there is a general belief that this challenge like the previous three can be met. In the context of fostering effective webs of cross sectoral functional interests, it will be essential to do so.

Towards Webs of Interests

Defining Webs

In 2022, the Robotics Growth Partnership developed the Cyber-Physical Infrastructure (CPI). Its purpose was to find new solutions for solving problems in sectors including agriculture, manufacturing, healthcare and logistics.

> Its relevance for those concerned with data sensitivity and inclusivity, however, begins with its flexible, interactive processes that bring together virtual and physical infrastructures on an ongoing basis for dealing with complex problems... . The CPI is based upon networked interactions between AI and humans on an-ongoing basis. It is not locked into any particular system or framework, but grows spontaneously and organically rather than being the result of a fixed, time-bound plan. No single sectoral specialist determines the nature and objectives of 'the product', but rather researchers, private sector engineers and society, more generally, take the lead in *on-going networks*.[47]

As one of the lead developers of the CPI told this author, the initiative to produce it stemmed from a very loose cluster of private sector, research institutes, governmental and intergovernmental organisations concerned with the impact of artificial intelligence on their respective areas of interest. They, in his words, had formed a cluster of interested parties.

From this perspective, clusters can result in *webs* of actors to address problems or maximise opportunities or both. In that sense, clusters may serve as bridges, a kind of identification-phase, into more enduring functional relationships. Those relationships reflect patterns of connectedness stemming from intertwined interests, and they take various forms. From projects and forums to regular information exchange and agreed institutional arrangements, from endorsements to fund raising, webs generally consist of hybrid components and their boundaries determined principally by functional interests.

The webs formed by clusters may be local or global. What they are not is centralised or hierarchical or necessarily permanent. Webs are about closer alignments among cluster components. They make possible interlinkages, overlaps, interactions and interplay, and increase the prospect that 'achieving common goals becomes more plausible; disruptive fragmentation less so'.[48]

Increasingly they are formed and sustained by communication systems such as the internet and internet-dependent communications networks. Clearly blending the virtual and physical has intensified opportunities for collaboration among hybrid multisectoral collections of actors. Such webs of interests may be non-binding and voluntary, but in a world where multilateral fragmentation is increasingly evident, webs have a growing role.

Some have seen webs as potential 'risk sharing pools'. 'All the actors of the risk-sharing domain,' noted Cambridge University's Institute for Sustainability Leadership, be they 'tax -based and premium-based, from community programmes to multinational level are inclined to be integrated in a public-mutual risk sharing continuum'.[49] It is interesting to note that, according to one extensive analysis of diverse actors dealing both with climate change and Covid-19, that

> variation in climate actions by actor type and lack of strong connections may not necessarily suggest that the global climate governance system is characterized by "fragmentation and functional overlaps" rather than by coherence and hierarchy.[50]

The coherence which creates functional webs of interests is often attributed to information and data flows. Exchange of both, including individual plans of action, are recognised drivers that can lead to consolidated webs of agreed action. Here, dealing with climate change again offers examples where different types of actors that have control over their own sectors may actually result in greater efficiencies in action. This conclusion is certainly in line with what one analyst imagined a polycentric governance system could achieve.[51]

Fostering Webs

Webs reflect the consequence of mobilising recognised interdependencies. They are the result of state and non-state actors moving from clusters to an acceptance of interconnected interests.

Building upon Recognised Mutual Self-Interests

In order to foster coherence, consistency and agreement on plausible risks and threats across a wide range of interacting clusters, promoting shared knowledge is and increasingly will be vital.[52] There are, for example, United Nations' initiatives created to establish a digital governance framework which among other things could guide global, regional, and national approaches for sharing information about risk and response priorities.[53]

The UN recognised from the outset that such objectives required extensive knowledge and data exchange with a wide range of multisectoral private and public organisations, many of which would see types of risks and response priorities from differing perspectives. In this case, extensive knowledge and data exchange were seen as essential starting points for arriving at some form of consistency about the elements of the proposed digital framework. It is also why such initiatives as the UN's annual Digital Cooperation Forum were regarded as indicative of the importance attested to the knowledge and data exchange processes.

In a related vein, the United Nations Development Programme, the World Bank and the International Monetary Fund were enthusiastic supporters of UNESCO's efforts to promote the importance of knowledge and data exchange about global threats and mitigation measures. The objectives of this exchange are, for example, 'to help Ministries integrate disaster risk reduction in school curriculum',[54] review military as well as non-military approaches for risk and threat identification,[55] and to foster public 'intelligence assemblies' through, for example, the International Telecommunications Union.[56]

Others which to date have been at the forefront of information and data exchange include the Digital Data Organisation, bringing together 'international ecosystem leaders', willing to share their expertise and learned experiences. According to the OECD, many governments by 2018 were increasing data exchange with the private sector and the private sector certainly acknowledges its heavy reliance on quick and seamless exchange of data across international borders.

Knowledge and data exchange has clearly been enhanced through scientific and technological innovations, and these are and increasingly will be reflected in various types of anticipatory webs, including

- ***Computational diplomacy*** – Digitally gathered data when given increased access to machine learning algorithms will result in mechanisms that will enable policy planners and decision-makers to solve real-world problems collaboratively and enable them to measure the potential success or failures of actions that might be taken;
- ***Large-scale collaboration*** – Collective intelligence, certainly by 2033, will be applied to solving big global challenges such as climate change, access to water and pandemic response. Organisations such as the Intergovernmental Panel on Climate Change will embrace new tools that use a combination of AI and Collective Intelligence to better organise scientific knowledge and bring in perspectives from a wide range of diverse groups;
- ***Earth systems modelling*** – Earth systems models will become sufficiently reliable and sensor networks sufficiently extensive to use real world data to make predictions about imminent ecosystem tipping points. In so doing, scientists will achieve detailed global analyses and forecasts of species movements and ecosystem shifts;
- ***AI enhanced political forecasting*** – Superforecasters, prediction markets and artificial intelligence work together to create forecasts for systems that otherwise cannot be easily modelled over a range of timescales. This approach will be as well established for political and economic domains as they will have been for weather forecasting and climate modelling. It is predicted that they will be used at the highest levels of decision support;
- ***Disease control and early warning systems*** – An integrated global pandemic early warning system will be developed, based upon technologies that will integrate disease surveillance in humans and animals, ecosystem monitoring (including land use change and biodiversity) and tracking human-animal contacts.

Such webs of information and data exchange feed directly into the issue of how they will affect responses for identifying, monitoring and responding to humanitarian threats. The answer will be through swarms of actors, or, in other words, through diverse multisectoral and multidimensional groupings that reflect an awareness of mutual self-interests

Those actors deemed to be 'traditional humanitarians' will have to recognise that their roles will have to accommodate interventions and involvement of those not deemed to be so. In so doing, they will also have to accept that the latter's assessments of vulnerabilities and response may in a variety of instances differ, and that a starting point to accommodate such differences is – once again – data and knowledge exchange. The sheer willingness to do so is a step towards recognising areas of agreement as well as disagreement, comparative advantages and alternative capacities.

At the same time, traditional humanitarians will have to accept that they cannot assume automatic lead roles. They may on occasion take lead roles, but then again, they might just be parts of swarms under the guidance of others or they might not even be included in a particular swarm at all.

From that perspective, policy planners and decision-makers will have to take into account two interrelated factors. The first is how best to ensure that existing structures, including standard humanitarian organisations, will be sensitive and appropriately responsive to emerging webs of multisectoral and multidimensional actors. The second is to resist the seemingly automatic temptation to create new systems and structures to deal with the increasing complexity underpinning more and more humanitarian crises.

Reflecting on the past, there has always been a tendency to create more organisations and organisational systems to deal with unanticipated types of complex problems. Yet, adding more and more organisations to an already institutionally inundated world could further compound complexity, if not cynicism, to efforts, in this instance, for dealing with humanitarian threats. A more positive challenge would be to use what already exists more effectively: focus on the dynamics of webs as much if not more so than on their structures, and recognise that the agreed objectives of swarms of multiple actors can be effectively facilitated based upon improved but existing constructs.

Facilitating Swarms

Creation of webs of recognised interests and agreed courses of action clearly interrelate. The processes are interactive and can fluctuate strategically and operationally. Therefore, in moving from webs to swarms, the challenge in the first instance will be to bring together 'autonomous groups to align activities to sponsor particular events and deliver targeted services in pursuit of compatible goals'.[57] The results, one would hope, is what Pierre Levy has described in the concept of 'collective intelligence', *viz*, the art of simultaneously maximising creative freedom and collaborative efficiency.[58] In an ever more complex, polylateral world order, it begins to answer the need for new types of collective problem solving.[59]

Mobilising collective intelligence, or focused engagement on a particular issue or set of issues, is the way the metaphor, swarms, is used here. Granted, the metaphor might not be always situationally sensitive, but at least it does suggest a kind of momentum where diverse groupings come together to achieve a particular objective or objectives. The momentum that moves webs into swarms is not necessarily dependent upon pre-existing structures or agreements but rather upon that common awareness of risks and the utility of risk-sharing.

The creation of the GAVI (Global Vaccine Alliance) in 2000 suggests how a cluster of actors convened around an agreed objective and a web of solutions, i.e. vaccination programmes for developing countries, which eventually evolved from a swarm to a formal alliance. From a loose-knit cluster of private and public sector actors to a well-recognised alliance, GAVI included representatives from state-based systems but was not dependent on them. It was described as innovative, effective and far less bureaucratic than multilateral government institutions such as the World Health Organization. It was not locked into an election cycle, rightly noted one analyst.[60] In other words, structure and convention, per se, did not determine initial inputs or outputs.

Project ECHO (Extension for Community Healthcare Outcomes), too, reflects a swarm to the extent that it reflected an 'unconventionally structured global health and community services initiative' to deal with the Covid-19 challenge, 'operating at scale to reach some of the world's most vulnerable populations'.[61] This non-profit networked body emerged at a time when multilateral structures were finding it difficult to adapt to the complexity of the crisis, when, according to two social entrepreneurship experts, the World Health Organization and the US federal government, among others, 'struggled to meet the challenge of the disease'.[62]

More and more, non-conventional swarms of different types of actors have been emerging to deal with complex crises.

Take, for example, the Za'atari refugee camp in Jordan. Established in 2012 for Syrians fleeing conflict, it was unofficial, refugee-led and consisted principally of informal supply networks that provided vitally-needed assistance. Humanitarian needs were met through an 'aggregate of predominantly illicit—yet legitimate—channels and social relationships that support[ed] the economic exchange of goods and services between distinct actors or actor groups'.[63]

On a regional level, the creation of the Humanitarian Think Tank Network (HUT) in 2022 is a good example of a cluster evolving as a swarm of informal partnerships. Founded against the backdrop of 'persistent reform deficits in international humanitarian policies and practices', leading European think tanks came together to enhance

> the impact of engaged think tanks by increasing cross-national collaboration to pursue synergies, exchange know-how and expertise, cooperate in thematic areas of joint interest, avoid duplications and work jointly on the strategic advancement of our think tanks in an increasingly complex humanitarian context. Currently, the network primarily focuses on European members and policies but is also open to engaging in thematic collaborations with non-European partners.[64]

When *syndemics*, or, in other words, concurrent or sequential epidemics were testing the fates of millions of refugees between 2019–2020, it became evident that new combinations of actors were emerging to provide assistance. A 2021 study concluded that all three borderlands under focus – Mexico and the United States, Bangladesh and Myanmar, Colombia and Venezuela – benefited from the collective intelligence of new actors. Though in some instances, governments, INGOs and NGOs were involved in humanitarian interventions on those borders, in all three instances, a diverse range of actors from the corporate sector, local communities and households, religious and educational institutions, social networks and temporary 'non-state actors' were all part of response swarms.

The Dynamics

In a 2021 OECD report on anticipating health crises, it was noted that observational data could be facilitated by global policy observatory that should be linked to national policy tracking systems which for the most part already exist.[65] That is not to suggest that what exists and the ways that they exist should be deemed to be sacrosanct. Rather, it is to say that there are interesting constructs and methods of engagement that evolve in myriad ways. They evolve either through formal linkages or as loose knit networks. The former includes functional, time-bound 'alliances' as well as more enduring collaborative commitments, while the latter suggests a constellation of multiple components that interact in ways less formal and structured than systems.

Both will most likely come together in what has been described as 'global solution networks' (GSN).[66] Such networks reflect increasing interconnectedness across a wide and fluid amalgam of actors, from individuals to well-established organisations, that generally share information, seek partnerships and opportunities for collaboration. When it comes to threats,

> emerging non-state networks of civil society, private sector, government and individual stakeholders are achieving new forms of cooperation, social change and even the production of global public value. They address every conceivable issue facing humanity from poverty, human rights, health and the environment, to economic policy, war and even the governance of the Internet itself.[67]

Such networks when combined with more standard regional and international organisations, here, will be described as platforms. Already, platforms are emerging and increasingly will. They foster and facilitate cluster identification and web development and frequently enhance what already exists. They, too, can also serve as means to engage the public and increase the prominence of issues of regional and global concern such as climate change and disaster risk reduction.[68]

Take for example, the Sendai Framework Voluntary Commitments (SFVC) online platform which enables stakeholders to inform the public about their work on disaster risk reduction. The SFVC online platform serves as a tool to let followers know who is doing what and where for implementing the Sendai Framework. One of its main purposes is to foster collaboration among stakeholders, including the private sector, civil society organisations, academia and media as well as local and regional organisations. All can use the platform to submit their intentions or reports dealing with their respective progress and deliverables on DRR, and all interested in the SFVC have easy access to potential clusters and webs for DRR action.

Another example is the Leading Edge Programme (LEP), a global initiative of the United Nations Office for the Coordination of Humanitarian Affairs (OCHA). The LEP acts as a worldwide community of practice and offers a unique space for year-round collaboration between networks and technical experts in crisis preparedness and response cooperation. Its model is one of continuous cooperation to achieve tangible results based upon a collectively set agenda. It is not an organisation, but instead a platform for engagement and facilitation.

In other words, the systems, coalitions, networks, alliances or social movements form webs for sharing information and data in the pursuit of a particular objective or sets of objectives or to identify and pursue. compatible goals.[69] Yet, whatever specific outcomes result from what here are referred to as platforms, there is one consistent theme, namely, that all reflect forms of consensus and feedback loops and interconnectedness.

That, of course, is not to suggest that such linkages always have strategically and operationally effective processes and outcomes. There certainly are instances when interconnectedness and interrelationships may trigger forms of collaboration that are duplicative or even counterproductive or inconsistent.[70] Nevertheless, all will increasingly reflect a recognised need to coalesce, stimulated in no small part by that growing awareness of interdependencies.

Of course, that emerging reality is not to suggest that perceived interests and interdependencies, or, mutual self-interests, alone will be the sole determinants of humanitarian action. However, in an increasingly polylateral world order, diverse groupings of actors, or, clusters, are and more and more will be at the core of crisis prevention, preparedness and response, and it can already be assumed that

1. Conventional humanitarian organisations, including government agencies, INGOs and NGOs, as well as actors not deemed to be part of the humanitarian sector increasingly recognise interdependencies based on degrees of mutual self-interests when it comes to humanitarian action;
2. Intervention by conventional humanitarian organisations when it comes to dealing with potential or actual humanitarian threats cannot be assumed, and that on occasion they will be replaced by different types of actors that normally would not be considered to be humanitarian – particularly those crises deemed to be politically complex;
3. The diversity of actors have already and increasingly will undertake humanitarian action often based upon different types of expertise (e.g. access to different types of data) and greater financial flexibility;
4. It is increasingly evident that recipient institutions, including governments, as well as donor institutions have become increasingly dependent upon unconventional 'humanitarian actors' – whether formally recognised or not;
5. On many occasions those deemed to be unconventional humanitarian actors achieve their objectives by bypassing formal state-based systems, including intergovernmental organisations.

Platforms for Facilitation

In anticipation of the UN's *Summit of the Future: What Would it Deliver?*, the UN Secretary General stressed that in light of increasing complex global shocks of significant scale, the standing authority of the Secretary General should be used 'to convene a time-bound Emergency Platform that would add value through high-level, multi-sectoral coordination, advocacy, and accountability for the contributions of participating actors. This would not displace or duplicate existing mechanisms.'[71]

Conceptually and operationally, his proposal reflects a perspective that needs to be borne in mind as one looks to present and future humanitarian challenges and opportunities. Nevertheless, while the Secretary General's 2023 proposal remains important, particularly its emphasis on greater inclusivity, its more enduring value will depend in no small part upon how the plethora of systems, networks, alliances, coalitions and social movements can best coalesce as webs and swarms to deal with increasingly complex humanitarian threats.

Here, the focus should be on building mainly upon platforms that already exist and where vertical and horizontal interests should and will become increasingly interdependent and interactive.

Maximising the Impact of Existing Platforms in a Polylateral World. There are myriad actors that do and can be prime movers – swarms – when it comes to triggering humanitarian action. States, of course, will remain of continuing importance as will INGOs and NGOs. However, too little attention has been given to the interaction between those and existing regional organisations (ROs) and interregional organisations (IROs). Nor, has the full potential of clustering those bodies with non-state actors such as private sector confederations, research councils, religious movements and subnational groupings been adequately explored.

In part this is due to the sheer growth in their numbers[72] and in part due to a belated appreciation of their present and potential synergies and, of course, to the sheer complexity of bringing such widely dispersed sets of actors into more interactive webs and swarms.

All three challenges return the reader to the issues of mapping, horizon scanning and data and information exchange.

What earlier had been called 'mapping' is essential for the global community to have a much clearer idea about the potential amalgam of actors that can contribute to identifying possible areas of vulnerabilities and means to offset them on an on-going, real-time basis. The capacities to do so will to a significant extent depend upon unprecedented flows of data and information, generated to an exponentially increasing extent through artificial intelligence. Nevertheless, to generate the webs and swarms necessary for humanitarian action should ultimately depend upon existing institutions appreciating and responding to the changing environment in which they are operating.

In other words, neither mapping nor data and information exchange should be seen as rationales for new institutions to be created. Rather, they should be regarded as means to enhance the capacities of those actors that already exist, and that they, too, could help facilitate efforts to establish and maintain cross sectoral and cross institutional collaboration. So closely related to this last step is that more attention has to be given to less top-down and more horizontal approaches for identifying, monitoring and preparing ways for mitigating humanitarian threats – a 'merge map' process.

Here, one example is the importance of strengthening the capacities of established regional organisations (ROs) as platforms for generating clusters and developing webs and swarms of humanitarian actors. But, why build upon ROs?

In the first place, ROs reflect an emerging reality in the foreseeable future that 'the global multilateral set is no longer the sole framework for institutionalized cooperation [and that] the balance between the regional/ interregional level of governance and the global level is shifting in favor of the former'.[73] Already by 2006, two UN Secretary Generals, Boutros-Ghali and Kofi Annan, had stressed the emerging importance of regionalism and interregionalism as essential for helping prevent or manage conflicts and establish economic cooperation.

While ROs are subject to similar criticisms to those aimed at global IOs, they are

> often regarded as suitable arenas for effectively tackling problems of cross-border nature and contributing to the solution of today's global governance challenges since they tend to be smaller than IOs, more homogenous in terms of their member states, and consequently in a better position to agree on common policies and activities.[74]

It is that level of access and accessibility which would make ROs in the first instance more highly effective platforms for a more diverse group of actors to explore and gauge potential humanitarian threats, and in turn gain general agreement on regional strategies and operations.[75]

Regional organisations would also spread their perspectives, information and data as well as strategic and operational plans across regions, or, in other words, through interregional regional organisations (IROs). One reason is that

> interregional networks connect knowledge resources and possibly compensate for weak or missing knowledge production capabilities between regions, which is particularly helpful in increasing less advanced regions' ability to generate knowledge. Interregional linkages give access to complementary and additional capabilities as long as they are related to existing ones. Such linkages enhance regions' ability to diversify, particularly that of peripheral ones.[76]

A second reason for the potential importance of ROs and IROs in a humanitarian context is that they would be able to adjust more readily – not always but more often than not – to accommodating more diverse clusters than their international counterparts. However, that assumption is based upon the premise that ROs and IROs will have to comprise not only government institutions but also those across a wide spectrum of actors, including those at community levels, the private sector and other non-governmental interests groups. Hence, it will be that diversity which will underpin RO's and IRO's potential value, and here, the proposition is that ROs and IROs will be able to bring together such diverse interests more readily than established IOs.

Underpinning this assumption is that ROs and IROs will be seen as more accessible and more immediate risk sharing pools. Greater geographical, cultural and employment proximity will lead towards more tangible webs of agreements that will be compatible with the interests of neighbouring ROs.

Also at those levels, humanitarian issues of common concern can be regularly explored – and, it is here where the importance of horizon scanning becomes key. How best to institutionalise foresight should be of paramount importance in the facilitating functions of ROs and IROs as platforms. In other words, it is not only the immediate vulnerabilities that should be identified through a multisector lens but also possible 'what might be's' from 10-, 15-, 20-year perspectives.

In so doing, the multisectoral and multidisciplinary approach to horizon scanning may well lead to underexplored or unexplored vulnerabilities as well as innovative practices that could mitigate them. 'Diversity tends to generate better ideas.'[77]

Certainly by 2021, on-going collaboration between global level actors and those at regional levels, had already 'grown exponentially',[78] and with that in mind, a critical function of the United Nations 'at headquarter levels' should be to serve as a single, integrated facilitating platform to link ROs, IROs, confederations of non-state actors and, of course, governments as part of a process for identifying threats at the global level. Beyond the UN as a vehicle for international cooperation, it should also be vehicle for promoting and facilitating new forms of collaboration in a distributed way.

That level of analysis would include, for example, the humanitarian consequences of disruptive space exploration, global pandemics, global financial collapse and what earlier had been referred to as 'synchronous failures'. These would come together as part of on-going process of information and data exchange, leading to appropriate strategic and operational plans at global levels.[79]

All would be tested regularly based not only upon on-going data and information flows, but also upon regular capacity assessments, including inputs from horizon scanning. However, this central platform would only play a tertiary role when it came to humanitarian action at community, state or regional levels. In other words, those platforms for actually facilitating prevention, preparedness and response would be based upon arrangements agreed at RO and IRO levels – depending upon the nature and dimensions of the threat. And, here, the role of the UN would be principally to seek financial and non-financial resources to do so, when requested.

At a Critical Juncture

The reader by now must feel that the global architecture outlined here for dealing with humanitarian threats reflects a world in chaos, or at least an unlikely amalgam of global and cross-regional webs and swarms in what appears as an increasingly fragmenting and cantankerous world order.

Such perspectives, however, fail to take into account the positive potential of increasing entanglements and growing multisectoral interdependencies. Nor, do they reflect already evident growing patterns of interaction at RO and IRO levels, or the plethora of efforts by clusters of multilateral institutions and non-state actors to be more anticipatory and explore possible longer-term futures.

The importance of the conventional humanitarian sector should by no means be diminished. However, when it comes to preparing to deal with future threats. far more attention needs to be given to ways to bring diverse actors together. Multisectoral and interdisciplinary actors need to come together for data and information exchange, for sharing existing plans of action or for developing them, and interact with those institutions – principally the United Nations with the support of the Bretton Woods organisations – to facilitate on-going anticipatory, strategic and operational planning vertically and horizontally.

That said, the swarms reflected in the proposed architecture for dealing with humanitarian threats will of course have to contend, for example, with political objections, with contending interpretations of objectives and risks, let alone a reluctance to share too much.

These are all acknowledged, but it is also assumed that many of these potential stumbling blocks will increasingly be circumvented or overcome as the interrelated and interactive consequences of humanitarian threats become ever more evident. One critical factor in making that assumption is the nature of 'the organisation'. To what extent might organisational behaviour undermine efforts to manage global 'threats'? Indeed, might organisational behaviour be a threat, in and of itself?

That concern leads to Chapter 7 *The Humanitarian Organisation for the Future.* Its purpose is to provide insights for those organisations determined to effectively manage humanitarian threats in an increasingly polylateral world.

Notes

1 Relief Web – UN OCHA, *Our common agenda: Report of the Secretary-General*, 10 September 2021.
2 Ibid.
3 Ibid.
4 https://news.un.org/en/story/2021/09/1099522
5 Don Tapscott. 'Introducing global solution networks: Understanding the new multi-stakeholder models for global cooperation, problem solving and governance', *Innovation*, 9 (1–2), 2014, p. 3.
6 Steve Waddell, 'Societal change systems: A framework to address wicked problems', *Journal of Applied Behavioral Science*, 52 (4), 2016, pp. 422–449.
7 J. Forrester, R. Taylor, L. Pedoth and N. Matin, 'Wicked problems', in H. Deeming, M. Fordham, C. Kuhlicke, L. Pedoth, S. Schneiderbauer and C. Shreve (Eds), *Framing community disaster resilience: Resources, capacities, learning, and action*, John Wiley & Sons, 2018, pp. 61–75.
8 The UN 'system was constitutionally unfit to deal with transnationality and that "sovereign" states…, even acting in concert, were unable to address a host of transnational problems such as… technological disasters and systems collapse, pandemics, opioid proliferation, resistance to antibiotics,… and, of course, climate change and its cortege of threats to survival'. Antonio Donini, 'UN 2.0', *Global Governance 26*, 2020, p. 266.
9 The Sustainable Development Goals (SDGs), also known as the Global Goals, were adopted by the UN in 2015 as a universal call to action to end poverty, protect the planet, and ensure that by 2030 all people enjoy peace and prosperity. They comprise a global action plan composed of 17 Sustainable Development Goals (SDGs), 169

targets and 232 indicators to advance sustainable development by 2030. For more information, see Sustainable Development Goals, www.un.org/sustainabledevelopment/, accessed 27 May 2022.

10 IISD, SDG Knowledge Hub, 'Are we serious about achieving the SDGs? A statistician's perspective', 14 January 2020.

11 Michael D. Watkins and Max H. Bazerman, *Predictable surprises: The disasters you should have seen coming and how to prevent them*, Harvard Business School Press, 2004, p. 99. See also Daniel J, Clarke and Stefan Dercon, *Dull disasters? How planning ahead will make a difference*, Oxford University Press, 2016, p. 53.

12 Systems tend to get disassembled if they are dealing with unlikely risk and the crises that gave rise to them… They will focus on recurrent risk and not on exceptional exogenous risk'. Randolph C. Kent et al., *Towards an international architecture for managing global threats*, Royal United Services Institute, 2021, p. 14.

13 Raphael Baumler, Maria Carrera Arce and Anne Pazaver, 'Quantification of influence and interest at IMO in maritime safety and human element matters', *Marine Policy*, 133, November 2021. See also Harilaos N. Psaraftis and Christos A. Kontovas, 'Influence and transparency at the IMO: The name of the game', *Maritime Economics and Logistics*, 22, March 2020) pp. 151–172.

14 Randolph C. Kent et al., *Towards an international architecture for managing global threats*, Royal United Services Institute, 2021, p. 15.

15 Mark Bowden and Angela Penrose, *The evolution of the humanitarian marketplace and NGO financing models*, www.nuffield.ox.ac.uk/media/5567/the-evolution-of-the-humanitarian-marketplace-and-ngo-financing-models.pdf. See also R. Baumler, M. C. Arce and A. Pazaver, 'Quantification of influence and interest at IMO in maritime safety and human element matters', which notes that '42.5% of Member States attending the meetings do not actively participate. Additionally, it seems that the ownership of maritime assets determines the influence.'

16 Shabtai Gold, 'G-20 report says that MDBs are holding back 100s of billions', DEVEX Exclusive, 20 July 2022.

17 Henry Kissinger, Eric Schmidt and Daniel Huttenlocher, *The age of AI: And our human future*, John Murray Press. Kindle Edition, 2021, pp. 81–92.

18 OECD, *OECD science, technology and innovation outlook 2021: Times of crisis and opportunity*, OECD Publishing, 2021, https://doi.org/10.1787/75f79015-en.

19 James Ball, *The system: Who owns the internet and how it owns us*, Bloomsbury Publishing, 2020. The author suggests that efforts to constrain social media have been growing. China and the United States, for example, embarked on measures intended in varying ways to define acceptable roles for social media organisations. And, in the aftermath of Russia's invasion of Ukraine, Facebook (renamed, 'Meta') had been blocked entirely by Russian authorities, while Twitter (renamed X) was almost completely cut off. In parallel, companies such as TikTok withdrew from Russia, which now had been seen as 'joining the likes of Iran as a digital pariah state'.

20 Douglas Yeung, 'Social media as a catalyst for policy action and social change for health and well-being: A viewpoint', *Journal of Medical Internet Research*, 20 (319), March 2018: 'Social media remains a relatively untapped source of information to catalyze policy action and social change. However, the diversity of social media platforms and available analysis techniques provides multiple ways to offer insight for policy making and decision-making. For instance, social media content can provide timely information about the impact of policy interventions. Social media location information can inform where to deploy resources or disseminate public messaging. Network

analysis of social media connections can reveal underserved populations who may be disconnected from public services.'

21 Randolph C. Kent et al., *Towards an international architecture for managing global threats*, Royal United Services Institute, 2021. See, also, *A systems compendium*. Royal United Services Institute, August 2021

22 See NCD Alliance, https://ncdalliance.org/, accessed 27 May 2022.

23 Maud H. Deves et al., 'Why should the IPCC evolve in response to the UNFCCC bottom-up strategy adopted in Paris? An opinion from the French Association for Disaster Risk Reduction', *Environmental Science and Policy*, 78, December 2017, pp. 142–148.

24 AI technologies are delivering remarkable results in highly specialised fields such as cancer screening and building inclusive environments for people with disabilities. They also help combat global problems like climate change and world hunger, and help reduce poverty by optimising economic aid. But the technology is also bringing new unprecedented challenges. We see increased gender and ethnic bias, significant threats to privacy, dignity and agency, dangers of mass surveillance, and increased use of unreliable AI technologies in law enforcement, to name a few. Until now, there were no universal standards to provide an answer to these issues. See UNESCO, 'Recommendation on the ethics of artificial intelligence', https://en.unesco.org/artificial-intelligence/ethics, accessed 27 May 2022.

25 Patricia Lewis, *Create a global code of conduct for outer Space*, Chatham House, 12 June 2019, www.chathamhouse.org/2019/06/create-global-code-conduct-outer-space

26 UNDP, Accelerator Labs Network, Qatar Fund for Development, United Nations / Multilateral body #SDGAction33432.

27 Op. cit. #21, Kent et al.

28 ALNAP, *The state of the humanitarian system*, ALNAP Study, ALNAP/ODI, 2022, p. 6.

29 Geoff Mulgan, *Thinking systems: How the systems we depend on can be helped to think and to serve us better,* 1 STEaPP Working Paper Series, Department of Engineering and Public Policy, University College, London, 2021, steapp.communications@ucl.ac.uk, p. 5

30 Lisa Dreir, David Nabarro and Jane Nelson, *Taking action on complex challenges through the power of networks*, Harvard Kennedy School, 2019. www.hks.harvard.edu/centers/mrcbg/programs/cri

31 Explicit in this instance is the assumption that a cluster has a defined set of actors with a relatively defined set of activities that in principle should be regarded as interconnected, e.g. activities triggered either by a UN Humanitarian Coordinator or by a government of an affected country or both to deal with a complex crisis. *UNHCR Emergency Handbook, Cluster Approach*, 15 July 2022, defines a 'cluster' as 'an IASC …system-wide mobilization in response to a sudden-onset and/or rapidly deteriorating situation in a given country or region and is declared when national or regional capacity to lead, coordinate and deliver humanitarian assistance does not match the scale, complexity, and urgency of the crisis'.

32 OECD, *Enhancing the competitiveness of SMEs in the global economy: Strategies and policies – local partners, clusters and globalisation*, Conference for Ministers responsible for SMEs and Industry Ministers, Bologna, Italy, 14–15 June 2020.

33 Gareth Priday, *Global Swarm*, Action Foresight, 2020. https://actionforesight.net>global-swarm

34 United Nations, *Integrity Matters: Net zero commitments by businesses, financial institutions, cities and regions: report from the high-level expert group on the net zero emission commitments of non-state entities*, 8 November 2022.
35 These included clusters of religious organisations and community groups, such as *No More Deaths*, groupings of community and faith groups such as *Border Links*, *Derechos Humanos*, *Humane Borders*, and *Healing Our Borders*. Then, too, were institutions such as the *Border Action Group* and *TeleECHO* which directly relied upon the policy support of universities to accomplish their humanitarian objectives.
36 Alina Rocha Menocal, Social Movements as Contentious Politics, GSDRC Applied Knowledge Series #50, September 2016
37 Annette N. Markham, 'Bricolage', in Eduardo Navas, et al., *Key words in remix studies*, Taylor & Francis, 2018.
38 An example can be found in Khiam Jin Lee, Sanna K. Malinen and Venkataraman Nilakant, 'The dynamics of cross-sector collaboration in disasters', *Disaster Prevention and Management*, 32 (2), 12 July 2023, ISSN: 0965-3562: The authors show that although the command-and-control model was dominant, organisations also attempted to improve disaster management efficacy through collaborative approaches. Central institutional agencies and their wider external partners are capable of using cross-sector collaboration as a strategy to tackle the complex problems post-disaster. However, pre-disaster relationship building will likely help organisations to collaborate more effectively when a disaster occurs.
39 Op. cit., #18, OECD.
40 For the issue of 'inflection points', see, for example, Paul Berkman, 'The pandemic lens focusing across time scales for local-global sustainability', *CellPress*, 1 (8), 13 November 2020.
41 Independent Panel for Pandemic Preparedness and Response, *Covid-19: Make it the last pandemic, 2020*, 20 May 2021.
42 OECD, *Scientific advice in crises: Lessons learned from Covid-19*. Summary report of a GSF virtual workshop held on 3–4 March, 2022, Science and Policy Technical Division, DSTI/STP/GS.
43 Shahar Avin, Bonnie C. Wintle, Julius Weitzdörfer, Seán S. Ó. Héigeartaigh, Martin J. Rees, *Classifying global catastrophic risks*, https://doi.org/10.1016/j.futures.2018.02.001Get(Not accessible as of [2024/06/12]) rights and content
44 Op. cit., #29, Mulgan, p. 19.
45 Such integrated data results in sets such as genomics, proteomics and metabolomics.
46 See, for example, Alice Obrecht, *Imagining future urban landscapes from a 2050 perspective*, Humanitarian Futures Programme, 2013, www.humanitarianfutures.org Library
47 Robotics Growth Partnership (RGP), *Vision for cyber-physical infrastructure (CPI)*, 11 February 2022.
48 Angel Hsu and Ross Rauber, 'Diverse climate actors show limited coordination in a large-scale text analysis of strategy documents', *Communications Earth and Environment*, 2 (30), 2021.
49 Ana Gonzalez Pelaez, Geoff Summerhayes and Nigel Brook, 'Risk-sharing in the climate emergency', University of Cambridge, Institute for Sustainability Leadership, 2021.
50 Gian Maria Campedelli and Maria R. D'Orsogna, 'Temporal clustering of disorder events during the COVID-19 pandemic', *PLOS*, 22 April 2021, https://doi.org/10.1371/.journal.pone.0250433

51 E. Ostrom, 'Polycentric systems for coping with collective action and global environmental change', *Glob. Environ. Change*, 2010, https://doi.org/10.1016/j.gloenvcha.2010.07.004
52 Toby Ord, Angus Mercer and Sophie Dannreuther, *Future proof: The opportunity to transform the UK's resilience to extreme risks*, Centre for Long-term Resilience, June 2021, www.longtermresilience.org/futureproof?s=03
53 United Nations, *Summit of the Future: What would it deliver?*, www.un.org › summit-of-the-future
54 To fulfil its mandate, UNESCO performs five principal functions: (1) prospective studies on education, science, culture and communication for tomorrow's world; (2) the advancement, transfer and sharing of knowledge through research, training and teaching activities; (3) standard-setting actions for the preparation and adoption of internal instruments and statutory recommendations; (4) expertise through technical co-operation to Member States for their development policies and projects; and (5) the exchange of specialised information.
55 One example of this sort of exercise emerged from workshops held with representatives of the Singapore military, civil servants and NGOs in March 2021 at the S. Rajaratnam School of International Technology, Nanyang Technological University, Singapore
56 Inter-Agency Working Group on Artificial Intelligence, UN System Chief Executives Board for Coordination, March 2021. See also, Geoff Mulgan, *Big mind: How collective intelligence can change our world*, Princeton University Press, 2018.
57 Merry Rutledge, 'A framework and tools to strengthen strategic alliances', *OD Practitioner*, 43 (2), 2011, p. 23.
58 Paul Levy, *Collective intelligence: Mankind's emerging world in cyberspace*, Plenum Press, 1997.
59 Rolf K. Baltzersen, 'What is collective intelligence' (Chapter 1) *in Cultural-historical perspectives on collective intelligence: Patterns in problem solving and innovation*, Cambridge University Press, 3 February 2022, online https://doi.org/10.1017/9781108981361.001
60 Katerini T. Storeng, (). 'The GAVI Alliance and the "Gates approach" to health system strengthening', *Global Public Health*, 9 (8), 14 September 2014, pp. 865–879, doi:10.1080/17441692.2014.940362. PMC 4166931. PMID 25156323.
61 Tamara Kay and Jason Spicer, 'A Non-profit Networked Platform for Global Health', *Stanford Social Innovation Review*, Winter 2021
62 Op. cit. It should be noted that the authors also included NY's Mount Sinai Queens and Elmhurst Hospitals as 'other notable examples' along with WHO and the US federal government..
63 Ismail Abushaikha, Zhaohui Wu and Theodore A. Khoury, 'Towards a theory of informal supply networks: An exploratory case study of the Za'atari refugee camp', *Journal of Operation Management*, 67 (7), 8 June 2021, https://doi.org/10.1002/joom.1151
64 See HUT description on Centre for Humanitarian Action website. Centre for Humanitarian Action (CHA) is a Berlin-based think tank founded in 2018. chaberlin.org
65 OECD Global Science Forum, 'Priority setting and coordination of research agendas: Lessons learned from Covid 19' – 4–5 October 2021 Workshop Summary, Directorate for STI, 20 January 2022, p. 10.

66 Kenneth W. Abbott and Thomas Hale, 'Orchestrating global solutions networks: A guide for organizational entrepreneurs', *Innovations*, 9 (1/2). www.mitpressjournals.org/doi/pdf/10.1162/inov_a_00209

67 Dan Tapscott, 'Introducing global solution networks: Understanding the new multi-stakeholder models for global cooperation, problem solving and governance', *Innovation*, 9 (1–2), 2014, p. 3.

68 Robert Sakic Troglic et al., 'Science and technology networks: A helping hand to boost implementation of the sendai framework for disaster risk reduction 2015–2030', *International Journal of Disaster Risk Science*, doi: 10.1007/s13753-017-0117-x, 27 March 2017.

69 Merryn Rutledge, 'A framework and tools to strengthen strategic alliances', *OD Practitioner*, 43 (2), 2011, p. 23.

70 In preparations for COP28 in Dubai, the president of COP was also Chairman of Dunai's largest petroleum consortium, and prior to the COP had been in discussions with other energy companies about trading arrangements. This 'duality' was condemned, but it underscores a point made by the systems analyst, Stephen Waddell seven years before that 'one of the best examples [ed. of such duality is] renewable energy trade associations that are actively promoting change in the system, and at the same time its members include companies conventionally producing electricity'. See Stephen Waddell (Acrobat – 423): Downloaded from jab.sagepub.com on 21 October 2016. swaddell@networkingaction.net

71 *Summit of the future: What would it deliver?* United Nations www.un.urg>sites>un2.un.org>files

72 According to the ALNAP study, op. cit., #28, Humanitarian Outcomes estimated that there were an estimated 5000 NGOs and INGOs, numbers which increased between 2012 and 2022 by 1/3rd and 1/5th. In all likelihood, the numbers of local NGOs was underestimated since many 'escalate and then subside'.

73 Mario Telo, 'Regional organizations and inter-regional relations: Competitive models or a bottom-up change of global governance?', National Committee of Geography of Belgium, Société Royale Belge de Géographie, 11 November 2020, http://journals.openedition.org/belgeo/43943. The author goes on to note that a growing number of scholars suggest that 'all in all, the development of multipurpose regionalism and interregionalism also can be seen as the only way possible to revive and reform global multilateralism, by enhancing not only its efficiency but also its legitimacy, because regional governance often plays the role of a bottom-up support of global governance'.

74 Diana Panke and Anna Starkmann, 'Trajectories of regional cooperation: A comparative analysis', *Comparative European Politics*, 19, 2021.

75 This point was particularly evident in a study concerning 'Waters of the Third Pole' which focused on the Hindu Kush-Himalayan (HKH) region, one of the world's greatest sources of natural hazards, when the diversity, types and dimensions of such hazards are all taken into account. *Humanitarian Crisis drivers of the future: Preparing now for the what-might-be – a synthesis report.* See: www.humanitarianfutures.org.

76 Adi Weidenfeld, Teemu Makkonen and Nick Clifton, 'From inter-regional networks to systems', *Technological Forecasting & Social Change*, 171, 2021, p. 120904. www.elsevier.com/locate/techfores

77 Charles J. Gomez and David M. J. Lazar, 'Clustering knowledge and dispersing abilities enhances collective problem solving in a network', *Nature Communications*, 10 (5146), 2019.

78 'In times of global crises, collaboration between regional organizations, United Nations has "grown exponentially", Secretary-General tells Security Council', Press Release, SC/14498, 19 April 2021.

79 It is worth noting that UNOCHA already produces a Global Humanitarian Overview. According to UNOCHA, 'the Global Humanitarian Overview (GHO) is the world's most comprehensive, authoritative and evidence-based assessment of humanitarian need. In essence, it is a global snapshot of the current and future trends in humanitarian action for a large-scale resource mobilization effort as well as for exploring opportunities to deliver humanitarian assistance better.' The GHO is the ultimate outcome of a one-year process known as the Humanitarian Programme Cycle. The HPC consists of a set of inter-inked tools to assist the Resident Coordinator/Humanitarian Coordinator (RC/HC) and the Humanitarian Country Team to improve the delivery of humanitarian assistance and protection through better preparing, prioritising, steering and monitoring the collective response based on evidence.

Bibliography

Abbott, Kenneth W. and Hale, Thomas, 'Orchestrating global solutions networks: A guide for organizational entrepreneurs,' *Innovations*, 9 (1/2). www.mitpressjournals.org/doi/pdf/10.1162/inov_a_00209

Abushaikha, Ismail, Wu, Zhaohui and Khoury, Theodore A, 'Towards a theory of informal supply networks: An exploratory case study of the Za'atari refugee camp', *Journal of Operation Management*, 67 (7), 8 June 2021, https://doi.org/10.1002/joom.1151

ALNAP, *The state of the humanitarian system*. ALNAP Study, ALNAP/ODI, 2022.

Avin, Shahar, Wintle, Bonnie C., Weitzdörfer, Julius, Héigeartaigh, Seán S. Ó., and Rees, Martin J., *Classifying global catastrophic risks*, https://doi.org/10.1016/j.futures.2018.02.001Get rights and content

Ball, James, *The system: Who owns the internet and how it owns us*, Bloomsbury Publishing, 2020.

Baltzersen, Rolf K., 'What is collective intelligence', in *Cultural-historical perspectives on collective intelligence: Patterns in problem solving and innovation*, Cambridge University Press, 2022. https://doi.org/10.1017/9781108981361.001

Baumler, Raphael, Arce, Maria Carrera and Pazaver, Anne, 'Quantification of influence and interest at IMO in maritime safety and human element matters', *Marine Policy*, 133, November 2021.

Berkman, Paul, 'The pandemic lens focusing across time scales for local-global sustainability', *CellPress*, 1 (8), 13 November 2020.

Bowden, Mark and Penrose, Angela, *The evolution of the humanitarian marketplace and NGO financing models*, www.nuffield.ox.ac.uk/media/5567/the-evolution-of-the-humanitarian-marketplace-and-ngo-financing-models.pdf

Campedelli, Gian Maria and D'Orsogna, Maria R., 'Temporal clustering of disorder events during the COVID-19 pandemic', *PLOS*, 22 April 2021. https://doi.org

Clarke, Daniel J. and Dercon, Stefan, *Dull disasters? How planning ahead will make a difference,* Oxford University Press, 2016.

Deves, Maud H., Lang, M., Bourrelier, P. H. and Valerian, F., 'Why should the IPCC evolve in response to the UNFCCC bottom-up strategy adopted in Paris? An opinion from the French Association for disaster risk reduction', *Environmental Science and Policy,* 78, December 2017.

Dreir, Lisa, Nabarro, David and Nelson, Jane, *Taking action on complex challenges through the power of networks*, Harvard Kennedy School, 2019. www.hks.harvard.edu/centers/mrcbg/programs/cri

Gold, Shabtai, 'G-20 report says that MDBs are holding back 100s of billions', *DEVEX Exclusive,* 20 July 2022.

Gomez, Charles J. and Lazar, David M. J., 'Clustering knowledge and dispersing abilities enhances collective problem solving in a network', *Nature Communications,* 10 (5146), 2019.

Gonzalez Pelaez, Ana, Summerhayes, Geoff and Brook, Nigel, 'Risk-sharing in the climate emergency', University of Cambridge, Institute for Sustainability Leadership, 2021.

Hsu, Angel and Rauber, Ross, 'Diverse climate actors show limited coordination in a large-scale text analysis of strategy documents', *Communications Earth and Environment*, 2 (30), 2021.

Humanitarian Futures Programme, *Humanitarian crisis drivers of the future: Preparing now for the what-might-be's: A synthesis report.* See: www.humanitarianfutures.org.

IAIS Strategic Plans 2020–2024 www.iaisweb.org

Independent Panel for Pandemic Preparedness and Response, *Covid-19: Make it the last pandemic*, 2020 [covid19 make it the last pandemic. Pdf]

Inter-Agency Working Group on Artificial Intelligence, UN System Chief Executives Board for Coordination, March 2021.

Kay, Tamara and Spicer, Jason, 'A non-profit networked platform for global health', *Stanford Social Innovation Review*, Winter 2021.

Kent, Randolph et al., *Towards an international architecture for managing global threats*, Royal United Services Institute, 2021.

Kissinger, Henry, Schmidt, Eric and Huttenlocher, Daniel, *The age of AI: And our human future*. John Murray Press. Kindle Edition, 2022.

Lee, Khiam Jin, Malinen, Sanna K, and Nilakant, Venkataraman, 'The dynamics of cross-sector collaboration in disasters', *Disaster Prevention and Management*, 32 (2), 12 July 2023.

Letwin, Oliver, *Apocalypse now: Technology and the threat of disaster*, Atlantic Books, 2020.

Levy, Paul, *Collective intelligence: Mankind's emerging world in cyberspace*, Plenum Press, 1997.

Lewis, Patricia, *Create a global code of conduct for outer space*, Chatham House, 12 June 2019, www.chathamhouse.org/2019/06/create-global-code-conduct-outer-space

Markham, Annette N., 'Bricolage', in Eduardo Navas, et al. (Eds), *Key words in remix studies*, Taylor & Francis, 2018.

Menocal, Alina Rocha, *Social movements as contentious politics*, GSDRC Applied Knowledge Series #50, September 2016.

Mulgan, Geoff, *Thinking systems: How the systems we depend on can be helped to think and to serve us better,* 1 STEaPP Working Paper Series, Department of Engineering and Public Policy, University College, London, 2021, steapp.communications@ucl.ac.uk

Mulgan, Geoff, *Big mind: How collective intelligence can change our world*, Princeton University Press, 2018.

NCD Alliance, https://ncdalliance.org/, accessed 27 May 2022.

Nicholson, Jack E., Challenges for the Insurance Industry in the Future, 2019 @National Association of Insurance Commissioners. Also see B3is Blockchain Platform, re: Major re/insurers and brokers complete complex placements on B3i's blockchain platform.

Obrecht, Alice, *Imagining future urban landscapes from a 2050 perspective*, Humanitarian Futures Programme, 2013, www.humanitarianfutures.org Library

OECD, *Enhancing the competitiveness of SMEs in the global economy: Strategies and policies – local partners, clusters and globalisation*, Conference for Ministers responsible for SMEs and Industry Ministers, Bologna, Italy, 14–15 June 2020.

OECD Global Science Forum, 'Priority setting and coordination of research agendas: Lessons learned from Covid 19' – 4–5 October 2021 Workshop Summary, Directorate for STI, 20 January 2022.

OECD, *OECD science, technology and innovation outlook 2021: Times of crisis and opportunity*, OECD Publishing, 2021, https://doi.org/10.1787/75f79015-en

OECD, *Scientific advice in crises: Lessons learned from Covid-19*. Summary report of a GSF virtual workshop held on 3–4 March, 2022, Science and Policy Technical Division, DSTI/STP/GS.

OECD, *Technology and innovation in the insurance sectors*, OECD, 2017.

Ord, Toby, Mercer, Angus and Dannreuther, Sophie, *Future proof: The opportunity to transform the UK's resilience to extreme risks*, Centre for Long-term Resilience, June 2021. www.longtermresilience.org/futureproof?s=03

Ostrom, E., 'Polycentric systems for coping with collective action and global environmental change', *Glob. Environ. Change*, 2010, https://doi.org/10.1016/j.gloenvcha.2010.07.004

Panke, Diana and Starkmann, Anna, 'Trajectories of regional cooperation: A comparative analysis', *Comparative European Politics,* 19, 2021.

Priday, Gareth, *Global swarm*, Action Foresight, 2020. https://actionforesight.net>global-swarm

Psaraftis, Harilaos N. and Kontovas, Christos A., 'Influence and transparency at the IMO: The name of the game', *Maritime Economics and Logistics,* 22, March 2020.

Rachman, Gideon, 'Europe is an Alliance, not a union of values: Internal pressures are less powerful than the external pressures of keeping members together', *Financial Times*, 21 January 2019.

Relief Web – UN OCHA, *Our common agenda: Report of the Secretary-General*, 10 September 2021.

Robotics Growth Partnership (RGP) *Vision for cyber-physical infrastructure (CPI)*. 11 February 2022.

Rutledge, Merry, 'A framework and tools to strengthen strategic alliances', *OD Practitioner*, 43 (2), 2011.

Skinner, Paul, *Collaborative advantage: How collaboration beats competition as a strategy for success*, Robinson, 2018.

Storeng, Katerini T., ' The GAVI Alliance and the "Gates approach" to health system strengthening', *Global Public Health*, 9 (8), 865–879, 2014. doi:10.1080/17441692.2014.940362. PMC 4166931. PMID 25156323 (14 September 2014).

Tapscott, Don, 'Introducing global solution networks: Understanding the new multi-stakeholder models for global cooperation, problem solving and governance', *Innovation*, 9 (1–2), 2014.

Telo, Mario, 'Regional organizations and inter-regional relations: Competitive models or a bottom-up change of global governance?', *National Committee of Geography of Belgium, Société Royale Belge de Géographie*, 11 November 2020. http://journals.openedition.org/belgeo/43943

UNDP, Accelerator Labs Network, Qatar Fund for Development, United Nations / Multilateral body #SDGAction33432.

UNESCO, 'Recommendation on the ethics of artificial intelligence', https://en.unesco.org/artificial-intelligence/ethics, accessed 27 May 2022.

UNHCR Emergency Handbook, *Cluster approach*, 15 July 2022.

United Nations, *Integrity matters: Net Zero commitments by businesses, financial institutions, cities and regions: Report from the high-level expert group on the net zero emission commitments of non-state entities*, 8 November 2022.

United Nations, 'In times of global crises, collaboration between regional organizations, United Nations has "grown exponentially", Secretary-General tells Security Council', Press Release, SC/14498, 19 April 2021.

United Nations, *Summit of the future: What would it deliver?* www.un.org › summit-of-the-future

Waddell, Steve, 'Societal change systems: A framework to address wicked problems', *Journal of Applied Behavioral Science*, 52 (4), 2016.

Watkins, Michael D. and Bazerman, Max H., *Predictable surprises: The disasters you should have seen coming and how to prevent them,* Harvard Business School Press, 2004.

Weidenfeld, Adi, Makkonen, Teemu and Clifton, Nick, 'From inter-regional networks to systems', *Technological Forecasting & Social Change*, 171 (2021), 120904. www.elsevier.com/locate/techfore

World Benchmarking Alliance, *Measuring what matters most: Seven systems for benchmarking companies on the SDGs*, July 2019.

Yeung, Douglas, 'Social media as a catalyst for policy action and social change for health and well-being: A viewpoint', *Journal of Medical Internet Research*, 20 (3), 19 March 2018.

7 The Humanitarian Organisation for the Future

As head of Joint Special Operations Command in Iraq (JSOCI), General Stanley McCrystal began to wonder why with all the sophisticated training and material and technical advantages of the US and coalition forces in country, Al Qaeda in Iraq (AQI) always seemed to evade the clutches of the JSOCI. Worse than that, from his point of view, in too many instances they achieved military objectives which his forces should have been able to prevent, but didn't. One critical answer to his concerns was that, despite all its advantages, the JSOCI was trapped in an organisational model that had decreasing relevance. The solution: We had to tear down familiar organisational structures and rebuild them along completely different lines, swapping our sturdy architecture for organic fluidity because it was the only way to confront a rising tide of complex threats.[1]

The Humanitarian Organisation for the Future

Intensifying entanglements and a paradigmatic shift away from multilateralism to polylateralism will all be reflected in the nature of organisations, be they physical or virtual. For the purposes of *Humanitarian Futures: Challenges and Opportunities*, this emerging reality concerns those organisations that are and most likely will assume roles for identifying, monitoring and mitigating humanitarian threats. Undoubtedly, their impacts and effectiveness will depend to a very significant degree upon their resources and professional capacities. Here, however, the focus will be on the sorts of organisational structures and behaviour patterns that will enable 'the organisation' to respond effectively and sensitively as a humanitarian actor.

Of course, in this context, one needs to be clear about what one means by an organisation – including those that have indirect as well as more direct humanitarian roles. In any event, the overarching theme underpinning this search for the humanitarian organisation for the future is concerned with five essential criteria. To what extent are those organisations inherently anticipatory and how adaptive as organisations are they? How do they collaborate with those deemed to be principally humanitarian focused and those who are not? How innovative is the organisation, and, if it is, then is the driver for innovation principally concerned with

DOI: 10.4324/9781003471004-8

problem solving or something broader? And, what should leadership look like in an organisation for the future that assumes humanitarian responsibilities?

What Do We Mean by an Organisation?

Chapter 6 *Managing Threats in a Polylateral World* sought to define and assess the strengths and weaknesses of a range of structures that comprised the global architecture. Systems, alliances, coalitions, networks and social movements all were seen as having strengths and weaknesses, and in various ways all shared degrees of commonality. Perhaps not surprisingly one key common characteristic was that each generally consisted of various types of organisations. In that sense, an increasingly diverse range of organisations, intentionally temporary or intended to be permanent, is a central feature of a polylateral world. They will comprise the clusters, webs and swarms that will inevitably be at the heart of humanitarian action.

That said, as an astute analyst made very clear, defining an organisation is not without its complexities and inherent contradictions.[2] There has, for example, been an assumption that an organisation has 'common objectives' and that there is a structure to their contributions which are intended to achieve a shared purpose. Yet, frequently, common objectives do not necessarily mean 'commonly understood' objectives. Nor, for that matter, does structure mean 'a physical manifestation', for an organisation can be virtual, temporary and possibly have very fluid, fluctuating boundaries. And, very obviously, there are organisations that evolve over time. Like various 'start-ups' in California's Silicon Valley, they may begin as small, dynamic, driven, non-hierarchical and innovative but eventually assume more standard, hardened patterns of organisational behaviour.[3]

Here, however, by-passing what has been referred to as the definitional complexities of 'Aristotelianism',[4] the concept of an organisation will be assumed to have identifiable operational boundaries and – though not necessarily rigid – hierarchical in its structure. Organisational objectives might not always be clear or consistent, but the importance of the organisation's survival is generally assumed to be fundamental by those within it.

Normally, the organisation will have sub-systems, or specialised components, informally referred to as 'silos'. These are generally staffed by specialists whose expertise justifies their organisationally distinct roles.

A frequent criticism of organisations is that they tend to resist fundamental adjustments to their strategic objectives or operational *modus vivendi*. Such criticisms may be overstated, but in any event, essential adjustments to strategic and operational objectives are often only made at the point of self-evident failure. In other words, essential adjustments are made when weaknesses are threatening the organisation as a whole or at least some of its essential subcomponents. Conversely, perceived success can narrow organisational interest in exploring new ways to achieve their objectives and, hence, avoid the need, for example, to adopt potentially transformative innovation.

As for leadership, there are inevitably different types and levels of decisions which are required for an organisation to achieve its objectives. Generally, those decisions perceived as essential for the overall objectives of an organisation are made at the top of organisational hierarchies. They then are transmitted down and interpreted according to the particular responsibilities of the organisation's subcomponents. Of course, that does not mean that decisions and related organisational requirements go uncontested. Frequently, the subcomponents seek clarification and modifications of the decisions passed down. In that sense, an organisation can be seen as an interacting 'collective' where individuals have an ongoing relationship and have varying degrees of mutual dependencies. There is a structure to their contributions and broadly speaking institutional commonalities in their goals.

Finally, the organisation which will be explored below also has characteristics that relate to what has been defined as a 'complex system'. One way or another, all share the following characteristics.[5] The organisation

- normally involves multiple numbers of interacting elements;
- involves interactions that are nonlinear, and minor changes can produce disproportionately major consequences;
- is greater than the sum of its parts, and solutions more often than not arise from circumstances. This is frequently referred to as *emergence*;
- has a history, and the past is integrated with the present; the elements evolve with one another and with the environment; and evolution is irreversible;
- finds it difficult to escape its past – hindsight – when attempting to understand and anticipate the future.

The Organisation That Plans from the Future

According to a growing number of analysts, policy planners and decision-makers have all too often become 'collectively short-sighted', succumbing to a kind of 'future blindness' in which potential implications of transformative change and complexity are ignored.[6] Today, a considerable number of organisations and certainly those found in most governmental bodies are deemed to be relatively insensitive to substantive change. As organisations, they have been described as inherently linear, siloed and reductionist in approach when it comes to defining solutions and problems.

This proposition had been reenforced in a 2023 report, *Defining the Path to Zero Hunger in an Equitable World*, in which the authors highlighted the fact that 'current conditions have brought us to a crossroads', but still the global community and certainly humanitarian organisations reflect

> intricate and long-standing silos and a preoccupation with short-term horizons that have for many years shaped the foreign assistance sector.
>
> Silos, in this context, have come to mean groups of stakeholders or institutions that have separated and segregated themselves from each other, and/or operate without sharing decisions, information, processes, or communication. [There, too] is the prevalence of short-term initiatives that address specific problems for a finite time period. Rarely do these projects coordinate with each other, often

housed across multiple bureaus, agencies, programs, and initiatives, without an eye on the larger picture.[7]

In discussing evolution as a 'failure of the less fit' rather than 'the survival of the fittest', a well-known British economist noted that 'disconcertingly, given our instinctive belief that complex problems require expertly designed solutions, [evolution] is completely unplanned'.[8] For policymakers, the randomness and unpredictability of the source and solutions of complex problems can indeed be disconcerting. In that sense they probably would get little comfort from the fact that modern social and natural sciences increasingly assume that most phenomena in the universe are somewhere between random and deterministic, and that science has come to accept the messy and the indeterminate.

Policymakers, however, generally have not accepted either, and instead seek solutions that are unambiguous and readily implementable. That, in the context of theories of complexity and uncertainty, goes against perceived reality. In this instance, those who are responsible for humanitarian policy will have to adjust to an operating environment in which crisis drivers, triggers and causation are not readily apparent, and where consequences are uncertain and solutions potentially evasive.

By no means is this a call for passive circumspection. To the contrary, those who will guide humanitarian action will have to take approaches that go beyond the certitudes of the past and present. In this sense, using hindsight as a starting point for fostering and implementing foresight undermines the objectives of the latter. Those who appreciate the importance of foresight for identifying and achieving the overarching mission of the organisation will have to actively seek ways to identify, monitor and mitigate a growing number and types of threats that may have few precedence.

Mechanisms will increasingly be needed that are able to integrate information and respond to a fluid external environment beyond the capacities of conventional organisations. Increasingly, the sheer speed and access to information and interdependence of the modern environment leave little time for conventional constructs. For highly complex problems to be solved, 'shared consciousness' – i.e. extremely transparent information sharing – and 'empowered execution', pushing decision-making and ownership to the right level for every action will begin to mitigate some core failings of conventional behaviour.[9]

As one looks to creative and effective approaches for dealing with such threats, five positive and interrelated challenges come to mind: anticipation, adaptation, innovation, collaboration, and strategic leadership. Each of these involves structural and institutional change, and, perhaps even more significantly, each requires changes of 'mind sets' and attitudes.

The Art of Anticipation

It was back in 2012 when this author gave a talk to a mixed group of business and humanitarian organisations in Toronto. The talk was about the importance of organisations in general to have a commitment to be more speculative about increasingly complex and uncertain futures. A willingness to explore 'the plausible and implausible' should be regarded as an inherent part of their strategy formulation processes.

The presentation seemed to be well received. In fact, a member of the audience stood up spontaneously and enthusiastically thanked me for 'extremely interesting insights'. In fact, he said, the talk was invaluable, 'but unfortunately now I have to get back to work'. To which, I replied, 'If you don't see this as an inherent part of your work, then you've missed my point.' A slight smirk went across the room.

The art of anticipation needs to be seen as an essential part of an organisation's ethos. A willingness to be sensitive to potential changing contexts, to rarely considered vulnerabilities and solutions should be a central feature of a futures-sensitive organisation. A key objective is to challenge preconceptions – 'not to predict the future, but to give an array of future worlds that seem to flow from these assumptions'.[10]

However, all too often the term assumes that anticipation is about prediction. For organisations that have to deal with ever increasing complexity and uncertainties (and this is increasingly the case for those concerned with humanitarian issues) it is not about prediction. Rather it is about a willingness to explore an array of future worlds in order to test the organisation's capacities and indeed its willingness to think more creatively and adapt accordingly. An effective organisation must avoid becoming trapped in the assumptions of the present, let alone those of the past.

Exploring the 'what might be's' is a recognised asset for the objectives of the organisation and its ensuing policies. The organisation has to be sensitive to the possibility that it will have to contend with the unforeseen and that its conventional standard operating procedures and repertoires will not necessarily be adequate to do so.

Such breakthroughs, of course, will in various ways enhance anticipatory capacities.[11] Nevertheless, no matter how effectively transformative technologies and algorithmic calculations might deal with complexity, there will always be those 'black swan' events – those unknown unknowns. The organisation needs to be sensitive to that reality, and appreciate that prediction, *per se*, is not the primary objective of fostering anticipatory capacities. Rather, the abiding objective of anticipation is to have an organisation accept the importance of challenging the conventional, its standard operating procedures and institutionally accepted norms. Without an ethos of anticipation, the organisation will tend to rely on well-engrained norms, without questioning their relevance or suitability.

Since the 1960s, so-called 'futures studies' have emerged, and many continue to focus on methods for identifying plausible risks and threats and possible ways to deal with them.[12] However, it is evident that neither the concept of anticipation nor its purpose emerges from futures study methodologies in any consistent way. They veer from prediction to speculation, and there certainly is a lack of a common language when it comes to scale, scope and methodologies for looking into the future.[13]

That is not to say that a considerable range of future-exploring techniques has not emerged over the years. No doubt, artificial intelligence will enhance their effectiveness exponentially. Examples of such techniques include,

- ***Environmental scanning*** – monitoring and analysing the external environment to identify emerging trends, risks and opportunities;
- ***Delphi method*** – structured forecasting technique involving panels of experts providing their opinions and predictions on future trends, which are then aggregated and analysed to identify potential future developments;
- ***Scenario planning*** – developing multiple plausible futures scenarios based on different assumptions and drivers of change, and then determining necessary strategies for dealing with each;
- ***Trend analysis*** – analysing historical data and patterns to identify trends an extrapolate them into the future;
- ***Technology road mapping*** – methodology focuses on mapping the development and adoption of technologies over time to help organisations understand their potential impacts;
- ***Weak signal detection*** – actively scanning for weak signals or early indicators of potential future developments.

Though there are many types of anticipatory tools, there is one common objective which underpins most, namely, the need to foster a willingness to think in more systematic ways about the 'what-might-be's'. One failure to do so was made evident with the onset and response to the 2020 coronavirus pandemic, and explains the 2021 Independent Panel for Pandemic Preparedness and Response's call for more creative and adaptive approaches for dealing with pandemics.[14]

Both as a concept and as practical planning devices, anticipatory methodologies are rarely assumed to be means for accurate predictions. Even for those who do, there is a general assumption that the results will normally be compelling probabilities. Ultimately, one of the most important results of anticipatory objectives should be to have the organisation 'think outside the box' and to recognise the value of 'mind-shifting exercises'.

This sort of thinking was reflected in the *Museum of the Future* where its designers concluded that of fundamental importance in futures thinking was *not to maintain mental and emotional constructs that ensured certitude* but rather to promote a degree of cognitive flexibility and challenge the conceptual security protected by 'knowledge shields'. Instead, the designers emphasised, it was intended

> ... to offer insights not as a template for delivering a way of making policy about the future to policymakers but rather as an ethically self-reflexive speculation about how to approach the problems and opportunities of future policy; how to set about effecting an institutional shift in behaviours and practices of futures-thinking and -making; and how to undertake a meaningful assessment of what futures thinking is – and could be – in an institutional context ripe for change.[15]

At the same time, if used effectively, such approaches should provide 'high-level descriptions that help to clarify very long-term strategic direction, threats and opportunities'[16] and methodologies for fostering perspectives and capacities that can strengthen ways to anticipate and adapt to potential risks and threats.[17][18] Here can be added the Center for Science and Imagination, mentioned in the *Introduction*, which also uses stories, for example, those from Africa, to anticipate positive aspects of the Continent's future.

Anticipatory methods can also provide opportunities to recognise inter-dependencies 'at local-global levels, short-term to long-term, before-through-after the inflection point…'[19] It, too, can foster an ethos of exploration across organisations, networks and systems. This certainly was the case for Singapore's Centre for Strategic Futures (CSF). Based in the Prime Minister's office, the CSF developed planning processes that helped to integrate foresight work on a whole-of-government level.

> Regular national-level scenario exercises and horizon scanning work help the government maintain the discipline of examining assumptions, applying new perspectives and ensuring that the long-term context is considered when developing medium-term priorities and plans.[20]

As organisations, including those who have or will have humanitarian roles and responsibilities, begin to prepare for the future, it is worth considering six insightful suggestions made by the Institute of Risk Management about the importance of anticipation practices and methodologies:[21]

- to deepen the understanding of the driving forces affecting future development of a policy or strategy area;
- to identify gaps in understanding and bring into focus new areas of research required to understand driving forces better;
- to build consensus among a range of stakeholders about the issues and how to tackle them;
- to identify and make explicit some of the difficult policy choices and trade-offs that may need to be made in the future;
- to create a new strategy that is resilient because it is adaptable to changing external conditions;
- to mobilise stakeholders to action.

For an organisation that is determined to be responsive to change in timely and effective ways, it will understand and appreciate the words of a scientist from a previous century:

> we are now emerging into another cultural epoch [where] it seems futile to suggest what lies in store fifty years into the future. However, there is a way to prepare for the unexpected so that the appropriate transition is facilitated even if it cannot be foreseen.[22]

The Adaptive Organisation

It was another talk. This time in front of a large audience from a distinguished NGO known principally for its humanitarian involvement in conflict situations. The lecture was about futures and the importance for such organisations to be inherently adaptive. In other words, even the most respected organisations had to have in-built flexibility to enable it to adapt effectively and efficiently when confronted with plausible change. It could no longer be mired in standard operating procedures or past assumptions when its very operational environment was changing.

I thought that my remarks made sense, but the meeting's chair was becoming slightly irritated. I sensed his fingers drumming on the desk by the speaker's podium. Then, in a slightly condescending way, he said, 'Randolph, why do you think we have a policy department?' 'Oh', I replied, 'but do the cleaners know?' The chair then just shook his head and raised his eyes to the ceiling.[23]

No truly effective organisation should ignore the fact that its adaptive capacities will ultimately determine the utility of its anticipatory competencies and what below will be discussed in an organisational context, namely, *collaboration, innovation and leadership*. The fact that 'the cleaners should know' was a point made to emphasise that when confronted with uncertainties all who are part of a truly adaptive organisation should understand the direction of the organisation, the adjustments that have to be made to deal with rapidly evolving strategic and operational contexts and be sensitive to the importance of such organisational adjustments for themselves and for the institution as a whole.

This was a point clearly recognised by the International Committee of the Red Cross when a representative spoke of the ICRC's rationale for introducing anticipatory programming:

> What we… have learned over the course of the development and implementation of this initiative is that any organization's ability to innovate stems from its innovation system. And this system must be made up of coherent and interdependent processes that dictate how we search for novel problems, how we recognize possible solutions, when we should synthesize ideas into concepts and why we choose which initiatives go forward. Our current focus is to empower every interested and motivated ICRC staff member with the knowledge and tools to pursue any potential innovative solution. We are there to support and guide, not manage or control the outcome.[24]

In this regard, the ICRC is not alone. A growing number of organisations with humanitarian roles and responsibilities have been making efforts to be more adaptive by planning and developing longer-term strategies on an organisational-wide basis. While one might question whether such planning and strategising are sufficiently long-term or adequately speculative,[25] there is nevertheless a clear effort by many to set out objectives that reflect assumptions about the values that the organisation wishes to pursue, the context in which such values will be pursued and the organisational adjustments required to do so.

In this context, the difference between an adaptive and a maladaptive organisation is indicated by five 'tests':

- the extent to which plans and strategies are understood within and across the organisation;
- the degree to which such plans and strategies relate to the organisation's operational activities;
- the extent to which the assumptions that underpin plans and strategies are regularly reviewed;
- a willingness to identify sceptics about proposed plans as well as supporters to fully appreciate potential downsides;
- the extent to which the results of reviews 'feedback' into operational activities.

The barriers to passing such tests are well known for all who have worked in even small, let alone large, organisations. It is worth reflecting on at least some of these barriers and some possible solutions. Clearly one is how to bring the multiple elements of the organisation together? How to foster shared experiences, needs and vision that will negate the downsides of competitive expertise, silos and lack of a common institutional language.

Cross-Systems Organisations

> Though most executives recognize the importance of breaking down silos to help people collaborate across boundaries, they struggle to make it happen. That's understandable: It is devilishly difficult. Think about your own relationships at work—the people you report to and those who report to you, for starters. Now consider the people in other functions, units, or geographies whose work touches yours in some way. Which relationships get prioritized in your day-to-day job? [26]

The value of horizontal teamwork is generally recognised in principle but less so in practice. Employees who can reach outside their silos to find colleagues with complementary expertise learn more and enhance their skills more quickly. As innovation hinges more and more on interdisciplinary cooperation, digitalisation transforms business at a breakneck pace and globalisation increasingly requires people to work across national borders, the demand for executives who can lead projects at interfaces keeps rising.[27]

Yet, the admission by one large US-based non-governmental organisation that there was no real cross-over between the organisation's vice-president for policy and the vice-president responsible for emergencies is indicative of the sorts of challenges that organisations face.[28] In this context, organisations may wish to look at recent business experiments with knowledge networks and communities of practice. These two types of structures mesh, based upon recognised needs to share information ('common ground') in order to achieve common goals, purposes, and objectives.

Knowledge networks and communities of practice are non-hierarchical, fluid, inter-active, and – as opposed to many aspects of organisational behaviour – non-judgmental. As Olson and Sarmiento had pointed out, the world of disaster risk reduction is a key theme for such networks. The field is changing so quickly, according to these authors, that one needs a far quicker and more interactive process than standard organisations can normally provide. Agility is vital.[29]

That agility, as a leading management consultancy firm underscored, can in part be achieved by fostering flat and fluid structures built around high-performing cross-functional teams, instituting more frequent prioritisation and resource-allocation processes building a culture that enables psychological safety, and decoupling technology stacks:

> Enterprise agility is thus a paradigm shift away from multi-layered reporting structures, rigid annual budgeting, compliance-oriented culture, separation of business and technology, and other traits dominating organizations for the past hundred years. If this is true, and not just hype, a discontinuity of this magnitude should provide an opportunity for organizations to turn their operating models into a competitive advantage.[30]

Promoting inter-disciplinary methodologies

In a related vein, it is highly likely that every humanitarian organisation that provides some form of technical assistance has experienced the gulf between its technical experts and its policymakers and decision-makers. It might be amusing when management – at headquarters or at field level – is teased for not understanding the implications of the 'techies' language. Those small groups of experts that only understand each other are important, but at the same time the conceptual and linguistic distance between them and others in the organisation can prove a serious constraint on broad-based organisational understanding – about the present and about the future.

Every effort at inter-disciplinary analysis faces the hardship of bringing to bear the full weight of relevant perspectives without over-simplifying or diluting the contribution of each individual discipline. It is a test rarely satisfied completely, except perhaps in the planning and making of policy on matters that are principally technical in nature.[31] All too often, though, even the concept of collaboration across the organisation poses a difficult initial barrier.

One fundamental problem that needs to be confronted in promoting inter-disciplinary methodologies is that of language. It is a well-known issue, yet continues to hamper, for example, the contribution of science to the planning process. The mutual challenge for the pure sciences, social sciences, and planners is to break down the technical language barriers that hinder the establishment of synergy, which is so necessary for understanding and responding to the dynamics of change. As noted in a 2022 OECD report on priority setting, language barriers frequently explain the lack of coordination between researchers and government authorities, which all too often impede the efficiency of the policy and research response.[32]

General approaches for overcoming language barriers reflect in various ways means to reduce the impacts of silos. For example,

- Both language and silos often reflect efforts to protect perceived expertise which in turn is deemed to justify departmental boundaries. It has been proven that when overarching common organisational goals are understood across an organisation, silos become more permeable and language reflecting different expertise less restrictive;
- Barriers between the sciences and policy planning and decision-making can present particularly difficult to surmount. Therefore, establishing consistent long-term mechanisms that fully engage science actors is particularly important when it comes to preparedness, let alone responsiveness to evolving priorities during crises;
- Organisations can break down silos and promote common language between departments by encouraging or requiring them to work together on projects. These projects provide specific goals for different departments to work toward together;
- When it comes to cross-departmental projects, organisations should have members with liaison roles to help establish consistent communications between departments to keep joint projects on target;
- Capacities need to be introduced to curate information from disparate public and private sources, to promote the collection, storage and analysis of such sources and to actively promote potential interoperability;
- In those instances where effective interoperability has emerged from a particular crisis response, efforts need to not revert to 'business as usual'.

Reducing the impact of unanticipated options

By 2020 in the wake of the Covid-19 crisis, it was becoming evident to authorities in Singapore that public as well as private organisations seemed increasingly focused on 'major changes and disruptions [which] lay ahead for the world'. There was an emerging propensity to explore ways to navigate what was seen as a 'novel environment'.[33] Similar concerns were also evident in a number of other governments and non-governmental institutions in ASEAN.

Exploring possible patterns of change is indeed an essential approach for enhancing the adaptive capacities of organisations. However, in exploring possible patterns of change, there was an issue that, too, was evident, namely, a tendency to ensure that 'the futures' being explored would not come as a surprise to those responsible for planning and decision-making. Herein, lies the paradox in attempting to reduce the impacts of unanticipated options.

On the one hand, policy planners and decisionmakers can gain a sense of going beyond the self-evident by being part of a process that puts new scenarios on the table; on the other hand, the unanticipated may be discarded because for the recipient they have no frame of reference. A way around the worst aspects of this paradox may seem obvious, but it does work.

Organisational behaviour should regularly include briefings for planners and decisionmakers on plausible future *portraits* as well as trends and their implications. Not always perfect, nevertheless by enhancing familiarity it can reduce the potential dissonance created by unanticipated analyses, options, and proposals. Its value is increased even further if those with those with overall planning and decisional roles explore the 'unanticipated' in joint departmental meetings.

Innovation and Innovative Practices

The importance of innovation and of adopting innovative practices has underpinned many aspects of the sorts of organisational dynamics considered so far. In 2008, it had been suggested that:

> Currently, humanitarian organizations – responsible for implementing projects over a relatively short time frame (usually 12 to 18 months) – have little time to observe and reflect on the profile and changing needs of their 'customers' and on the efficacy of their implementation of goods and services.[34]

That said, there is no doubt that a growing number of scientific and technological innovations have the potential to expand policymakers' and decision-makers' capacities to prevent as well as to anticipate and respond to ever more complex humanitarian crises. The challenge for those involved in humanitarian policy and practice is how to identify, prioritise, and implement innovation and innovative practices when the very nature of both – as the uncertainties presented by artificial intelligence continue to demonstrate – can be so unpredictable.

Despite this challenge, there are ways in which organisations can identify, prioritise and implement innovation and innovative practices more effectively than they do at present.

In the first place, most organisations with humanitarian roles and responsibilities need to devote more time to studying the nature of the problems that they wish to resolve. Second, most need to recognise the fact that innovations and innovative practices that might be relevant to their concerns and needs will probably come from sources well outside the conventional humanitarian sector, reinforcing the importance of what were referred to above as knowledge networks and communities of practice.

Finally, those seeking appropriate innovation and innovative practices will also have to go to those who, in a seemingly paradoxical way, understand innovation and innovative practices as well as, if not better than, most, namely the vulnerable. They are the ones who survive in extreme conditions very often because of their ability to innovate. As a founding director of the Center for the Advancement of Collaborative Strategies in Health emphasised, it is the innovative capacities of vulnerable populations in situations such as Hurricane Katrina in 2005 that are too often ignored by presumed experts.[35]

Again, in the context of innovation and innovative practices of humanitarian organisations, a very relevant study by NESTA, the UK's innovation agency, noted that innovative technologies were all too often presumed to be outside the capacities of those communities that were deemed to be 'local', including local and national NGOs. NESTA stated that such presumptions were wrong. Clearly, the exponential increase in the transfer of cash and the proliferation of mobiles in and across vulnerable communities suggested burgeoning capacities for using innovative technologies. However, according to NESTA,

> the failure to put AI in the hands of frontline humanitarian actors can be explained by organisational inertia and lack of leadership buy-in. Slow adoption of new tools and innovative methods is often a result of a lack of senior advocacy within major humanitarian organisations. Many of these organisations have traditional structures and approaches that have been ingrained through decades of practice, often resulting in 'organisational inertia'. Persistent scepticism about the value of community or frontline derived knowledge and data has resulted in top-down preference for traditional data sources and a lack of process shift and/or willingness to include participatory approaches into the workflows.[36]

In this context, organisations need to make greater efforts to identify and help scale up innovations and innovative practices that can be found within vulnerable communities. With that in mind, 'one method is to learn from the people most immersed in a problem'. This advice from a highly experienced former senior civil servant in the United Kingdom underscored the point that:

> anyone seeking to find an answer to the management of chronic diseases or alienation amongst teenagers may do best by looking at how people are themselves solving their problems, and starting from the presumption that they are 'competent interpreters' of their own lives.[37]

The challenge in this context is to ensure that organisations also accept the premise that 'customer-led' approaches are essential to adopting appropriate innovative practices. The potential range of innovations and innovative practices that stem from community-based initiatives is impressive, but too often overlooked by those very external actors who ostensibly have community interests at heart. Therefore, when it comes to vulnerability reduction and disaster preparedness,

> the anticipatory organization will be far more speculative not only about plausible though by no means certain crises, but also about the potential means to offset them. 'Exploration competence', or the ability to harvest ideas and expertise from a wide array of sources, is vital for staying on top of innovations and their implications, according to the authors of ***Radical Innovation***.[38]

All too often, innovation and innovative practices are 'internalised' and the essential external cross-fertilisation necessary to maintain focus and development of ideas is sacrificed to insular institutional interests.[39] Adaptive organisations will need to develop open information and communication linkages with new types of partners, institutionally (e.g. commercial, non-governmental organisations) as well as geographically. They will also need to find ways to institute 'a new kind of go-between', such as knowledge networks and communities of practice, that will be responsible for ensuring the exchange and incorporation into planning processes of trends and innovative ideas.[40]

The 'nexus approach' in Central Asia is a case in point. Created to assess how climate change might affect the region's water, energy and land resources, the nexus project has resulted in a multi-year regional programme to support the operationalisation of an integrated approach for the use of energy, water and land-use in the region's five countries.

It was at the outset understood that governments' planning processes had to go well beyond traditional sectoral thinking. Rather, the effectiveness of the nexus approach still continues a commitment to exchange a broad spectrum of information and data across the three sectors. Information and data are provided through an array of networks and state and non-state practitioners, and as a 2022 review of the imitative stressed, the nexus has overcome the decision-makers' propensity to identify options for governance arrangement and policy measures that are usually addressed in isolation.[41]

New Forms of Collaboration

The importance of the organisation when it comes to planning to deal with ever more complex and uncertain humanitarian futures will depend upon fundamental conceptual as well as operational change. Conceptually, the organisation able to effectively meet the challenges of the future will be part of inherently collaborative systems and networks. It will appreciate that its effectiveness and development will depend upon 'collaborative advantage' and less on competition, that positive change and innovation 'does not occur so much within firms as within the spaces between them'.[42]

In the previous chapter, reference was made to *clusters* of different types of actors principally concerned with problem-focussed processes . These can merge into *webs* of understanding about problem-solving which in turn could lead to relatively predictable and timely *swarms* of appropriate responses.

Humanitarian action reflecting those metaphors will involve a growing number of different sectors. The humanitarian sector on its own, as presently configured, generally lacks the full capacities needed to deal with the changing types, dimensions, and dynamics of humanitarian threats. Some in the sector find that competing objectives means that they lack the capacities to deal with them.[43] More generally, however, the sector has been perceived as reluctant to undertake initiatives that might be of considerable use but which are too expensive and potentially of high risk.[44]

With these and other significant constraints in mind, collaborative partnerships and networks are essential to ensure adequate capacities in order to deal effectively with future threats, to enhance anticipatory and adaptive abilities and to promote innovation and innovative practices.

Yet, the assumptions that humanitarian actors all too often make about the humanitarian potential of 'non-traditional humanitarian actors' creates unnecessary barriers. The former presume that the latter lacks awareness about the subtleties required, for example, to provide assistance to innocent civilians in times of conflict. They are presumed to be disparaging or at least insensitive to moral purpose. Conversely, the latter can be frustrated by what appears to be haphazard and often unclear approaches for developing clear strategies and implementing them.

Both sides often have 'language differences' which obviously complicates collaboration. Non-traditional and traditional actors have to have a clearer understanding about what the other means when it comes to engaging in humanitarian affairs. The issue of language can be as simple as the differences in terminology: for example, the private sector's use of 'continuity planning', which for many in the humanitarian sector translates into 'disaster risk reduction' and 'preparedness'.

Below such linguistic differences, however, lies a far more complex issue, namely that of perceived motives. In the case of private sector–humanitarian relations, the relationship remains fraught with suspicion about the motives of each.[45] In this regard, there is a crescendo of calls for platforms at community and national levels in which humanitarian policymakers, private sector representatives, and those from humanitarian and other concerned organisations can discuss openly what each has to offer.[46]

A second such hurdle involves understanding the intrinsic capacities of non-traditional actors, which too often are not recognised by humanitarian practitioners. It is interesting to note, for example, that discussions about the added value supplied by the military in humanitarian action normally boils down to logistics, lift capacities (in terms of humanitarian operations, the amount of weight that can be lifted normally from pallets or from the ground, usually by helicopters or fixed-wing aircraft) and protecting civilians in armed conflict.

While this sort of support can indeed be operationally important, for the twenty-first-century humanitarian organisation, the military's potential added-value should also include its strategic development and surge capacities (the ability to intensify operational resources to meet an unanticipated crisis) as well as its ability to undertake institution-wide transformation when it comes to adopting innovations and innovative practices.

The use of ASEAN member-states' militaries for disaster and emergency response is a case in point. Throughout much of Southeast Asia, the militaries' extensive anticipatory as well as response roles are clearly recognised.[47] Despite stronger civilian coping mechanisms, militaries continue to be seen as the primary responders in ASEAN states during crises and calamities. The military are also among the first to be mobilised when governments send or receive humanitarian assistance and disaster relief (HADR). However, as other commentators have recognised, there are gaps in what civilian bodies know about the military and *vice versa*. A lack of data and inadequate means for promoting common understanding clearly have negative impacts upon collaboration.[48]

In a related vein, there, too, is the assumption by conventional humanitarian actors that the 'non-traditional' do not understand the societal contexts in which humanitarian crises occur, let alone how to effectively engage with the variety of different actors who form part of loose networks or disparate groupings. As noted in the previous chapter, a case in point is provided by diaspora-based communities. The dependence in many vulnerable countries upon the flow of remittances from families residing overseas is well known. As the World Bank noted in 2021, 'As COVID-19 still devastates families around the world, remittances continue to provide a critical lifeline for the poor and vulnerable.'[49]

It is interesting to note, however, that, while remittances and diaspora phenomena are recognised for their importance, only recently have humanitarian organisations begun to establish formal links with diaspora organisations as early warning systems that indicate the onset of crises or as means to undertake support operations to provide assistance in complex relief settings.[50]

Alternatively, as evidenced by 'the corporates', non-traditional actors often have a very clear sense about the needs and attitudes of the crisis-threatened. And, the reason can in some instances reflect the dynamics of the commercial marketplace (e.g. mobile phones, enhanced fertilisers) and even insurance sales.

In other words, core business interests, disaster risks and social stability are increasingly not only inter-related but also integrated phenomena. In that sense there is a parallel between an emerging sensitivity to crisis risks and their 'business consequences'. between the private sector and the military. Fundamental to the sorts of collaboration which are intrinsic to evolving clusters, webs and swarms will be

- recognised mutual self-interests and a willingness to 'know yourself', including assessment of capacities, strengths and limitations;
- active efforts to have a clear understanding about the objectives, processes and 'language' of different types of actors who have shown interest in collaboration. For example, the definition of 'security' for the military differs from the ways that corporate actors might use the tern, let alone, those in the humanitarian sector;
- clarity and common purpose which could at the outset be triggered by data and information exchange as one step towards developing collective understanding;
- a clear appreciation about the present activities of potential and actual collaborating partners. In Indonesia, for example, the role of the military to anticipate and deal with coastal crises demonstrates important surge capacities which can prepare the way for humanitarian actors to provide assistance;
- the agreed use of collaboration-strengthening technologies such as those generated by artificial intelligence.

Strategic Leadership and the Enabling Environment

Of course, there are different types of situations and circumstances which may call for different types of leadership. There are immediate crisis threats which might require instant decisions and there are those where there is sufficient time to have a deeper and wider assessment of ways forward.

In either case, the leader will have to contend with the reality that his or her organisation will be far more fluid than conventionally assumed. The organisation will be far more porous. Rapidly changing types of communication will often mean that information necessary for decisions will access the organisation at different levels from external virtual and physical organisations, and will not automatically revert to the top of a hierarchy.

In that sense, it will be increasingly important to have a balance between self-management and hierarchy.[51] Perhaps, the Prussian Field Marshal Helmuth Von Moltke the Elder captured the emerging importance of decentralised decision-making when he famously said,

> No plan of operations extends with any certainty beyond the first contact with the main hostile force. Only through the closest cooperation of the leaders of the divisions and brigades, and through their own initiative, can the commander bring the battle to a successful conclusion.[52]

In Amartya Sen's review of William Easterly's *The White Man's Burden*, he borrows Easterly's distinction between 'planners' and 'searchers'.[53] The former incarcerate those whom they wish to assist in pre-set planning frameworks and solutions, while the latter are more willing to listen and understand local conditions and needs, and what might be wanted and when. In a world in which complexity and interconnectedness make top-down strategies obsolete, the planner is not an appropriate strategic leader, and the searcher is.

Strategic leadership in the 21st century needs, in the first instance, to change present approaches to planning and to focus upon three broad issues:

- new-style planning processes reflecting a range of key uncertainties likely to be faced in obtaining core value-driven goals;
- diffuse and 'flatter' forms of leadership, where strategic leadership does not collide with 'managerialism', and is sustained by different leaders at various levels;
- blending of traditional leadership strengths with new dimensions of leadership.

Strategic leaders, now and certainly in the future, will need to position themselves at the node where different networks connect, or where there is maximum overlap between the elements of a collaborative Venn diagram. They will need skills to build multisectoral collaborative networks, and also to enable others to learn from them.

The strategic leader will have the ability to identify and seize opportunities for innovation, and through stakeholders' net assessments will be better able to understand the value that he or she brings to stakeholders and the value that they in turn bring. Future strategic leaders will have to move beyond their traditional comfort zones and embrace the ambiguity that reflects reality, and consequently will have to develop appropriate anticipatory and adaptive skills.

Strategic leadership in the humanitarian sector will therefore require at least six competencies for enhancing the overall value and purpose of the humanitarian sector in general and humanitarian organisations in particular:

- envisioning, or the ability to identify and articulate value-driven goals that have overarching importance for the leader's own organisation and a wider community;
- posing the critical question, or the ability to challenge certitudes and seek alternative explanations;
- externalisation, or networking on a multi-sectoral and interactive basis;
- communication, or disseminating value-driven goals in ways that become deeply embedded in the objectives of the organisation as a whole;
- listening, or the confidence never to pass up the opportunity to remain silent;
- recognising that the role of a leader will include that of a mentor, particularly in the aftermath of a subordinate's failure.

Strategic leaders and the organisations that they seek to guide will understand that the emerging agenda that will enable them to be relevant in a rapidly unfolding and ever more complex humanitarian future will not be merely an extension of the past. Not dissimilar to the lessons learned by the US Task Force in Iraq in 2004, if organisations rely on conventional, standard organisational and inter-organisational behaviour in ever more complex settings, they will eventually lose their relevance and advantages as effective actors.

In Chapter 4 *Towards the Brink*, readers were provided with 'portraits of the future' in part to enable them to assess their organisations' capacities for identifying, adapting and responding to rarely considered humanitarian threats. Such speculative portraits of the future should have raised some fundamental questions about what needs to be done now to prepare for a rapidly changing humanitarian future. How will our understanding of crisis threats, humanitarian action and what defines a humanitarian actor have to change? How will myriad institutions across the globe play effective mitigation roles, and what changes in organisational behaviour will be vital for identifying, monitoring and responding to crisis threats, now as well in the future?

All of these are fundamental issues which should provide a broad framework for those with humanitarian leadership roles and responsibilities. Leadership in the future will require a much greater capacity to listen, to speculate, to network and ultimately to be responsive to rapidly changing events and contexts.

It will certainly require critical elements of *planning from the future*. If there are any doubts, practical steps which the leader needs to consider are proposed in the next and final chapter – Chapter 8 *The Helenus Alternative*.

Notes

1 Stanley McChrystal et al., *Team of teams: New rules of engagement for a complex world*, Portfolio/Penguin, 2015, Kindle copy pages 17 ff.
2 Paul Griseri, 'What are organisations?', *An introduction to the philosophy of management*, Sage Publications Ltd, 2013, p. 11.
3 That may not be inevitable. There are those who regard many of such companies as perpetually 'transformative', that have, in other words, the ability to anticipate challenges and to adapt. However, it is worth noting that in the US alone, 49 per cent, 49.7 per cent of new businesses have disbanded within the first five years of their formation.
4 Op. cit., #2, p. 21 – 'Once we focus on the essence of an organisation relating to intentions then these go away, for this makes the essence of an organisation more of an idea than an object, and ideas do not have beginnings and endings, or insides and outsides. Note that we said 'more of' – organisations would not be purely ideas: they have physical aspects, such as the people, documents, buildings etc. referred to previously. But following Aristotle's style of thinking, we might say that these are accidental aspects, and the underlying reality of an organisation is its idea.'
5 The relationship between a 'complex system' and an 'organisation' is the assumption of the author and taken from David J. Snowden and Mary E. Boon, 'A leader's framework for decision-making', *Harvard Business Review*, November 2007/Revised 2011,
6 Farhad Manjoo, 'Why we need to pick up Alvin Toffler's torch', *New York Times*, 6 July 2016.
7 Catherine Bertini, Peggy Tsai Yih, Roger Thurow and Gloria Dabek, *Defining the path to zero: Hunger in an equitable world*, Chicago Council on Foreign Relations and the Rockefeller Foundation, 30 March 2023.
8 Tim Harford, *Adapt: Why success always starts with failure*, Little, Brown, 2011, p. 13.
9 These propositions had been described in Frederick Laloux's *Reinventing organisations: A guide to creating organisations inspired by the next stage of human consciousness*, Nelson Parker Publishers, 2014.
10 Liz Else, 'Opinion interview: Seizing tomorrow', *New Scientist*, 1 December 2001, pp. 43–44.
11 Examples from the *GESDA 2023 science breakthrough radar* (www.gesda.global) include *Computational diplomacy* (SBR – p. 215), *Large-scale collaboration* p. 56), *Earth systems modelling* (SBR – p. 135), *AI enhanced political forecasting* (p. 192), *Disease control and early warning systems* (p. 167).
12 An interesting variation of horizon scanning is 'threatcasting', which combines future scenarios transmitted via augmented reality. See, for example, Brian David Johnson and Natalie Vanatta, 'What the heck is threatcasting?', *Future Tense*, Arizona State University, 2017.
13 'The various disciplines that have contributed to horizon scanning have resulted in a variety of views of what it is. Furthermore, the inconsistency of application means the term horizon scanning is widely used and, in many cases, misused. You should define your terms and meanings.' John Carney, 'Futures and foresight planning', Principal Scientist within the Systems Thinking and Consulting Group of the Defence Science and Technology Laboratory (Dstl), 8 March 2018.
14 Independent Panel for Pandemic Preparedness and Response, *Covid-19: Make it the last pandemic*, May 2021, p. 20. See, also, Oliver Wyman LLC Forum, *Leading in a permacrisis*. 'It's striking that most companies did not have a crisis management team when COVID-19 hit. Even more striking is the fact that a majority still don't have crisis

playbooks at the ready – or test them. That won't cut it in today's permacrisis world.' oliverwymanforum@e-mail.oliverwyman.com

15 Emily Spiers, Will Slocombe, Jim Maltby, Tim Dedopulos, Greg Stolze, Paul Goodenough, Richard Claridge, Lucy Mason, James Biggs and Jack Norris, 'Estrangement, immersion and the future: Designing the speculative environments of the virtual reality: "Museum of the Future"', *Elsevier Futures*, 138, 102922, 2022.

16 Hugh Courtney, *20/20 Foresight: Crafting strategy in an uncertain world*, Harvard Business School Press, 2001, p. 1.

17 Emily Spiers et al., 'Estrangement, immersion, and the future: Designing the speculative environments of the virtual reality "Museum of the Future"', https://doi/10.1016/j.futures.2022.102922(Not accessible as of [2024/06/12]).

18 In a related vein, see: The importance of interconnectedness and its conceptual dimensions is noted by Paul Berkman, 'Science diplomacy and its engine of informed decision-making: Operating through our global pandemic with humanity', *The Hague Journal of Diplomacy*, 15, 2020, p. 445.

19 Op. cit., #12 (1) 'Don't think that Horizon Scanning is about predicting the future – this is a common misconception. The value of Horizon Scanning is in using it to change mind-sets, challenge assumptions and provide more options. (2) Don't look for "what you know or want" – scanning is not the same as searching. This may seem contradictory, but it is one of the hardest commandments to get your mind around as either a practitioner or a client. Horizon Scanning is more about asking the "unasked questions" or identifying the "unknown unknowns" (after Donald Rumsfeld).'

20 *Conversations for the Future* (vol. #3, 2023), Centre for Strategic Futures, Prime Minister's Office. www.csf.gov.sg

21 Innovation Special Interest Group, *Horizon scanning: A practitioner's guide, institute of risk management*, 2018, pp. 7 ff.

22 Brian Goodwin, 'In the shadow of culture', in J. Brockman (Ed.), *The next fifty years: Science in the first half of the twenty-first century*, Vintage Books, 2002, p. 42.

23 In a related vein, Randolph C. Kent discusses over-siloed organisational structures in his introduction to Tim Harford's book *Adapt: Why success always starts with failure*, part of an ODI public event held in London on 13 June 2011 – available on ODI YouTube, 2011.

24 ICRC's Strategic Foresight Initiative, Contribution to the Panel on Innovation – Presented at the Geneva Innovation Movement Workshop – 24 March 2022, www.humanitarianfutures.org See: News – March 2022.

25 The problem for many planners is that they assume that a plan must reflect relatively firm and fixed steps for a defined period of time. Hence, when one busy executive argued that anyone nowadays with a five- or ten-year plan is 'probably crazy', he implied that to plan one had to be relatively certain about the environment in which one was operating. Op. cit., #16, H. Courtney, p. 160.

26 Amy C. Edmondson, Sujin Jang and Tiziana Casciaro, 'Cross-silo leadership', *Harvard Business Review*, May–June 2019, p. 130.

27 Op. cit., #18.

28 This is based upon a consultancy dealing with preparing for pandemics undertaken by this author in 2005.

29 Richard S. Olson and Juan Pablo Sarmiento, 'Communities of practice and disaster risk reduction', *Natural Hazards Informer*, Issue 5, University of Colorado Natural Hazards Research and Applications Information Center, 2012. See also A. M. Aslam Saja, S. M. Lafir Sahid and M. Sutharshanan, 'Capacity-building strategy for creating disaster- and

climate-risk-sensitive development plans: A case study of multi-stakeholder engagement in Sri Lanka', *Integrated Research on Disaster Risks*, Springer Nature, February 2021; and Etienne C. Wenger, 'Communities of practice: A brief introduction', 2008. www.researchgate.net

30 Wouter Aghina, Christopher Handscomb, Olli Salo and Shail Thaker, 'The impact of agility: How to shape your organisation to compete', A survey, McKinsey & Co., 25 May 2021.

31 An interesting and positive example of inter-disciplinary methodologies stems from the NGO, Concern Worldwide's evaluation of its 2017–2018 Multi-sectoral Emergency Response for Conflict-Affected and Food Insecure Populations in South Sudan programme. Due to effective cross-organisational planning, Concern was able to provide assistance in the sectors of health, nutrition, WASH, food security and livelihoods as well as shelter and non-food items in the three former states of Northern Bahr el Ghazal, Unity, and Central Equatoria (Juba). Overall, the evaluators found the program to be highly *relevant* and fit for purpose, *efficient* in terms of budget utilisation and adaptability, *appropriateness* of the intervention, *timely* delivery and *effective* synergies with other programs and – though a humanitarian program intended to be life-saving and short-term in nature – there were elements of **sustainability.** See: Knowledge Hub/Multi-sectoral Emergency Response for Conflict-Affected and Food Insecure Populations in South Sudan – Final Evaluation 2019.

32 OECD Global Science Forum, Report on Workshop on 'Priority setting and coordination of research agendas: lessons learned from COVID-19', 20 January 2022, DSTI/STP/GSF(2021)21/FINAL.

33 Op. cit., #20, *Conversations for the Future*.

34 Stacey White, 'Turning ideas into action: Innovation within the humanitarian sector – a think-piece for the HFP Stakeholders Forum', Humanitarian Futures Programme, King's College, London, 2008, available at: www.humanitarianfutures.org/sites/default/files/InnovationsThinkPiece.pdf

35 Roz Lasker, *The expert's blindspot* at: www.humanitarianfutures.org/tools/mediacent/film/expertblindspot

36 NESTA, *Collective crisis intelligence for frontline response*, 15 September 2021, This report provides the first analysis of how an emerging innovation approach, 'collective crisis intelligence' (CCI), is being used to improve anticipation, management and response in the humanitarian sector. CCI combines methods that gather on-the-ground human intelligence from crisis-affected communities and frontline responders with artificial intelligence (AI).

37 Geoff Mulgan, *The art of public strategy: Mobilizing power and knowledge for the common good*, Oxford University Press, 2009.

38 Richard Leifer, et al., *Radical innovation: How mature companies can outsmart upstarts*, Harvard Business School Press, 2000.

39 John D. Wolpert, 'Breaking out of the innovation box', *Harvard Business Review*, Special Innovation Edition, 80 (8), August 2002, p. 78.

40 Op. cit., #1, McCrystal, pp. 81 ff.

41 OECD, *Benefits of regional cooperation on the energy-water-land use nexus transformation in Central Asia*, OECD Green Growth Papers 2022–1, May 2022. The countries involved were Kazakhstan, Kyrgyzstan, Tajikistan, Turkmenistan and Uzbekistan. See https://oe.cd/NexusTashkent2021 for further information.

42 Paul Skinner, *Collaborative advantage*, Little Brown Book Group, 2018, p. 66.

43 An interesting example of contending objectives is that between 'localisation' and the Sustainable Development Goals, as noted by Nonso Jideofor Localizing Humanitarian Action, UNHCR Innovation Service, 2020–2021, unhcr.org/innovation @unhcrinnovation

44 The considerable number of constraints which other types of organisations could address include the humanitarian sector's frequent lack of understanding about the full range of innovations that could be used and the lack of hands-on capability for supporting or enabling innovation to scale. See Elrha, *Spring impact, and science practice, too tough to scale: Challenges to scaling innovation in the humanitarian sector*, Elrha, 2018.

45 Joanne Burke and Randolph C. Kent, *Commercial and humanitarian engagement in crisis contexts: Current trends, future drivers*, Humanitarian Futures Programme, King's College, London, June 2011, available at: www.humanitarianfutures.org

46 See, for example, Humanitarian Futures Programme, *Platforms for private sector-humanitarian collaboration*, King's College, London (no date). www.humanitarianfutures.org; Humanitarian Futures Programme, *The virtuous triangle and the fourth dimension: The humanitarian, private and military sectors in a fragile world*, 2014. www.humanitarianfutures.org

47 Tom Abke, *ASEAN militaries can play even bigger roles in disaster response*, Indo-Pacific Defense Forum, 18 May 2021.

48 Angelo Paolo Trias and Alistair D. B. Cook, *HADR in Southeast Asia: Unpacking the military's humanitarian role*, RSIS Commentary at RSISPublications@ntu.edu.sg

49 World Bank, 'Defying predictions, remittance flows remain strong during COVID-19 crisis', Press release, 12 May 2021.

50 Shabaka, *How international NGOs can support diaspora humanitarian actors and a stronger localised humanitarian sector – Blog 2 of 3*, (no date) '…Delays in, not to say failures of, the established humanitarian system have highlighted the need to seek alternatives and/or recognise those that already exist, which includes the key and complementary role played by local organisations and diaspora groups, who delivered vital aid in Northwest Syria and in Sudan. However, local NGOS and diaspora organisations are still being neglected in the distribution of international humanitarian resources, particularly funding. This limited access to resources risks making local and diaspora humanitarian responses less sustainable at a time when they are needed more than ever before.' Generally speaking, the value of the role of the diaspora was only really recognised after the issue of the Grand Bargain, including 'localisation', emerged out of the 2016 World Humanitarian Forum. Only since 2020 had, for example, the International Organisation for Migration introduced *Consolidating and operationalizing a framework for diaspora's engagement in humanitarian assistance – Phase II* in 2023. The Red Cross also introduced a Diaspora Humanitarian Partnership Programme with similar objectives as the NGO consortium, ReliefWeb, introduced a funding programme for diaspora organisations, DEMAC, in 2015.

51 Arne de Vet and Filip Lowette, *The fluid organisation: An ideal mix of self-management and hierarchy*, De Vet Management bvba, 2019.

52 Helmuth von Moltke, *Oxford Essential Quotations*, 4th Edition, Oxford University Press, 2016.

53 Amartya Sen, 'The man without a plan', *Foreign Affairs*, March/April 2006.

Bibliography

Aghina, Wouter, Handscomb, Christopher, Salo, Olli and Thaker, Shail, 'The impact of agility: How to shape your organisation to compete', A survey, McKinsey & Co., 25 May 2021.

Berkman, Paul, 'Science diplomacy and its engine of informed decision-making: Operating through our global pandemic with humanity,' *The Hague Journal of Diplomacy,* 15, 2020.

Bertini, Catherine, Yih, Peggy Tsai, Thurow, Roger and Dabek, Gloria, *Defining the path to zero, hunger in an equitable world*, Chicago Council on Foreign Relations and the Rockefeller Foundation, 30 March 2023.

Burke, Joanne and Kent, Randolph, *Commercial and humanitarian engagement in crisis contexts: Current trends, future drivers*, Humanitarian Futures Programme, King's College, London, June 2011. www.humanitarianfutures.org

Carney, John, 'Futures and foresight planning', Principal Scientist within the Systems Thinking and Consulting Group of the Defence Science and Technology Laboratory (Dstl), 8 March 2018.

Courtney, Hugh, *20/20 Foresight: Crafting strategy in an uncertain world*, Harvard Business School Press, 2001.

de Vet, Arne and Lowette, Filip, *The fluid organisation: An ideal mix of self-management and hierarchy*, De Vet Management bvba, 2018, 97890829810.

Edmondson, Amy C., Jang, Sujin and Casciaro, Tiziana, 'Cross-silo leadership', *Harvard Business Review*, May–June 2019.

Elrha, *Spring impact, and science practice, too tough to scale: Challenges to scaling innovation in the humanitarian sector,* Elrha, 2018.

Else, Liz, 'Opinion interview: Seizing tomorrow', *New Scientist*, 1 December 2001, pp. 43–44.

GESDA *2023 Science breakthrough radar*, www.gesda.global

Goodwin, Brian, 'In the shadow of culture', in J. Brockman (Ed.), *The next fifty years: Science in the first half of the twenty-first century*, Vintage Books, 2002.

Griseri, Paul, 'What are organisations?', *An introduction to the philosophy of management*, Sage Publications Ltd, 2013.

Harford, Tim, *Adapt: Why success always starts with failure*, Little, Brown, 2011.

Independent Panel for Pandemic Preparedness and Response, *Covid-19: Make it the last pandemic,* May 2021.

Jideofor, Nonso, *Localizing humanitarian action*, UNHCR Innovation Service 2020–2021 unhcr.org/innovation @unhcrinnovation.

Johnson, Brian David and Vanatta, Natalie, 'What the heck is threatcasting?', *Future Tense*, Arizona State University, 2017.

Knowledge Hub/Multi-sectoral Emergency Response for Conflict-Affected and Food Insecure Populations in South Sudan – Final Evaluation 2019 at: www.humanitarianfutures.org/sites/default/files/InnovationsThinkPiece.pdf.

Laloux's, Frederick, *Reinventing organisations: A guide to creating organisations inspired by the next stage of human consciousness*, Nelson Parker Publishers, 2014.

Roz Lasker, *The expert's blindspot,* www.humanitarianfutures.org/tools/mediacent/film/expertblindspot

Leifer, Richard et al., *Radical innovation: How mature companies can outsmart upstarts*, Harvard Business School Press, 2000.

McChrystal, Stanley et al., *Team of teams: New rules of engagement for a complex world*, Portfolio/Penguin, 2015.

Manjoo, Farhad, 'Why we need to pick up Alvin Toffler's torch', *New York Times*, 6 July 2016.

Mulgan, Geoff, *The art of public strategy: Mobilizing power and knowledge for the common good*, Oxford University Press, 2009.

NESTA, *Collective crisis intelligence for frontline response*, 15 September 2021.

OECD Global Science Forum, Report on Workshop on 'Priority setting and coordination of research agendas: lessons learned from COVID-19', 20 January 2022, DSTI/STP/GSF(2021)21/FINAL

OECD, *Benefits of regional cooperation on the energy-water-land use nexus transformation in Central Asia*, Green Growth Papers 2022–1, May 2022. See https://oe.cd/NexusTashkent2021 for further information.

Oliver Wyman LLC Forum, *Leading in a permacrisis*, oliverwymanforum@e-mail.oliverwyman.com.

Olson, Richard S. and Sarmiento, Juan Pablo, 'Communities of practice and disaster risk reduction', *Natural Hazards Informer*, Issue 5, University of Colorado Natural Hazards Research and Applications Information Center, 2012.

Saja, A. M. Aslam, Sahid, S. M. Lafir, and Sutharshanan, M., 'Capacity-building strategy for creating disaster- and climate-risk-sensitive development plans: A case study of multi-stakeholder engagement in Sri Lanka', *Integrated Research on Disaster Risks*, Springer Nature, February 2021.

Sen, Amartya, 'The man without a plan', *Foreign Affairs*, March/April 2006.

Skinner, Paul, *Collaborative advantage*, Little Brown Book Group, 2018.

Snowden, David J. and Boon, Mary E., 'A leader's framework for decision-making', *Harvard Business Review*, November 2007/Revised 2011.

Spiers, Emily, Slocombe, Will, Maltby, Jim, Dedopulos, Tim, Stolze, Greg, Goodenough, Paul, Claridge, Richard, Mason, Lucy, Biggs, James and Norris, Jack, 'Estrangement, immersion and the future: Designing the speculative environments of the virtual reality: "Museum of the Future"', *Futures*, 138, 2022.

Trias, Angelo Paolo and Cook, Alistair D. B., *HADR in Southeast Asia: Unpacking the military's humanitarian role*, RSIS Commentary at RSISPublications@ntu.edu.sg

Wenger, Etienne C., 'Communities of practice: A brief introduction', 2008. www.wenger-trayner.com/introduction-to-communities-of-practice

Wolpert, John D., 'Breaking out of the innovation box', *Harvard Business Review, Special Innovation Edition*, 80 (8), August 2002.

World Bank, 'Defying predictions, remittance flows remain strong during COVID-19 crisis', Press release, 12 May 2021.

8 The Helenus Alternative

Planning from the Future

Over the previous chapters, the reader joined this author on a journey – *an odyssey* – to see the ways that the humanitarian past might fit into a humanitarian future. Certainly the past, beginning with that 'famine of biblical proportions' in 1984, launched an expedition that by the 2020s showed the sector's mounting strengths as well as weaknesses. The critical issue, as the reader no doubt will recall, is how either would be reflected in efforts to deal with ever more complex humanitarian threats?

The answer began with taking the reader along a route where the transformations in the nature of human agency, governance and resource allocation could lead to humanitarian crises that were unprecedented but perhaps plausible. The purpose, however, was not to predict the future, but rather to let the reader explore *portraits of the future* to test the extent to which the humanitarian sector, relevant organisations and individuals had the conceptual and operational wherewithal to anticipate and adapt to increasing humanitarian uncertainties.

Whatever the conclusion, the fact of the matter is that the reader would have to take into account very evident systems and organisational dynamics that will most likely frame efforts to plan for an ever more complex humanitarian present and future. These clearly include the intensifying interrelatedness of the global community – that entanglement nexus. So, too, will increasing polylateralism determine ways that a multiplicity of actors are already becoming engaged in managing global threats. And, of course, the extent to which organisational behaviour will stimulate or constrain such efforts remains of utmost concern.

At this stage of the odyssey, the reader should appreciate that the perspectives and propositions laid out in the previous chapters present profound challenges. At the same time, they also point to significant opportunities to surmount them. Rather than ignoring such opportunities – as all did when it came to Cassandra's predictions – the reader should assume the role of her brother, Helenus, who not only understood the issues at hand, but recognised ways to address them.

For this reason, readers need to test their assumptions about the humanitarian implications of an increasingly entangled world construct. How would they identify,

DOI: 10.4324/9781003471004-9

monitor and mitigate complex humanitarian crises in an increasingly polylateral world? Who will they presume to be 'a humanitarian' and why? And, whatever the organisation, are those upon whom so many of the potentially crisis threatened will depend, adequately anticipatory, adaptive, innovative and collaborative and has its leadership broken away from the conventional?

With these questions in mind, Chapter 8: *The Helenus Alternative* offers a series of practical measures as first steps towards answering those questions. The measures that follow are based upon 'tools' and processes that have been developed in collaboration with governments, intergovernmental, regional and non-governmental organisations in Africa, the Americas, Europe, South and Southeast Asia and the Pacific region between 2004 and 2020.

All can be found on the Humanitarian Futures Toolkit website: www.humanitarianfutures.org.

Tools for the Future: The Humanitarian Futures Toolkit [HFT]

The *Humanitarian Futures Toolkit* has been designed to provide those with humanitarian roles and responsibilities with measures to strengthen their abilities to deal with increasingly complex and uncertain humanitarian crises. They offer ways to translate concepts into strategic and operational action.

There are four key components outlined, below, all of which have been tested in organisations in the humanitarian sector and in organisations that seek to support the sector.

While each offer different perspectives and objectives, in their totality they all offer tested and effective measures to *plan from the future*, which in practice means that

- Strategy formulation and planning need to be seen as a dynamic, ongoing process and not as one-off outputs.
- Dealing with uncertainty and complexity requires greater efforts to develop contending scenarios that can lead to a common set of propositions.
- Greater attention must be given to horizon scanning that will reflect different assumptions about *futures* perspectives.
- Bringing together the views of a wide range of non-traditional humanitarian actors – the private sector, the military, social and scientists – broadens the scope and depth of plausible futures.
- Collaborative efforts to promote solutions to complex problems should also focus on 'problem-solving' networks, namely, representatives of different sectors that have mutual self-interests in finding solutions to complex problems.
- *Futures* lenses can be enhanced by exploring innovations and innovative practices that may not have direct humanitarian application.
- Myriad organisational constraints hinder *futures*-oriented strategic planning, even for those who recognise the importance of looking for alternative approaches. Yet, these constraints can be overcome in various ways by promoting the anticipatory and adaptive organisation.

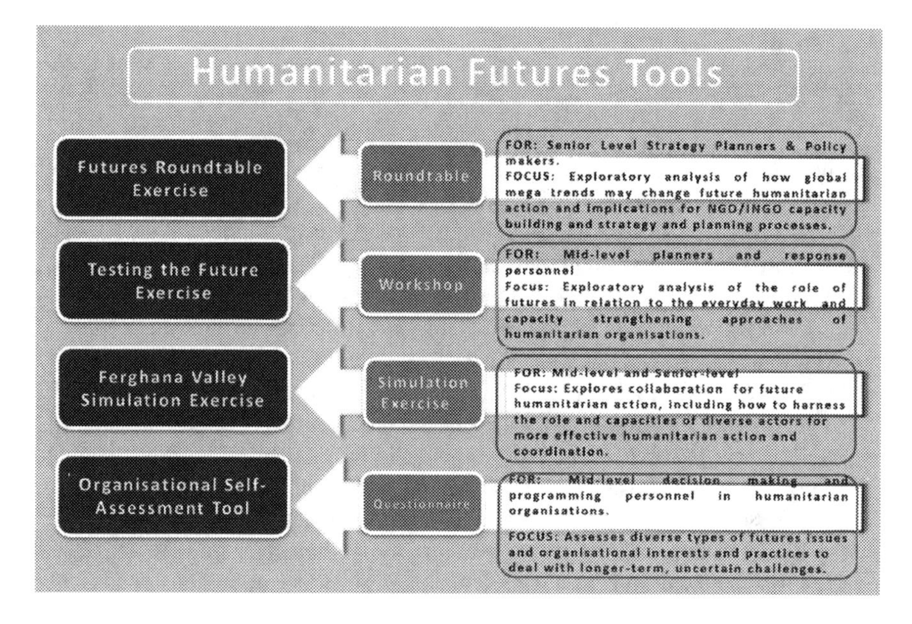

Figure 8.1 Humanitarian Future Tools

Source: https://www.humanitarianfutures.org

With these broad objectives in mind, the HFT has four specific tools: *The Futures Roundtable Exercise*, *Testing the Future Exercise*, *Ferghana Valley Simulation Exercise* and the *Organisational Self-Assessment Tool.*

Futures Roundtable Exercise (FRE)

FRE uses a roundtable format to bring senior level humanitarian decision-makers and policy planners together with natural and social scientists in order to develop global *portraits of the future*, and to consider the sorts of organisational transformations that must be taken now to deal with that future.

Overall Objectives

- Demonstrate the types of vulnerabilities and challenges which the humanitarian sector will have to consider for the future and therefore also to prepare for the present.
- Identify the capacity of the present humanitarian sector to prepare, prevent and respond to such threats and opportunities in order to elicit what sorts of transformations might be required to meet these.
- Test the usefulness of the Futures Roundtable approach for helping the humanitarian sector prepare for an ever more complex and uncertain humanitarian

future. In so doing, to provide recommendations on ways that the approach can be strengthened.

Key Features

- The FRE begins with a process intended to suggest plausible portraits of the world from at least a two decade perspective.
- These portraits reflect an amalgam of different disciplines that together describe what society might look like from a longer-term perspective, including perspectives from the global economy, transformative technologies and security to political and social structures, demographic patterns and the nature of livelihoods.
- Exercise includes focus on societal transformations and their impacts on societal resilience, vulnerabilities, disasters and emergencies.
- Participants are discouraged from looking to the past or identifying trends to explore the future. Instead, an FRE is about abandoning assumptions about the past, and looking to the 'what might be's' in the longer term.
- An FRE encourages the use of participatory methods to stimulate active and frank engagement and exchange. It includes a variety of formats such as the fishbowl technique, café-style conversations as well as small group and plenary discussions.

Outcomes

- Creative capacities for identifying multi-sector sources of information and research.
- Analytical tools necessary for identifying and anticipating plausible longer-term humanitarian threats.
- Measures for ensuring that futures perspectives – plausible threats and mitigation measures – are incorporated into strategic planning frameworks.
- Enhanced capacities for linking strategic plans into decision-making processes.
- Robust capacities for developing more integrated and anticipatory decision-making.
- Opportunities to reflect on the nature of humanitarian threats and ways to meet the challenges they present.

Testing the Future Exercise (TFE)

The TFE is a two-day exercise designed for an organisation's internal departments. It is targeted at those with roles in operational planning, in-country programme support, learning and development. The exercise encourages participants to reflect on a changing crisis landscape and to explore the types of organisational capacities required to identify and deal with future humanitarian crises.

Overall Objectives

- Explore what is meant by futures and its importance for a humanitarian organisation committed to being prepared for the future.
- Identify key global and societal patterns and transformative factors that may serve as drivers of change in the future.
- Consider how the impact of such global and societal patterns and transformative factors could trigger humanitarian risks, resulting in disasters and emergencies.
- Identify plausible implications of global and societal changes and transformative factors when it comes to strengthening organisational capacities for dealing with the future.
- Determine more specifically the types of capabilities that participants' organisation/s might require, and the sorts of challenges that could prevent implementation.
- Brainstorm follow-up ideas for enhancing organisational capability to prepare for an ever more complex future humanitarian landscape

Key Features

- Trend Mapping, Drivers of Change Analysis, STEEP (Social, Technical, Environmental, Economic, Political) Framework, Back casting and Scenarios are all means to identify factors that could influence societal change.
- Five capacities that are explored with the TFE are anticipation, adaptation, innovation, collaboration and strategic leadership.

Outcomes

- Insights into the types of trends and transformative factors that may shape and influence the future of humanitarian action and humanitarian organisations.
- An orientation to humanitarian futures, including key concepts, principles, terms, organisational barriers and challenges.
- An introduction and application of selected futures techniques and recognised approaches that can help humanitarian actors to understand and consider futures in a structured manner.
- Application of a five-capacity framework to support an organisation's efforts to be 'fit for the future'.
- A framework for participants in the TFE to consider practical options that could be introduced in their own work and that of their organisation as a whole to seed the idea of futures, and its organisational value and importance.

Ferghana Valley Scenario Exercise (FVSE)

Through a series of evolving scenarios, the FVSE explores methods for assessing and utilising the 'value-addeds' and comparative advantages of different types of organisations – e.g. the private, military and humanitarian sectors – for dealing with complex crises. In so doing it explores effective cross-sector collaboration.

Overall Objectives

- Demonstrate how a range of capacities from 'non-traditional' humanitarian actors can enhance the ways that the international community can prepare for, and respond to the growing number and types of future humanitarian crises.
- Identify capacities that can strengthen humanitarian action.
- Determine the extent to which sectoral differences in language, terminology, objectives, priorities and measures of success pose a constraint to participants in identifying such capacities.
- Itemise participants' respective comparative advantage and value added in regards to humanitarian action.
- Agree on methods by which the results of these tests can be reviewed, improved and implemented.

Key Features

- Diverse range of participants from multiple sectors, including the private sector, community authorities, the military and government departments, and humanitarian-focused.
- Complex scenario reflecting multiple factors that could trigger humanitarian crises affecting a particular area and various approaches for dealing with the ensuing crises.
- Participants to relate their potential value-addeds and comparative advantages, including those affected by transformative changes.
- Encourage participants to consider how they might respond to a particular complex scenario in a changing global context.

Outcomes

- Insights into different approaches for identifying vulnerabilities and resilience, including how different sets of participants (e.g. military, humanitarian, private sector) would respond and identify others and their own potential strengths and weaknesses regarding humanitarian crisis mitigation.
- Determine and how different sets of participants would assess possible strengths and weaknesses of the region under focus in terms of economic, social and political stability and growth potential.
- Determine perceptions of potential crises in order to see how different sets of participants prioritise them and generate contingency plans.
- Based upon the scenario, demonstrate the contributions that each sector could make towards a crisis response, the sorts of priorities that each establishes and ways that a coherent, integrated approach could evolve.
- Identify factors for which participants might not have been able to anticipate in order to capture the ways that participants respond to the complexities of an ever-changing crisis, including approaches to contingency planning.

Organisational Self-Assessment Tool (OSAT)

The OSAT is a questionnaire designed for individuals in humanitarian organisations interested in exploring the ways that their own capacities and those of their organisations would be able to deal with ever more complex humanitarian threats, both in the immediate and longer term. Its focus, though on the individual, is intended to identify possible interests, perceptions and constraints that can influence the ways that an organisation prepares for the future.

Overall Objectives

- Link systems and organisational perspectives with those individuals involved in the work of one or the other or both.
- Provide measures for individuals to assess their own and their organisation's anticipatory, adaptive, innovation, collaboration and leadership skills.
- Based on that assessment

The questions, broadly speaking, are divided into types. The first provides a list of possible threats that could lead to largescale humanitarian crises over a two-decade period.

Key Features

- The OSAT should be undertaken by individuals as part of a more general process. Particular departments of an organisation or even the organisation as a whole should be offered the opportunity to take the OSAT. It should not be seen to be a test of individual competences.
- The OSAT is based on a questionnaire format, designed for upper and middle management to explore (i) the types of longer-term humanitarian threats which respondents identify, (ii) the levels of interest and importance demonstrated by respondents' organisations to look to the longer term, (iii) the sorts of capacities, if any, the organisation presently has to focus on the longer term and (iv) the sorts of capacities that respondents' organisations deemed necessary to enhance their futures perspectives.
- Those organising an OSAT exercise should put the initiative in a context that emphasises that the exercise's purpose is to enhance the capacity of the organisation as a whole.

Outcomes

- The OSAT results will in the first instance be the basis of individual discussions, group meetings and workshops and possibly conferences to consider potential humanitarian threats, their possible impacts and ways that they should determine organisational structures and behaviour.

- The OSAT should be used as means to regularly assess progress being made throughout the organisation to achieve the sorts of structural and behavioural adjustments recognised from the initial and subsequent OSAT findings.

Testing, Exploring, Implementing

For those who appreciate the implications and importance of *planning from the future*, they can be assured that the sorts of tools found in the toolkit have generally been well received across a wide spectrum of organisations in many parts of the world.

How they were used and ultimately the impacts that they had varied. However, there were few occasions when participants and organisers did not benefit from 'lessons-leaned'. Generally, the HFT did trigger ideas and insights that those who will be using it should consider.

Of critical importance, though perhaps all too obvious, is the need for participants to understand that futures should be regarded as an important part of an organisation's ethos. That means not only what the exercises, *per se*, are seeking to achieve, but also how they will be used overtime to enhance and sustain the anticipatory and adaptive capacities of the organisation.

That said, from the outset, participants have to understand that the futures process might result in substantive organisational change. Some departments reduced, others integrated, new structures replacing old ones, new forms of leadership and decision-making authority – all could eventually be the result of that ethos. All, in one way or another, also has to reflect a very fundamental issue, namely, at the end of the day, who owns the process? Is it those who sit at the top of an organisational hierarchy, or those who in a much more latitudinal, cross-organisational way press for futures perspectives, or is it the interaction of both?

In terms of the substance of futures projections, it is essential to clarify whether the objective of the exercise was to explore uncertainty or probability. Obviously, the two interrelate. However, the objective of futures exercises in this context is to explore the unknowns and the rarely considered. If the search for plausibility is a term used to limit the sorts of scenarios which from the outset are deemed to be 'realistic', then the value of exploring the 'what might be's' becomes limited.

Perhaps one of the most persistent dilemmas that many participants faced was the tension between using time and resources for speculative thinking and the issue of accountability. Not only was the issue of immediate concern – 'why am I using my time this way, when I'm not paid for doing this?' – but for longer-term concerns that were seen as disrupting well defined and institutionalised organisational purpose. How could one account for the former when the latter had been the more defined and tangible purpose? And, given that the organisation's resources were normally provided for that purpose, how would one account for initiatives and perspectives that went beyond that? Accountability, according to one major government institution, was far more important than innovation.

More than once had the issue of 'triggering anxieties' arose. For those organisations that were dependent upon external funding or authorisation, there was a concern that essential accountability and acceptability would not necessarily be appreciated. The purpose of futures initiatives and concomitant structural changes and operations would have to be very clearly explained and accepted.

In a related vein, there were those, particularly in regional organisations, that wondered what the geographical boundaries of futures planning were. Of course, global perspectives might be interesting. However, of importance, too, were ways that the global and regional interrelated. For example, it would seem evident that the global issue of climate change would inevitably impact upon the regional and local. Yet, from an organisational perspective, where should the emphasis be placed?

The regional versus global quandary on occasion was reconciled by focusing on those countries and regions where the organisation had programmes. Would perspectives on the longer term also result in redefining those programmes? And, in any event, the purpose of HFT exercises is to have participants move away from the past and present as determinants and move to the far more speculative approach inherent in *planning from the future* for the future.

The issue of boundaries also had to address possible tensions between *humanitarian futures* and their relationship to what might be regarded as *development futures*. For those who accept the *normal life proposition*, as frequently referenced throughout this book, the answer is that from a futures perspective, they are intertwined and have to be acknowledged as such. However, that point has to be clarified, if not accepted, from the outset of the HFT process.

Of course, the consequences of the HFT process goes beyond issues of accountability, definitional consistency and geographical boundaries. In several instances, there were those who suggested that organisations should be restructured before testing the effectiveness of such changes through a *futures process*. There was considerable tension in one regional organisation between those who adamantly insisted that their organisation needed greater institutional change before introducing cross-directorate futures collaboration.

Such issues also introduced the question of what would trigger essential organisational change. There were those who believed that the sorts of change required for a more futures sensitive organisation would rest principally on the shoulders of the leader. Others responded that the nature of leadership would be secondary to the organisational dynamics that would ensue from changes in perceptions across the organisation – seen as one of the objectives of the HFT exercises.

One of the important dimensions of the HFT process is its reliance on sectors and specialisations that normally fall outside the scope of most organisations with humanitarian roles and responsibilities. Take, for example, the sciences – natural and social. The language and substance of unfamiliar specialisations have to be accessible to a wide range of competencies within the organisation. Those who are brought in from different backgrounds to help explore the future need to accommodate that diversity without being oversimplistic. This applies, for example, to the military and private sector as well.

And, what would be the consequences of one own's organisation becoming more futures oriented while its partners or systems in which it operated were far less inclined to do so? Sharing information and findings might be one way to begin to narrow these sorts of discrepancies. In the final analysis, though, these are indeed risks, and ultimately have to be accepted because those involved in the futures process believe in it.

The End of One Odyssey, the Beginning of Another

So, what will *Humanitarian Futures: Challenges and Opportunities* have given the reader by the end of this humanitarian odyssey? The author hopes that you, the reader, will ultimately have recognised the strengths and weaknesses of the systems that now determine and implement approaches for dealing with vulnerability and resilience on a cross-societal scale. He, too, hopes that if the reader will be willing to step back from a humanitarian world that is familiar into a world that is dramatically different, you and others will begin to ask if present systems and approaches – for all their strengths and weaknesses – are really adequate for dealing with ever more complex humanitarian threats?

And, with that last question in mind, has the book identified opportunities to meet future humanitarian challenges? If so, what do you, the reader, see are the ways forward?

Index

Printed in the United States
by Baker & Taylor Publisher Services